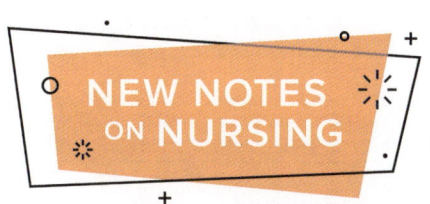

NEW NOTES ON NURSING

SUCCESSFUL CLINICAL PLACEMENTS IN NURSING

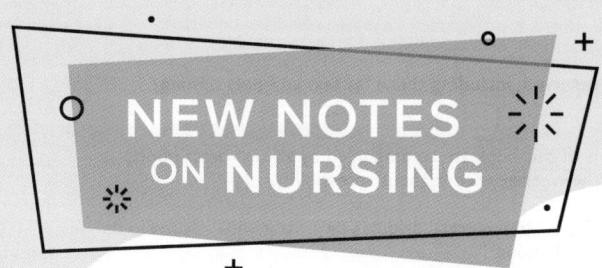

SUCCESSFUL CLINICAL PLACEMENTS IN NURSING

EDITOR

Natalie Elliott BA, BSc (Hons), RN

SERIES EDITOR

Teresa Chinn, MBE, RN, QN

CONSULTING EDITOR

June Girvin

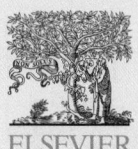

ELSEVIER

Notices

Practitioners and researchers must always rely on their own experience and knowledge in evaluating and using any information, methods, compounds or experiments described herein. Because of rapid advances in the medical sciences, in particular, independent verification of diagnoses and drug dosages should be made. To the fullest extent of the law, no responsibility is assumed by Elsevier, authors, editors or contributors for any injury and/or damage to persons or property as a matter of products liability, negligence or otherwise, or from any use or operation of any methods, products, instructions, or ideas contained in the material herein.

ISBN: 978-0-443-12722-9

Printed in India
Last digit is the print number: 9   8   7   6   5   4   3   2   1

Executive Content Strategist: Robert Edwards
Content Project Manager: Supriya Barua
Design: Miles Hitchen
Marketing Manager: Deborah J. Watkins

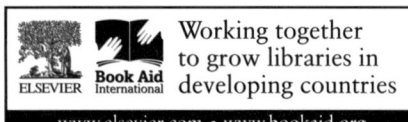

Working together to grow libraries in developing countries

www.elsevier.com • www.bookaid.org

LIST OF CONTRIBUTORS

Katie Anderson, BA Nursing (Child)

Paul David Jebb, OStJ, MA, BSc (Hons), DipHE

Matt Fallon, RN, DipHE, BSc, PgDip, FHEA

Richard Greensmith, FHEA, MSc, PGCAP, PGCE, NMCT, BSc, BA, Dip.N, RNA

Simon James, BSc, RN

Megan Kirk, BSc

Jessica Lister, DipHE, RNLD, PGDip, MBA, NMP

Hannah Louise Nicholls, BA, B Nurs, PGCHE, FHEA

Sarudzai Makaza, BSc (Hons)

Michelle McKinlay, BSc, MSc

Kelvin McMillan, BSc, PGCHE

Emily Mycock, BSc (Hons)

Christie Roberts, BSc Adult Nursing, MPH

Cameron Smith, MN, BN (Adult)

Steffi Ward, BaHons BSc PGCE RMN

Brian Webster, Cert HSC, BSc (Adult Nursing), PG Cert (Advancing Practice), RN

Elisha Woolf, BSc (Hons), PGCert, RN

TABLE OF CONTENTS

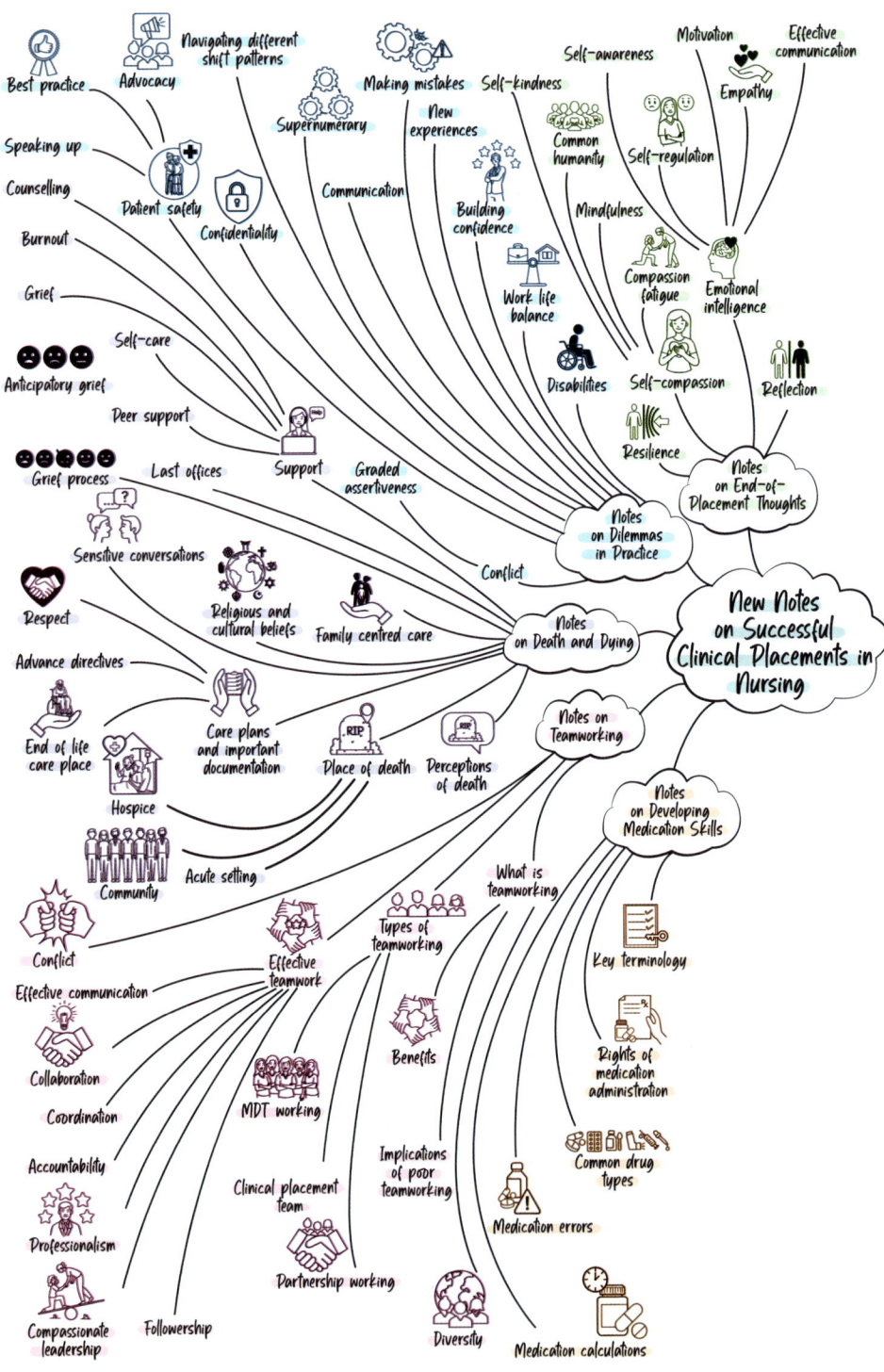

Best practice
Advocacy
Navigating different shift patterns
Supernumerary
Making mistakes
New experiences
Self-kindness
Self-awareness
Motivation
Effective communication
Empathy
Speaking up
Counselling
Communication
Patient safety
Confidentiality
Building confidence
Common humanity
Self-regulation
Burnout
Grief
Mindfulness
Work life balance
Compassion fatigue
Emotional intelligence
Self-care
Anticipatory grief
Peer support
Support
Graded assertiveness
Disabilities
Self-compassion
Reflection
Grief process
Last offices
Resilience
Notes on End-of-Placement Thoughts
Sensitive conversations
Respect
Religious and cultural beliefs
Family centred care
Conflict
Notes on Dilemmas in Practice
Advance directives
Notes on Death and Dying
New Notes on Successful Clinical Placements in Nursing
End of life care place
Care plans and important documentation
Place of death
Perceptions of death
Notes on Teamworking
Hospice
Notes on Developing Medication Skills
Community
Acute setting
What is teamworking
Conflict
Effective teamwork
Types of teamworking
Key terminology
Effective communication
Benefits
Rights of medication administration
Collaboration
Coordination
MDT working
Common drug types
Accountability
Implications of poor teamworking
Professionalism
Clinical placement team
Medication errors
Compassionate leadership
Followership
Partnership working
Diversity
Medication calculations

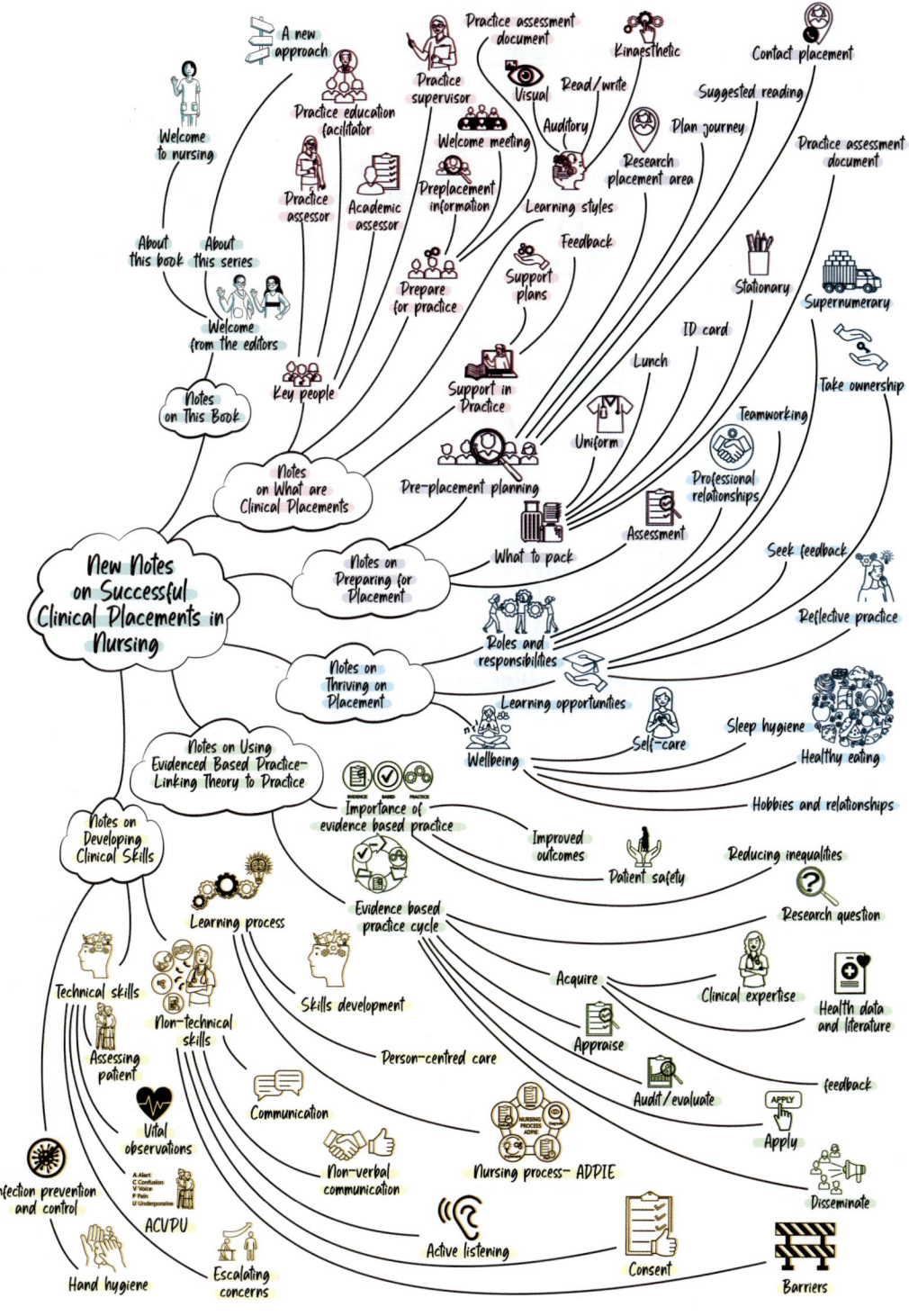

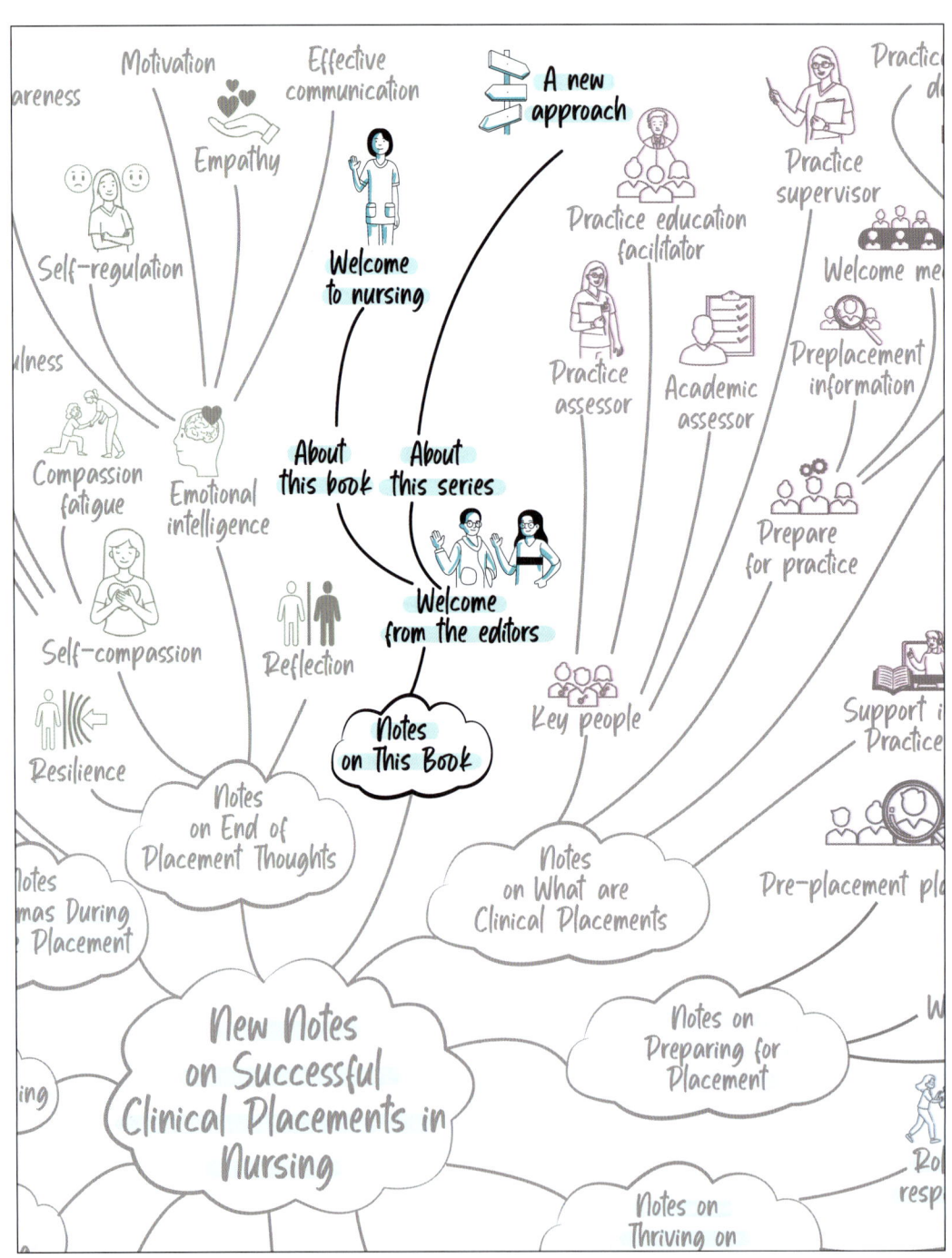

ABOUT THIS SERIES

Teresa Chinn (she/her) ■ **June Girvin (she/her)**

DEAR NURSING STUDENT,

We are so pleased that you have chosen this book from the other nursing books on the shelf! You may have noticed that it looks a little different to other books in the nursing section and there's a very good reason for that – it *is* different! This is the first in a series of books aimed at supporting you as a nursing student. The series combines a nursing book and a digital perspective, including the use of social media, that we hope will create a user-friendly and engaging approach to some of the fundamental topics and challenges in nursing.

The title for the series *New Notes on Nursing* is respectfully and humbly borrowed from Florence Nightingale's own writing. Her *Notes on Nursing* (1860), outlined a vision for health and wellness that encompassed social, political, economic and environmental determinants as well as public health and illness prevention – the bigger picture within which good nursing care must be grounded. We recognise that for many new nursing students, some of the concepts that inform nursing can be challenging and complex, and may not always appear immediately relevant. The *New Notes...* series seeks to address that. We have tried hard to present content in a friendly style, conversational as far as possible, and incorporating social media so that interacting with this book is not a solitary activity but one that can be shared with others who are using the same book and finding out about the same things – whether they are in your cohort or somewhere else in the United Kingdom.

We are trying new design approaches using colourful and engaging content that is aimed at helping you identify the information you need quickly and easily. We understand that sometimes you don't want (or need) to read a dense textbook from start to finish to pull out the most helpful information for your situation, but rather easily identify the bits that are relevant for you at a point in time. We think our colour-coding and infographics throughout the books will help you do just that. We have also included all sorts of helpful 'sidenotes'; again taking inspiration from Florence Nightingale's writing:

NMC

THE NMC SAYS

These show the part of the code that the text is relevant to, helping you to embed the code into every area of your practice and thinking.

SOCIAL MEDIA

'These are tweets from Registered Nurses and nursing students that share snippets of wisdom and perspective'

We have asked many people to contribute to the New Notes on Nursing books and we have included some long quotes from these people; these have been especially written for this series.

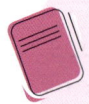

CASE STUDY

Case studies, both real and imagined, are a great way to put learning into context, so you will find plenty of them in this series.

Your notes are just as important as ours and you will find lots of space in *New Notes on Nursing* for your own notes.

_____

_____

_____

_____

_____

_____

_____

_____

We have created the books with neurodiversity in mind and have tried to ensure that there is a feeling of space and lightness to the book.

In addition to all of this, we really want to engage and support you on your nursing student journey, so we have created some social media resources for you to tap into. Please search #NewNotesOnNursing and #SuccessfulStN on SOCIAL MEDIA to find out more.

The team of Editors and Authors that we have asked to contribute to *New Notes on Nursing* are all practising health and care professionals, ranging in experience from nursing students and newly qualified Registered Nurses to registered professionals working in clinical and education settings with a wealth of experience. They all wanted to help you. By inviting a variety of voices to create these books, we are sharing many perspectives with you. We hope it helps you to develop well-rounded views on which to start your nursing career.

You are the latest generation of nursing students, and we are so pleased and honoured to be, in some small way, supporting you to flourish. We really hope you enjoy this book (yes, enjoy!) and that, at the end of your student journey, it contains lots of notes scribbled by you, the pages are dog-eared and the cover well-worn – a new generation of nursing texts for a new generation of Registered Nurses.

Today's nursing is socially complex, politically enmeshed and at times finding its way through conflict and controversy to give the best holistic, person-centred care. We think it's the best career in the world.

Best wishes

June and Teresa

The series is edited by:

'I've been a Registered Nurse since 1996 and have made my career in the social care sector. In 2012 set up the nursing Twitter community @WeNurses to help bring together nurses from diverse spheres of practice. I was awarded an MBE for services to nursing in 2014 and in 2018, I was named one of the 70 most influential nurses from 1948 to 2018 by the Royal College of Nursing. I communicate in many different ways in the UK and Europe, particularly on the use of social media in Nursing. I was made a Queens Nurse in 2022'.

Teresa Chinn, MBE QN @WeNurses

'I qualified as a Registered Nurse in 1976 and have spent a (very) long career in clinical and academic practice. I retired in 2017 and now work independently in roles committed to supporting individual nurses and nursing as a profession – writing, commentating, coaching, reviewing, etc. I was delighted to be asked to support the development of this new series of books and to work with the team of writers/editors and Elsevier'.

June Girvin @ProfJuneG

Space for reader's own reflection:

_____

_____

_____

_____

_____

_____

_____

_____

_____

_____

_____

_____

_____

_____

_____

_____

REFERENCE

Nightingale, Florence. 1860. Notes on nursing: what it is, and what it is not. London: Harrison. Harvard (18th ed.).

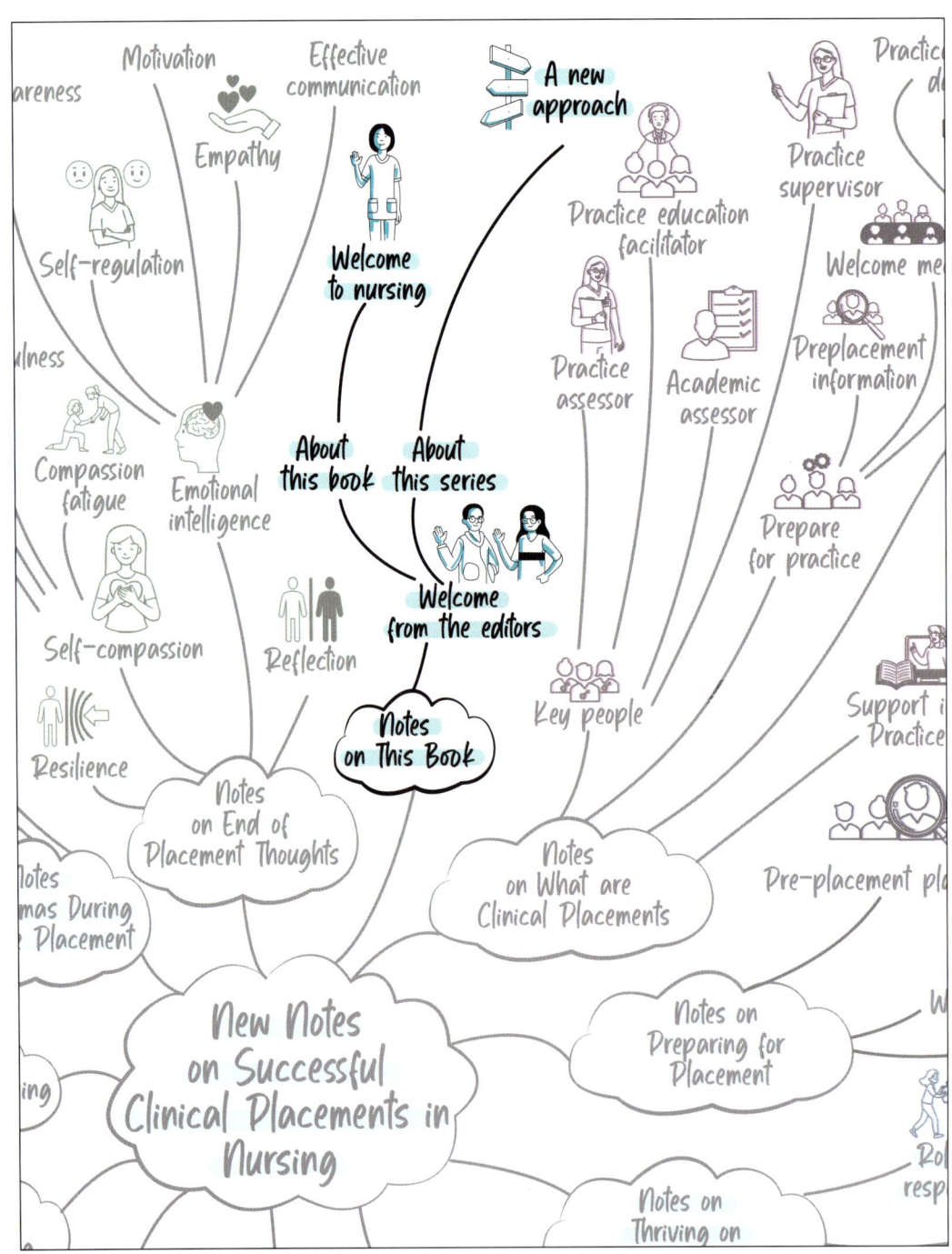

ABOUT THIS BOOK

Natalie Elliott (she/her)

DEAR NURSING STUDENT,

Hello and welcome to this book, *Successful Clinical Placements in Nursing*. You're probably reading this book because you are about to embark on your clinical journey, and within this book, you will be guided by the help of some experts in their fields. This will be real voices from real people who may be practising nurses, academics or nursing students—people who have been through this journey too. They will help steer you through some of the key elements of your clinical placement through storytelling, insights and invaluable advice to help you navigate the thrilling yet challenging world of clinical nursing placements.

Hopefully you see nursing as more than just a job. It's a privilege where you'll have the chance to bring comfort to those in pain, offer solace to the worried and celebrate small victories with your patients. It's one of the most amazing professions, which brings together knowledge and skills, in addition to providing compassionate care. Nurses are highly skilled, highly educated and highly trusted across the world. Its more than a privilege; it's also an exciting and dynamic profession, one in which we never stop learning.

> **Before we go any further, take a moment to write down how you are feeling about starting clinical placement.**
>
> _____
>
> _____
>
> _____
>
> _____

Let's consider the essence of nursing—the holistic care. It's not just about following protocols or administering medications; it's about understanding your patients on a person-centred level. Remember, every patient is more than their diagnosis or condition. They have a life story, dreams and fears. When you embrace the holistic care, you'll find that the most profound healing often comes from the smallest acts of kindness.

Your journey through clinical placements will undoubtedly come with its fair share of challenges. You'll face long shifts, complex medical cases and moments when you'll question your own abilities. But remember, it's in the middle of challenges that your strength and resilience are forged.

Clinical placement is where theory translates into reality and where things start to click into place. Imagine reading a recipe book but never cooking a meal—that's what nursing education would be without clinical placements. These hands-on experiences allow you to develop practical skills, gain confidence and bridge the gap between theory and practice.

But how can you make the most of your clinical placements and make the most of this learning experience? The secret lies in the 4 Ps of clinical placements: prepare, placement, ponder and practice.

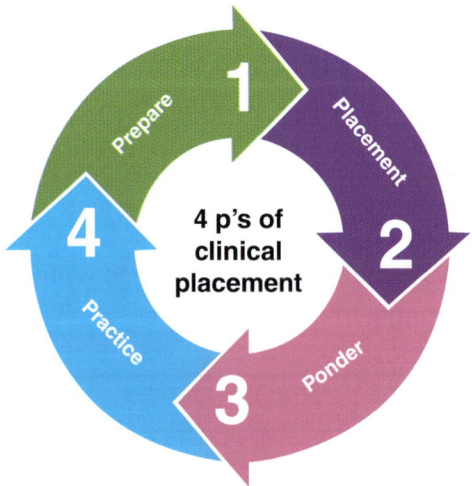

Fig. 1 Four Ps of clinical placements.

PREPARE: THE FIRST P

Imagine this: it's your first day of clinical placement. You're standing at the threshold of a brand-new adventure, dressed in your crisp uniform, practice assessment document in hand. It's a mix of nervous excitement and anticipation, and you wonder … 'Am I ready for this?'

THAT'S WHERE THE FIRST P COMES INTO PLAY: PREPARE

Preparing for a clinical placement is a crucial step for nursing students. It's more than just a routine task; you're laying the foundation for a successful clinical placement. Just like a builder starts with a strong foundation to ensure the stability of a structure, you're setting the groundwork for your nursing journey.

WHAT EXACTLY DOES 'PREPARE' ENTAIL?

Paperwork and logistics: First and foremost, get all your paperwork in order. Ensure you've completed all necessary health and safety checks, vaccinations and any mandatory training. This isn't just about ticking boxes; it's about ensuring your safety and the safety of your patients.

Uniform and equipment: Your uniform is more than just clothing; it's a symbol of your profession and a source of pride. Keep it clean and ready for each shift. Ensure you have all the necessary equipment, and keep it in good working condition.

Knowledge: Review what you've learned in the classroom. Refresh your memory on key nursing skills and procedures as well as any relevant medical knowledge. This preparation will boost your confidence when you're faced with real patient care situations.

TIPS

Reviewing textbooks, notes and online resources for the area you are going on placement is essential. This refreshes your theoretical knowledge, making you better prepared to apply it in real situations

Expectations: Understand what your placement will involve. What kind of clinical areas have you been assigned to? What are the expectations of your practice assessors and supervisors? Having a clear picture of what's ahead will help reduce uncertainty and anxiety.

PLACEMENT: THE SECOND P

The second P in your journey is placement. This is the heart of your clinical education, the space where you'll apply your knowledge, develop your skills and truly understand what it means to be a nurse.

During your placement, you'll have the opportunity to immerse yourself in the world of patient care. It's a pivotal phase, as it's where the theory meets practice and where your journey truly begins.

Here are some key aspects to consider:

Expectations: As you walk into your placement, it's essential to have a clear understanding of what's expected of you. Your practice assessors, practice supervisors, ward staff, peers and patients will all have expectations. Your role is to meet and exceed those expectations through your dedication, compassion and professionalism.

Professionalism: Your placement is your chance to shine as a future healthcare professional. Maintain punctuality, adhere to the dress code and exhibit the highest level of professionalism. Remember, your actions and attitudes reflect on both you and your nursing school.

Patient-centred care: Your patients are the heart of your placement. Embrace patient-centred care, which means seeing each patient as an individual with unique needs, fears and hopes. Listen to their stories, hold their hands and offer not just medical care but also emotional support. Remember nursing is more than the physical condition of a person, and we need to take a holistic approach to care.

PONDER: THE THIRD P

After every shift, every interaction, it's essential to take a moment to ponder. Remember that the learning doesn't stop after the placement.

This is the phase of reflection, where you consider your experiences, challenges and achievements. Seek feedback, and keep a journal to document your growth and challenges. This will be a great resource for your future self.

This introspection might seem simple, but it's a powerful tool for your growth as a nurse. It's where you learn not only from your successes but also from your mistakes. Here's how it works:

Reflect on your experiences: After each day of placement, take some time to reflect on what you've encountered. Think about the patients you've cared for, the procedures you've assisted with and the challenges you've faced. What stands out? What made you feel proud, and what made you question your skills?

Learn from your mistakes: It's important to understand that making mistakes is a natural part of learning. Rather than dwelling on them, use them as opportunities for growth. What could you have done differently? How can you avoid making the same mistake in the future?

Celebrate your successes: Don't forget to celebrate your successes, no matter how small they may seem. Did you successfully administer a medication, provide comfort to a distressed patient or assist in a complex procedure? Or was it simply walking through the front door when your anxiety levels were really high? Acknowledge these achievements and use them to boost your confidence.

PRACTICE: THE FOURTH P

The final P in your journey is practice. This is where you put all your learning into action. Once you have pondered, it's about identifying any gaps in your learning and honing your skills, embracing patient care and learning to work as a cohesive part of a healthcare team.

Why is practice so crucial? Not only because practice makes perfect but because humans are individuals. So what works for one patient may not work for every patient. The more you practise, the more you will build your exposure to situations and learn different methods of completing tasks. Here's how to make the most of this phase:

Skill development: Your clinical placements provide the perfect opportunity to practise and refine your nursing skills. Whether it's administering medications, taking vital signs or performing wound care, seize every chance to enhance your proficiency.

TIPS

If there is a specific skill you'd like to master, read the theory behind it before practising. For example, if you are on a community nursing placement and want to learn more about wound care, why not look at the anatomy of wounds and the healing process they go through?

Patient-centred care: Embrace the art of patient-centred care. Each patient is more than just their condition; they're individuals with unique needs and stories. Develop your communication skills to engage with your patients, listen to their concerns and ensure they feel valued and cared for.

Simulation labs: If you feel you need more practice in a specific area, practise your clinical skills in a safe environment. Simulation labs can be an invaluable resource to build confidence and competence. The more you practise, the better you'll perform in the clinical setting.

Lastly, one of the most important lessons in nursing is to care for yourself too. The demands of clinical placements can be physically and emotionally taxing. It's crucial to find time for self-care, whether it's a walk outdoors, a chat with friends or simply a moment of reflection. You can't provide the best care if you're running on empty.

As you journey through clinical placements, it's essential to celebrate your achievements, no matter how small they may seem. Whether it's mastering a new skill, helping a patient recover or simply making a fellow student's day brighter, your efforts matter.

In the chapters to come, we'll delve deeper into the world of clinical placements, offering practical advice and anecdotes to inspire and guide you. Your journey as a nursing student is just beginning, and the path ahead may be challenging, but it's also incredibly rewarding.

So get ready, stay curious and embrace your clinical placements with open arms. You're about to embark on a journey that will shape your future in healthcare. And let's not forget the essence of the four Ps of placement: prepare, placement, ponder, and practise. These four phases are your compass, guiding you through the intricate and rewarding world of clinical placements.

Kindest regards,

Natalie

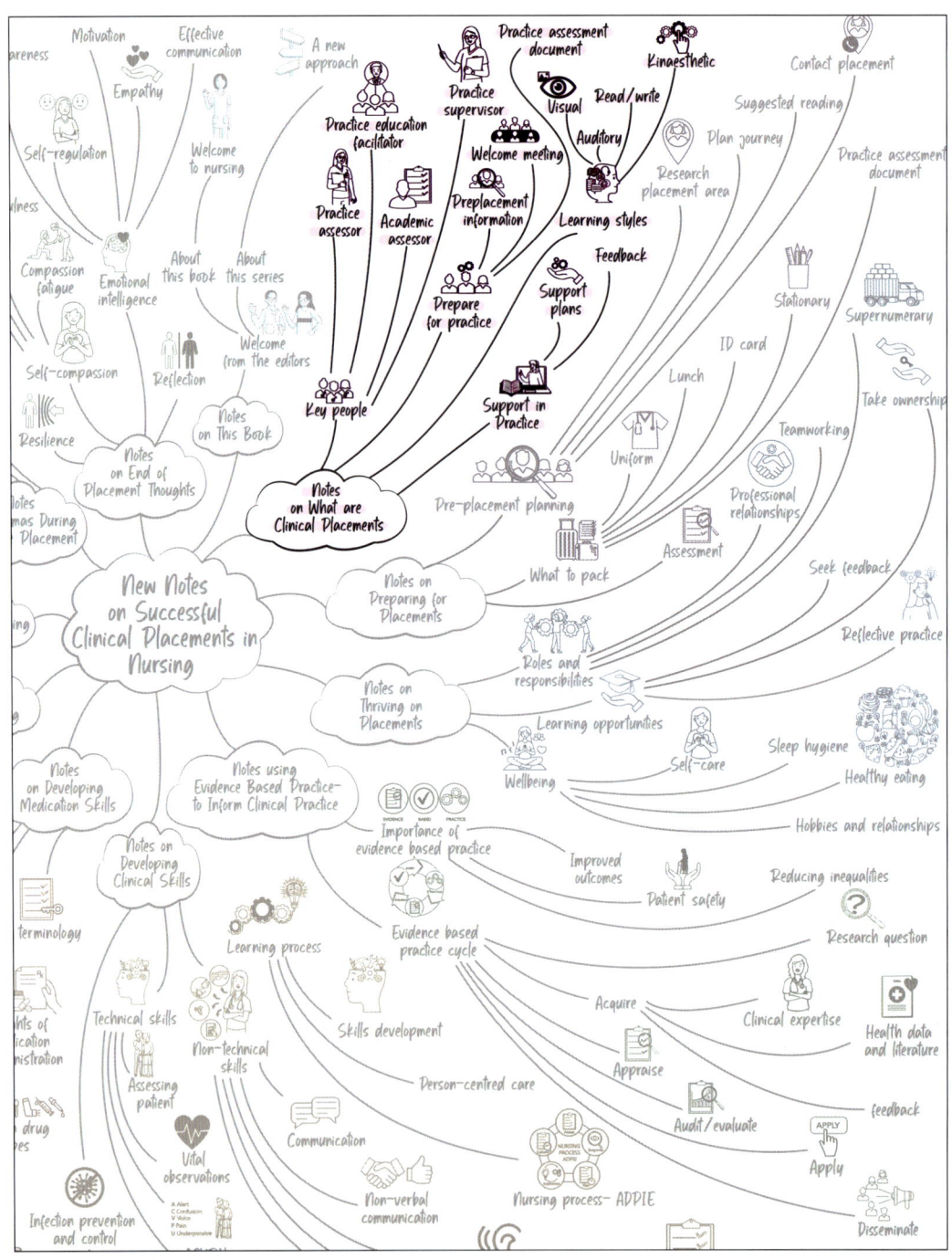

New Notes on Successful Clinical Placements in Nursing

NOTES ON WHAT ARE CLINICAL PLACEMENTS

Michelle McKinlay (she/her)

INTRODUCTION

Clinical placements are like stepping stones that bridge the gap between theory and practice in healthcare. Clinical placements provide nursing students with hands-on experience, working directly with patients and healthcare teams in a variety of different settings. These placements are where nursing students can apply their theory and knowledge to practise and consolidate learning. Clinical placements are also a great opportunity to learn and develop new skills, gain confidence and learn how to work effectively within different clinical settings. This chapter provides valuable insight into what clinical placements are, why they are important and what you can expect as a nursing student, with some helpful tips along the way.

What are clinical placements?

Clinical placements are an essential element of the nursing students' curriculum. Nursing students are allocated practice learning environments that offer various learning experiences throughout the programme. This allows the nursing student to link theory to practise and expand their knowledge and experience.

Half of the nursing programme is spent on placement, requiring students to complete 2300 mandatory hours. These hours count toward their evidence for entry into the Nursing and Midwifery Council (NMC) professional register.

Clinical placements give nursing students the opportunity to transfer theory into practice, learn new skills and achieve competencies (Royal College of Nursing, 2017).

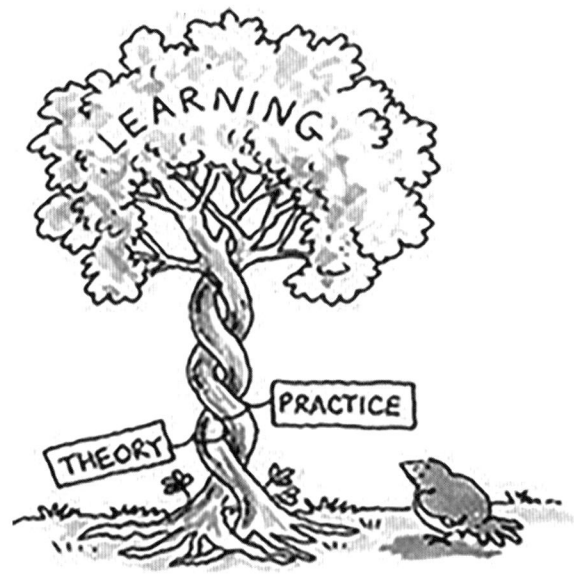

(Posthuma-Coelho, 2016)

Learning environments are diverse, providing varied experiences to ensure nursing students are experiencing different types of nursing in different environments. Practice placements are allocated; however, there may be occasions where the student can identify a preference. As a nursing student, you will learn valuable skills in each area, which will be transferable to other learning environments. You may find that the practice learning environment is not your preferred choice; however, you should embrace every learning opportunity and make the most of the experience. Your placement area may be within a hospital setting where there are adult health, mental health, children and young persons, and learning disability wards. Or your placement could be in community-based care, services which encompass community nursing, community mental health teams, care of the elderly or health visiting. Additionally, there are also placements made in care homes, mental health and psychiatry services, as well as childcare and services for young people.

These learning environments are essential for developing your fitness to practise and preparing you for the registered nurse role (Cant et al., 2021). Each clinical placement has different learning opportunities, levels of clinical activity and staffing issues. It is important during these times that you are supported and feel part of the team.

TIPS

There may be times that you feel the staff doesn't have time for you; however, this is not the case. Take a proactive approach and ask questions, offer to help and ask staff to show you what they are doing. They may have simply forgotten to ask if you want to come along!

As a first-year nursing student, you may be feeling anxious about your first practice placement. This is completely normal—remember all the nursing staff you will be working with have all been in your shoes at one point. It is important to remember that you are starting a new journey, so you are not expected to know everything. Do not be afraid to say 'I don't know'; staff are there to help you learn. There may also be other second- and third-year nursing students in the same learning environment who can also contribute to your learning. Nursing students starting their first placement have identified the need to feel that they belong in the practice area and worry that they may feel they are getting in the way (Doyle et al., 2017). Learning environments should be welcoming, inclusive, supportive and challenging and have clear and consistent expectations where nursing students feel valued and accepted (Cant et al., 2021).

The Willis Commission (2012) suggests that there are six characteristics of a good practice learning environment, as shown in Fig. 1.1.

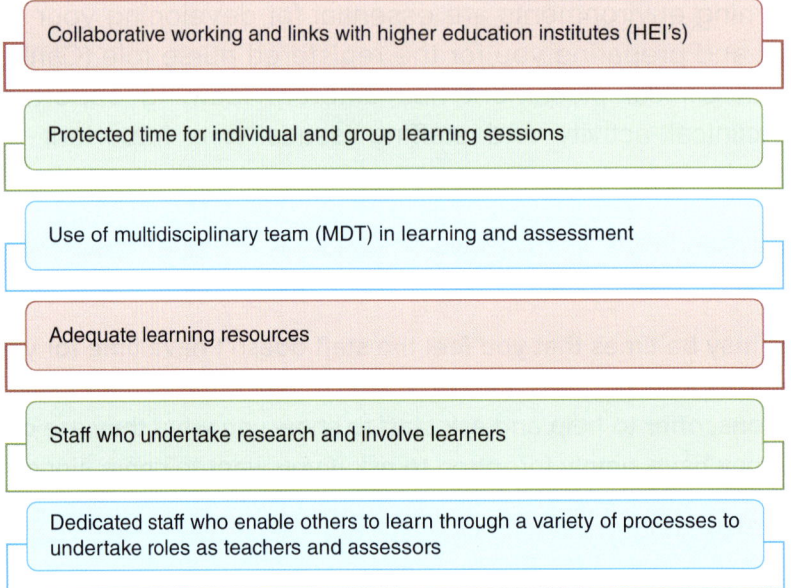

Fig. 1.1   Characteristics of a good practice learning experience.

'From my perspective as a clinical placement lead at an acute hospital, a good learning environment has many factors to achieve before it becomes a good practice learning environment. These factors are:

- *Enough practice assessors (PAs) and practice supervisors (PSs) in the placement area to ensure a positive learning experience for the student.*
- *A staff member who is identified as the placement's student lead and passionate about organising and planning the students off duty (shifts).*
- *Welcoming students to the placement, giving the students an intro- duction pack to their placement and prereading the students are expected to undertake before they start the placement, and holding an induction/orientation to the placement.*
- *Ensuring the placement clinical audit and online profile are current.*
- *Our trust has a large amount of practice development nurses; these nurses hold dedicated teaching sessions for students about the speciality.*
- *Having a board on the ward dedicated for students where students are encouraged to fill out a profile 'all about me' so the staff in the placement area can get to know the students' names and their likes and dislikes.*

Every placement you will attend as a student nurse will have a lot of learning opportunities; enjoy them all, even the challenging ones, as this will shape you to be a fantastic nurse'.

Hannah Welbourne, Clinical Placement Lead

POSITIVE LEARNING ENVIRONMENTS

Quality practice placement experiences within positive learning environments support the development of healthcare professionals to deliver safe and effective person-centred care (NHS Education for Scotland, 2008). Nursing students who have experienced positive learning environments have identified that the contributing factors were the manager's leadership style and staff demonstrating a positive attitude towards student learning and adopting an approach where mistakes are part of the learning process. Most importantly, students have identified that feeling welcomed and having a sense of belonging contributes to successful placements (Doyle et al., 2017).

'The staff were all helpful and made me feel comfortable from day 1. They all made me part of their team and made me feel safe in the environment'.

Anonymous nursing student

The culture of the practice learning environments also contributes to student success. It is important that practice areas demonstrate a positive work ethic and team morale, which contributes to a positive atmosphere. Staff members act as role models and should be aware of how their attitudes and behaviours can impact nursing students (Doyle et al., 2017). You will find role models along the way who you will remember throughout your career; these are the people who will help shape the nurse you will become.

The NMC (Nursing and Midwifery Council, 2018b) expects that practice learning environments are safe and effective, providing guidance for universities and health boards to adhere to. The standards for student supervision and assessment are designed to reinforce this, providing information regarding expectations and responsibilities for all involved in the practice learning experience, including:

- Learners
- Individuals supporting, supervising and assessing learners
- Managers and educators supporting practice learning
- Organisations providing practice learning experiences
- The educational institution

All practice learning environments must meet the expectations of the standards for student supervision and assessment. The quality of practice learning environments is integral to providing safe and inclusive places in which students can experience and learn healthcare (Hoy and George, 2018). All learning environments must be approved for use by using the educational audit. This process is completed in partnership with the higher education institute, the practice education facilitator (PEF) and the lead practitioner of the area in order to decide whether a learning environment is suitable for student learning. This process can be re-peated annually or biannually to ensure the placement area continues to be suitable for student learning (NHS Education for Scotland, 2020).

A crucial aspect of your practical learning involves your 'supernumerary status', indicating that you're not included in the staffing numbers re-quired for safe and effective care in that setting (Nursing and Midwifery Council, 2018c). According to the NMC (Nursing and Midwifery Council, 2018d), approved education institutes and practice learning partners must ensure students maintain this status. This ensures students are supported in their learning, even though they're not counted as part of the regular staffing. Despite not being 'counted in the numbers', you're still an integral part of the team and will contribute to patient care within the practice area. Your level of supervision will be tailored to your indi-vidual needs, with adjustments made as you progress and gain confi-dence (Nursing and Midwifery Council, 2018c).

Who is involved in practice placements, and what is their role in supporting students?

There are four key people who are involved in supporting students in practice placements, as shown in Fig. 1.2. This section will explain each role and what you can expect from them.

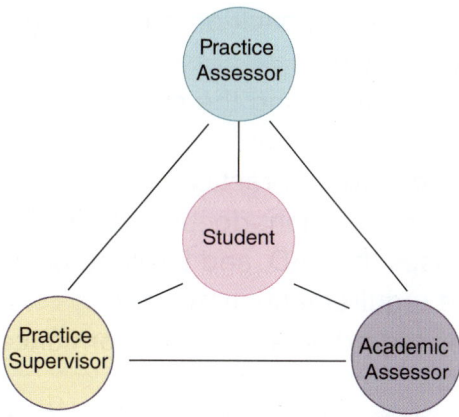

Fig. 1.2 People involved in practice placements.

Practice supervisor role

The PS is any registered health and social care professional working within the practice learning environment. PSs are supported and prepared to fulfil the requirements of the role and have knowledge and experience relevant to the nursing student. They supervise the nursing students in practice to help them learn and work towards achieving their learning outcomes and proficiencies by working in partnership with the PA and other staff within the learning environment (NHS Education for Scotland, 2019 & 2024, Nursing and Midwifery Council, 2018c). Each learning environment has an identified person who will allocate the nursing student a PS, which should occur before the student arrives.

What you can expect from your PS

- All nursing students are supervised while learning in practice.
- Supports learning in line with their scope of practice, having knowledge and experience of the area in which they are providing support.
- Contributes to the initial orientation to the learning environment, which is also part of the preliminary meeting where a learning development plan should be completed in collaboration with the student.
- Ensures that the learning environment is supportive and welcoming.
- Acts as a role model and practises in line with the NMC code of conduct.

- Provides constructive feedback on progress towards achievement of skills and proficiencies.
- Liaises with others supporting the student's learning journey, including the PA and academic assessor (AA) where required.
- Contributes to the student practice assessment document/ practice learning assessment document (PAD/PLAD). Please note: Scotland uses the PAD, and England and Wales use the PLAD; therefore requirements may vary.
- Raises concerns regarding student performance, conduct and competence.
- Supports the student using development support planning.
- Demonstrates an understanding of student proficiencies as per the PAD/PLAD.

(NHS Education for Scotland, 2019 & 2024; Nursing and Midwifery Council, 2018c)

The NMC requires approved education institutions and practice learning partners to ensure PSs receive ongoing support to prepare, reflect and develop to provide effective supervision and contribution to student learning and assessment. They must have an understanding of the proficiencies and expected programme outcomes they are supporting students to achieve (Nursing and Midwifery Council, 2018b).

Practice assessor role

The PA is a registered nurse who has knowledge and experience in the nursing students' field of practice. This role is different from the PS role, as the PA will receive feedback from the PS regarding the nursing students' learning, practice and conduct to inform the assessment. This will contribute to the decision making for progression to the next stage of the programme in collaboration with the AA (NHS Education for Scotland, 2019 & 2024; Nursing and Midwifery Council, 2018c). Each learning environment has an identified person who will allocate the nursing student a PA, which should occur before the student arrives.

What you can expect from your PA

- Supports learning in line with their scope of practice, having knowledge and experience of the area in which they are providing support.
- Understands student learning and achievement in theory.
- Contributes to the initial orientation of the learning environment. May also be part of the preliminary meeting, identifying learning outcomes and setting dates for the interim and final review meetings.
- Ensures continual support and coordination of supervision.
- Maintains contact and work in collaboration with the PS, AA and other staff members contributing to student learning.
- Participates in review meetings, agrees to the PS's contribution to this and draws on other sources to inform assessment.
- Conducts the student's assessment recording rationale for the outcome of the decision within the PAD/PLAD.
- Provides feedback to PSs on key aspects of their role.
- Raises concerns regarding student performance, conduct and competence.
- Supports the student using development support planning.
- Demonstrates an understanding of student proficiencies as per the PAD/PLAD.
- The PA can also carry out the PS role, but not for the same student.

(NHS Education for Scotland, 2019 & 2024; Nursing and Midwifery Council, 2018c)

Academic assessor

The AA is a member of staff from the student's university. They are a registered healthcare professional and have completed AA preparation or equivalent. The programme lead will allocate the nursing student an AA, who should be available to the student prior to commencing placement. The AA will participate in student assessments, working collaboratively with the AA in decision making for progression to the next stage of the programme (NHS Education for Scotland, 2019 & 2024; Nursing and Midwifery Council, 2018c).

What you can expect from your AA:

- All nursing students are assigned a different AA for each part of the programme who:
- Understands students' learning and achievement in theory.
- Works in collaboration with the practice learning environment to support the student.
- Liaises with others supporting the students' learning journey.
- Collaborates with PAs; this may be required once per clinical placement (this may vary between universities).
- Contributes to and conducts evidence-based assessments regarding student conduct, proficiency and achievement, providing rationale for the outcome.
- Collaborates with the PA and makes recommendations for progression to the next part of the programme.
- Supports students if conduct or competency issues are raised by practice learning environments.
- Demonstrates an understanding of student proficiencies as per the PAD/PLAD.

(NHS Education for Scotland, 2024; Nursing and Midwifery Council, 2018c)

Take a moment to reflect and consider what support you need from a PS and PA in practice learning environments.

_____

_____

_____

_____

_____

_____

Practice education facilitator

Practice learning environments may have an identified PEF (it may be known as something else in your area), and it is important that you establish who that is. The purpose of this role is to influence and improve the quality of the clinical learning environments by providing support, educational input and development activities for PAs/PSs and students.

Here is more information about the PEF role:

- Signposting and supporting adherence to the quality assurance of learning environments.
- Identifying and supporting the development of new learning environments and learning opportunities and increasing the capacity of student numbers.
- Supporting the development of PAs and PSs.
- Enhance the quality of the learning experience through encouragement, evaluation and feedback from learners and those supporting learning.
- Work collaboratively with higher education institutes, practice education providers, students, staff, service users and families.
- Provide support, information and development activities for staff and students.
- May also contribute to the development of preregistration and postregistration education programmes and continual professional development.

(NHS Education for Scotland, 2020)

The NMC future nurse: standards of proficiency for registered nurses highlights that nurses must support and supervise students in the delivery of care while promoting reflection, providing constructive feedback, and evaluating and documenting student performance (NMC, 2018a).

Nursing student

As you can see, there is lots of support available for nursing students in practice learning; however, as a nursing student, you also have responsibilities.

TIPS

- Approach your learning proactively by fulfilling learning development plans.
- Prior to starting your placement, ensure completion of prelearning activities listed in the assessment document (if applicable). These activities involve gathering information about your practice area, summarising it briefly, identifying learning opportunities, understanding the patient group you'll work with and considering best practice approaches.
- Familiarise yourself with the process for addressing concerns, knowing that support is available when needed.
- Keep your assessment document accessible to your PS/PA at all times. Though it's a bulky document, some placement areas offer safe storage options. If your university has transitioned to the Epad, check IT and computer access in your learning environment before arrival.
- Always seek consent from service users/patients before delivering care and treatment.
- Reflect on your practice placement, demonstrating how theory connects to practice.
- Share your learning evidence with your PS/PA, which may include additional learning opportunities such as collaborating with other professionals or departments.
- Ensure anyone making entries in your assessment document has completed the record of signatories for their respective roles.
- Collaborate closely with your PS/PA for all actions and entries.
- Accurately record all practice hours, including absences.
- Complete your assessment document fully before finishing the placement to avoid having to return for incomplete tasks later.
- Adhere to the allocated shift pattern specified by the practice learning environment, which you can verify beforehand.
- Participate in placement evaluation and provide anonymous feedback about your experience, aiding in identifying strengths and areas for improvement within the practice.

PREPARE FOR PRACTICE

Effective learning can start when the student is prepared for practice and ready to learn (Cant et al., 2021). Nursing students may be provided with a 'prep for practice' session prior to commencing clinical placements hosted by universities and clinical placement partners. The purpose of these sessions is to outline the expected values and behaviours of nursing students and to provide an awareness of policies and guidelines relevant to their practice. Fig. 1.3 shows the values which staff and nursing students are expected to adhere to. You must demonstrate these values and behaviours in practice at all times to ensure all care is delivered to a high standard in conjunction with staff, other disciplines, patients and families while promoting person-centred care.

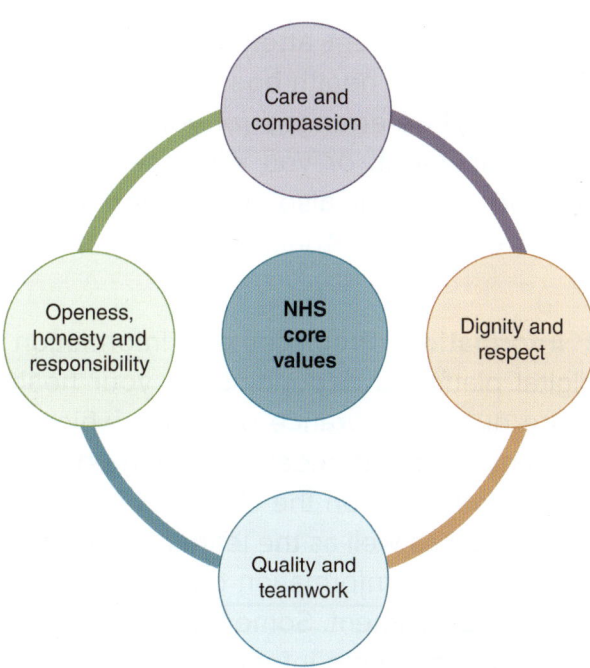

Fig. 1.3   NHS core values.

Topics covered by prep for practice

Professional image. It is essential to maintain a professional image; therefore please consider your values and behaviours outside of the practice learning environment, as this can have an impact on your position as a nursing student. It is important to adhere to the specified uniform policy and familiarise yourself with the sickness/absence policy as well as the use of mobile phones and social media.

Professional code. It is imperative that you adhere to the NMC code of conduct as well as university and health board/trust policies. If you make a mistake, the best thing to do is own up, as everyone has made mistakes in their careers; you will not be the only one! It is equally important to report any concerns you may have regarding the practice you witness. In this circumstance, please speak to your PS and/or assessor and follow the process for raising concerns outlined by your university.

IT access. As a nursing student attending a clinical placement, you will also require IT access to health board systems such as electronic patient records. This will be arranged for you and may be sent out to you prior to your placement, or you will receive these during your placement induction. You will also be notified of the process for reporting any IT access issues. Again, please comply with policies for IT use!

Preplacement information. Preplacement information will also be available on digital platforms depending on your health board area/country. These are quality assurance platforms which ensure that the practice learning environments meet the standards set by the NMC. Here, you will find information on the clinical placement you are going to and the care provided as well as the learning opportunities available. You can also find additional information on shift patterns, student support options and risk assessment. Some health boards may also attach a welcome pack, which can help inform your prelearning activities required for completion prior to attending the placement. Importantly, you will also find key contact information and your allocated PA and PS details. Some students like to contact the practice area prior to commencement of the placement to introduce themselves, which has been known to make a good first impression.

Welcome visit

As well as your prep for practice session, some practice learning environments may invite you to visit the clinical area prior to commencing your placement. Nursing students who have visited clinical areas before starting placements report that it was important to help them feel prepared for placement. Therefore appropriate induction enhances the quality of the student's experience, as it helps students fit in, reduce anxiety and focus on the learning outcomes they can achieve (Worrall, 2007). The students feel they are not being thrown in at the deep end; they feel more relaxed and less anxious when attending allocated placement areas.

'This placement was by far the best placement that I have attended. It presented many different opportunities for me. These opportunities allowed me to grow in confidence and most definitely expand my skills as a training nurse'.

Anonymous nursing student

TIPS
Here are some tips from second and third year nursing students

1. Keep on top of the PAD, and don't wait until the last week to get things signed off.
2. Stick with the nursing assistants until you get an idea of ward routine/layout.
3. Find someone you can talk to if anything is wrong, even if it is not your PA/PS.
4. Every practice area has a different note-writing process.
5. Don't be shy to offer to help out; staff always welcome the offer.
6. Don't be afraid to ask questions or ask to see how something is done.
7. Always leave contact details within the ward in case they need to get ahold of you.
8. If you're caring for the elderly, this can be tough, especially with personal care, but it can be rewarding.
9. Offer to make tea/coffee and take biscuits.
10. Enjoy the placements, as they fly by so quickly; before you know it, they will be finished, and you wish you had used your time better.

LEARNING STYLES

Learning styles refer to the different ways that individuals approach their learning to develop their knowledge and skills. Individual learning styles are based on how a person takes in and understands new information and how that information is processed and retained. Understanding your own learning style can enhance your learning experiences by applying different learning strategies that meet your needs.

Everyone learns differently; therefore it is important to be aware of your own learning style and preferences. Take a moment to consider how you learn considering the learning styles outlined in Fig. 1.4.

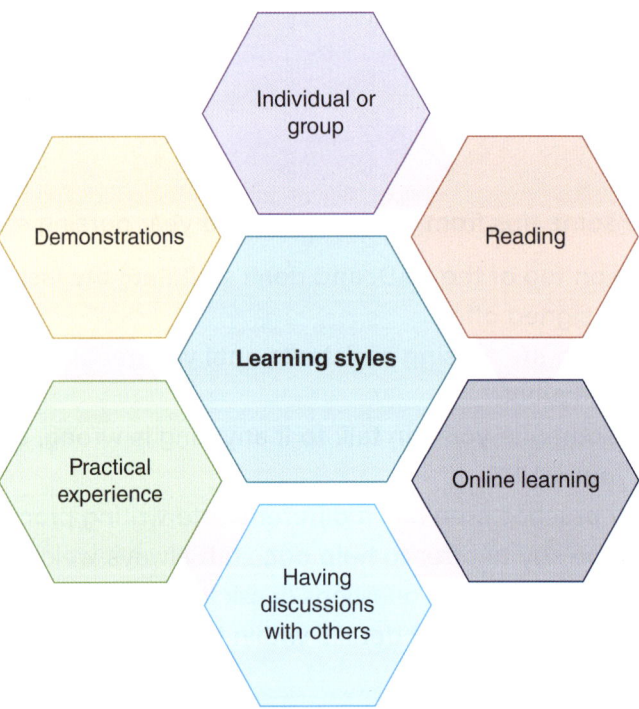

Fig. 1.4 Learning styles.

Take time to think about what your preferred learning method is.

_____

_____

_____

_____

_____

_____

Don't worry if you're not quite sure what you're learning style is at this stage, as there are useful tools that can help you to identify this. The visual, auditory, read/write, kinaesthetic (VARK) learning style model includes questions that can help you identify your learning preference. This model identifies four main types of learners, as shown in Fig. 1.5. However, you may be a person who learns through a combination of the four types. This is called a multimodel learning style (Fleming, 1987).

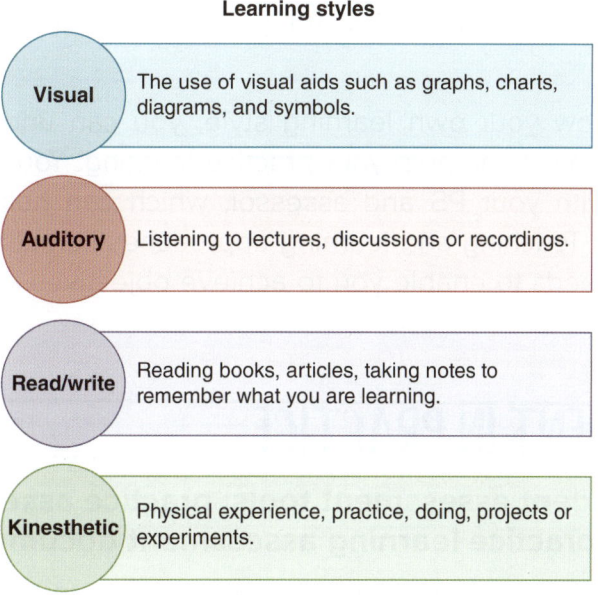

Learning styles

Visual	The use of visual aids such as graphs, charts, diagrams, and symbols.
Auditory	Listening to lectures, discussions or recordings.
Read/write	Reading books, articles, taking notes to remember what you are learning.
Kinesthetic	Physical experience, practice, doing, projects or experiments.

Fig. 1.5   Visual, auditory, read/write, kinaesthetic learning styles.

TIPS

Do an internet search to find a **VARK** questionnaire and discover your own learning style.

There are many factors that can affect the learning process. Firstly, it is important to maintain an open mind, recognising that even if the subject doesn't immediately capture your interest, there's always the opportunity to learn something new. Your motivation for learning something new can stem from intrinsic or extrinsic sources. Intrinsic motivation, driven by your personal desire to learn and improve, stands independent of external influences or rewards, while extrinsic motivation may be influenced by outside factors. Understanding the individual principle acknowledges that each student possesses various levels of proficiency and learns in unique ways. It's perfectly acceptable to approach learning differently from others. Active participation is fundamental for effective learning, encouraging engagement and comprehension. Within the affective domain, students have diverse personalities, including curiosity, emotions, boredom, and various degrees of motivation, all of which impact their learning journey. Recognising your preferred learning style, which may develop over time, empowers you to implement strategies that work best for you (Prithishkumar and Michael, 2014).

Once you know your own learning style, you can understand more about it and how it can help your practice learning. You can share this information with your PS and assessor, which can help inform your learning plan. Teaching and learning approaches can also be adapted to suit your needs to enable you to achieve objectives and reach your full potential.

ASSESSMENT IN PRACTICE

Nursing student assessment tools: practice assessment document, practice learning assessment document

Assessment is integral to practice learning to ensure nursing students meet the required professional standards to progress to the register.

Practice learning environments play an important part in developing the student's professional competence by ensuring students receive the support and experiences required to develop their knowledge and skills to become successful practitioners (Immonen et al., 2019). PSs, PAs and any other professional contributing to the learning experiences gather information regarding student performance and practice. This provides evidence that learning objectives have been met and demonstrates overall competence.

The (NMC, 2018b) states that assessment and confirmation of proficiency are based on an understanding of student achievements across theory and practice. Observation of practice also allows assessment of the student's performance of the skill, professional attitude and adaptability when placed in a variety of situations (Hand, 2006).

Forms of assessment

In practice, there are various different types of assessment. You may recognise this from your academic assessments.

In formative assessments, student performance and practice are observed and monitored in clinical placements. This informs feedback provided to the student during discussions with the PS/PA. This can help you and your PS/PA identify strengths, weaknesses and areas for development.

Summative assessments usually take place at the end of the clinical placement, which is your final review. This is the final decision on whether the student has achieved the required standard of proficiency and learning outcomes.

Another important form of assessment is self-reflection. The student should reflect on their own practice, identifying areas of strength and areas that require development. It is important to share this with the PS/PA to allow for further development opportunities.

Lastly, criterion referenced, the student's performance is measured against predetermined criteria, which is the (NMC, 2018d) standards, platforms and proficiencies.

Methods of assessment

Just like there are several forms of assessment, there are many ways to be assessed too.

Observation. All staff within clinical placements will be observing student practice and performance, which includes formal and informal interactions, participation in patient care, participation in meetings, carrying out practical skills and generally how the students present themselves.

Questioning. The student will be asked questions to determine their understanding of the practice learning environment, the care required for the service users/patient group and understanding of a specific diagnosis, clinical skills and procedures. Remember, it is ok to say 'I don't know'!

Discussions. It is good practice to have reflective discussions and talk things through. This may help the student understand things better, reflect on a clinical skill they have demonstrated and identify strengths and areas for development.

Written. Written assessments will be carried out within the PAD/PLAD at the interim and final review. This is in relation to the **seven platforms of proficiency** and should be discussed with the student.

Testimonies. Assessments involve the opinion of more than one person; they also take into consideration the opinions and observations of others within the learning environment. This ensures the assessment process is objective and fair, promoting validity and reliability (NHS Education for Scotland, 2020).

During practice placement, the student will have three mandatory meetings with the PS and/or PA (Practice Assessment Document, 2023).

The first meeting is part of the induction to the learning environment which the PS can facilitate. This is called the orientation and preliminary meeting. There will be a range of topics covered, including shift patterns, sickness/absence, reporting accidents/incidents, fire safety, health and safety, confidentiality, expected behaviours, raising concerns, students' needs, learning experiences available, uniform policy, mandatory training record, risk assessment and any previous assessments and development plans. During this meeting, the learning development plan will be discussed and put in place.

The next meeting is the interim/midway meeting. This is a formative form of assessment, and the meeting should occur halfway through the placement, which can be carried out by the PS; however, the PA and/or AA can also be present if required. At this point, the discussion will focus on the student's progress and review of the learning development plan, considering the seven platforms of proficiency.

The last meeting to be held is the final review. This is a summative form of assessment, and the meeting will take place near the end of the placement by the PA. However, the AA may also be part of this meeting. The PA will draw on evidence from the PS and others who have contributed to the students' learning considering the seven platforms of proficiency (outlined as follows).

Platforms of proficiency

The NMC sets out standards of proficiency that nurses must meet in order to practise safely and effectively, which also applies to nursing students. The seven platforms of proficiency is a framework that ensures nurses and students are competent and compassionate practitioners who prioritise the safety, wellbeing and dignity of those in their care. This is what the nursing student assessment process is based on.

Throughout their preregistration programs, students undergo a combination of theoretical learning, practical skills development and clinical placements to achieve proficiency in these areas. Fig. 1.6 shows what these are.

Part of the assessment also includes the PS and the student receiving feedback from the service users/patients, which is considered a valuable asset to the assessment process (Immonen et al., 2019). This is in relation to the student's ability to practise in accordance with and demonstrate the NHS core values.

Platform 1	Being an accountable practitioner
Platform 2	Promoting health and preventing ill health
Platform 3	Assessing needs and planning care
Platform 4	Providing and evaluating care
Platform 5	Leading and managing nursing care and working in teams
Platform 6	Improving safety and quality of care
Platform 7	Coordinating care

Fig. 1.6   Platforms of proficiency (Nursing and Midwifery Council, 2018a).

The student's participation in care differs at each stage of the programme. As a year 1 student, the expected level is dependent, which means working closely with the PS, who will direct and guide the student throughout the placement. Each platform identified has proficiencies that must be achieved at each level. You must achieve all of these before the end of each stage of the nursing programme. As the student progresses throughout the course, the level of participation would be expected to change.

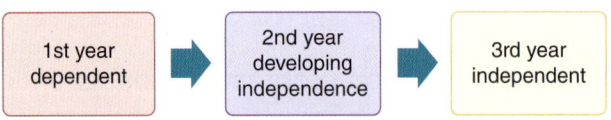

During all practice placements, the student will also demonstrate their communication and relationship management skills and nursing procedures (skills and procedures). It is important that all nursing students can perform these skills and procedures safely and effectively to progress to the NMC register. This can be demonstrated through practice (the student observes and then carries out the skill/procedure) or in exceptional circumstances through simulation (the student can demon-strate through knowledge and practical skills the ability to carry out skill/procedure).

TIPS

1. Take all learning opportunities offered; this will contribute to your knowledge and experience.
2. Keep practicing; just because you do something once doesn't make you an expert.
3. Take advantage of the learning environment: visit other departments. For example, if you are in a mental health ward in a hospital, visit other departments to meet physical health care proficiencies, skills and procedures.
4. Always seek service user/patient consent prior to carrying out care and treatment.
5. Always adhere to policy and procedures.
6. Familiarise yourself with the evidence base: why do we do this?
7. Don't follow bad practice, and avoid picking up bad habits. Always do things 'by the book'.

Development support plan

During any discussions about the student's progress, there may be areas identified for development. This will be documented in a develop-ment support plan, devised with the PS/PA and student to help achieve specific learning outcomes. Please remember that this is a supportive measure to help you progress; it is not a punitive measure.

The development support plan will identify the development needs and specific areas to be addressed. It will be related to a specific platform of proficiency and participation in care level. Actions and learning resources will be identified in collaboration with the PS/PA and the stu-dent. Student involvement is important, as this gives you the opportu-nity to identify what works for you. Evidence of achievement for each action is required, with an expected date specified. This is signed by the PS/PA, AA and student.

If a development support plan is created, it is useful to set SMART goals to clarify and focus on the areas for improvement. It also increased the chances of the goals being achieved. SMART is an acronym for specific, measurable, achievable, realistic and time bound. Fig. 1.7 explains SMART goals in more detail.

There are many common reasons why concerns may be raised in practice which are required to be addressed, such as behaviour and attitude (unenthusiastic, confrontational, lack of motivation, dishonesty); unwillingness to communicate with staff, patients and carers; repeated absence or lateness; lack of professional boundaries (inappropriate comments, oversharing personal information); noncompliance with uniform policy or inappropriate wear when uniform is not required; personal hygiene; failing to achieve learning outcomes; poor clinical per-

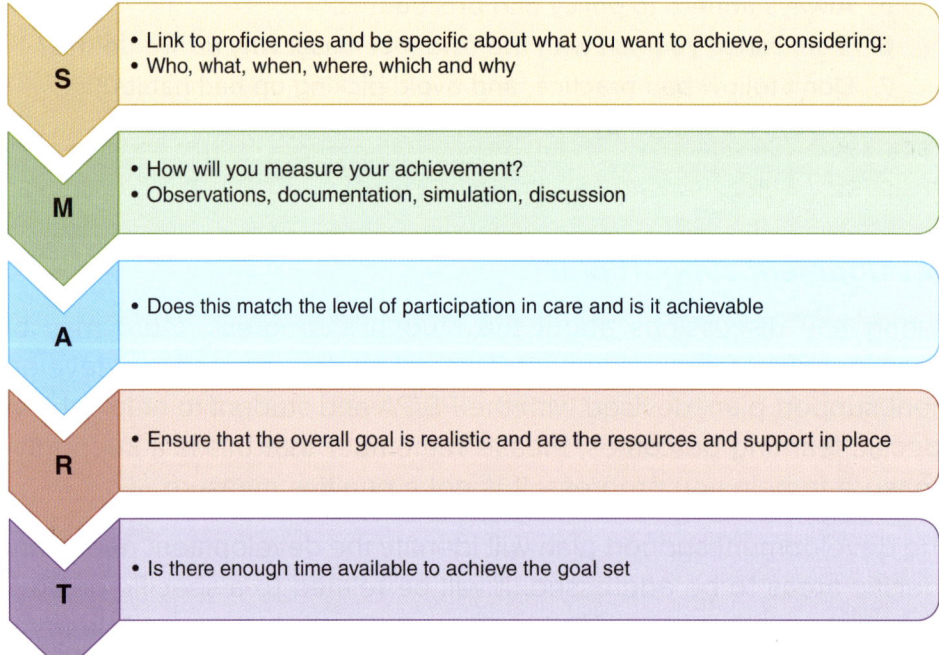

S
- Link to proficiencies and be specific about what you want to achieve, considering:
- Who, what, when, where, which and why

M
- How will you measure your achievement?
- Observations, documentation, simulation, discussion

A
- Does this match the level of participation in care and is it achievable

R
- Ensure that the overall goal is realistic and are the resources and support in place

T
- Is there enough time available to achieve the goal set

Fig. 1.7 Specific, measurable, achievable, realistic and time-bound (SMART) goals (NHS Education for Scotland, 2020).

formance; lack of insight into development; unsafe practice; inability to link practice to theory; avoidance of PS/PA and inability to take advice or feedback (NHS Education for Scotland, 2020). Any concerns raised should be discussed with the student in partnership with the PS/PA and AA. The student should be given the opportunity to work on any concerns raised where appropriate.

Reasonable adjustments

All students should have the opportunity to learn and have their needs met if they have a disability; therefore practice learning environments may be required to make reasonable adjustments to ensure the student is not at a disadvantage. It is at the student's discretion whether they want to disclose this information to practice, and they may choose not to. However, this may impact the learning experience, and staff members can't support something they know nothing about.

It is not easy to disclose to a stranger who is a professional that you have a disability due to the fear of stigma (Harris, 2018). However, these staff are in the caring profession, and you should not be judged for your disclosure. Students who have disclosed they have a disability have had support measures put in place to help them progress and achieve learning objectives, and they have flourished as a result. Please remember that some disabilities can impact the safety of yourself and others, depending on the environment you are in.

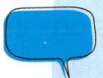

SOCIAL MEDIA
@christienursing

'It really helped me when there was a positive culture within the placement team and general support for students, including regular check-ins with supervisors- that's made me feel able to disclose my disabilities and set wheels in motion for putting support in place'.

SOCIAL MEDIA

@ChloJaconherMac

'I would say that giving students structure and pre-information to calm some pre placement nerves and thoughts. Taking time to listen and fill in entail paperwork to establish what the student would like to get from their placement. Exploring if the student has any reasonable adjustments and preferred learning styles so the mentors and team they work with can adapt to the students learning to harvest the best placement experience for the student. Patience and kindness is the two best approaches mentors can take with students. Disclosing any reasonable adjustments, disabilities or neurodivergent conditions can be challenging for some student nurses and speaking up for support can be tricky. It is important that mentors and placement areas build trust (a therapeutic relationship) just as you would with patients so to create a sense of safety for the student to speak up. Recognizing one's bias, both conscious and unconscious about a student can also be helpful to avoid judgment of students as this can formulate unfair ideas about students and influence important decisions. Please be patient and kind with students, especially those who do require a little further guidance or support. Find creative ways together to get the best from the students learning. From a student perspective I would say being prepared always helped me. Knowing what I have to achieve and finding creative ways to achieve hurdles was key to my success as a student. Being open to new learning at all times and showing an interest. Grabbing every opportunity possible'.

Having a disability does not mean that you cannot succeed as a nursing student. Many nursing students, nurses and other professionals have disabilities and continue to practice and have great careers. If you disclose your disability to your PS/PA, then a discussion should take place about how best to support you in practice, so it is important that you identify what works best for you. This can be documented within the development support plan. Tee et al., (2010) give some examples of support in practice, as shown in Fig. 1.8.

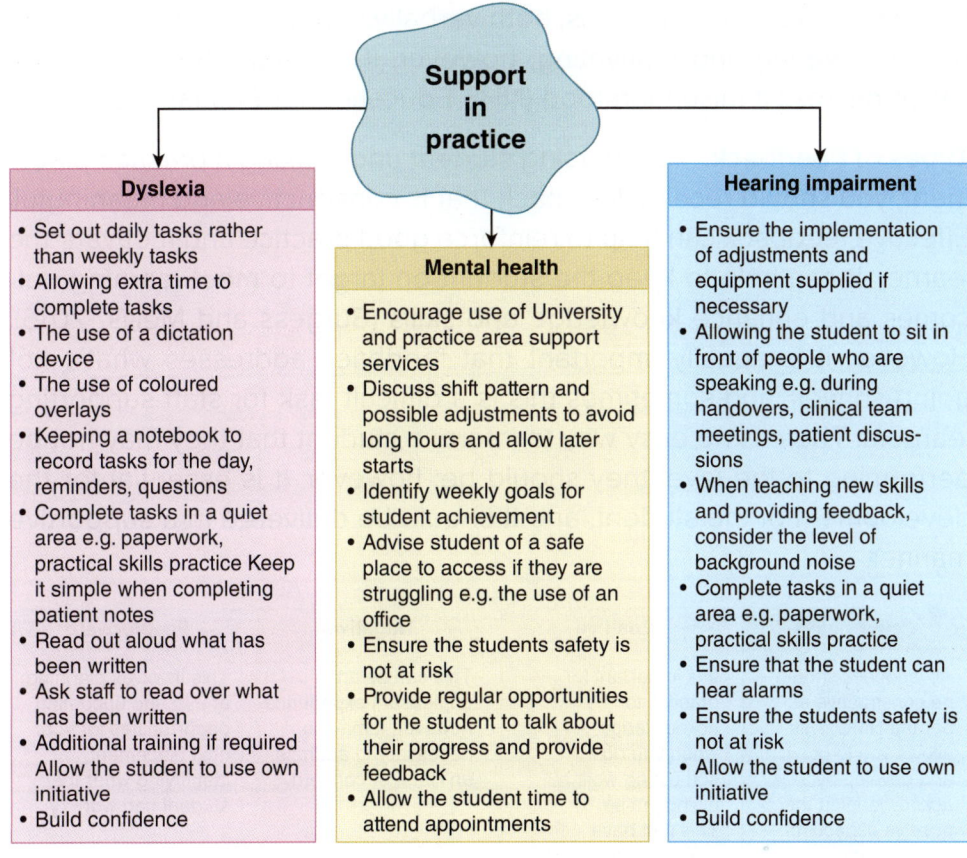

Fig. 1.8 Support in practice (Narayanasamy and Penney, 2014).

Nursing students who have a disability tend to have issues with communication, documentation, consistency and clinical skills; therefore it is imperative that effective support and additional time for learning are accommodated (Tee et al., 2010). If you feel you are not being supported, please report this to the PEF and/or the university.

Feedback

Feedback is a fundamental aspect of teaching and learning (Clynes & Raftery, 2008) and will help inform progression and assessment and identify strengths and areas for development. This is something that will be received on a routine basis, both verbally and written. Feedback can be empowering and motivating; however, it also has the potential to cause distress if misunderstood (NHS Education for Scotland, 2020).

Types of Feedback. As a nursing student undertaking a practice placement, you should receive feedback that is constructive and meaningful. Effective feedback can help to reinforce good practice and motivate the learner. It can help to keep the student on target to meet learning outcomes and enhance knowledge and skills (Burgess and Mellis, 2015). However, it is equally important that feedback addresses what's not going so well, and sometimes this is a difficult task for staff supporting learners. There is no easy way to inform a student that they may not be performing to the level they should be; however, it is essential for the development of the student, and it should be delivered in a supportive manner.

Constructive	Positive	Negative	Feedforward
All feedback should be constructive as per the NMC. This allows you to grow and develop by acknowledging the positive aspects of performance and providing suggestions as to how to further	It is important for practice to acknowledge when you do something well, giving praise. This can have a positive impact on your practice.	This can be an unpleasant experience however, it may be necessary to address an issue or concern.	This involves planning ahead and upcoming opportunities for your next placement, identifying what the student can work on.

Nursing students may also receive peer feedback from other students who may be in their second or third year and have been where you are now. This is perceived as beneficial for student learning and development (Burgess and Melis, 2015). Other students can provide hints and tips they have learned throughout their journey. However, it is important that peer feedback is honest and accurate. Some students may not want to provide honest feedback to peers, as it may impact the relationship; however, keep in mind that they are most likely trying to look after you and want you to succeed!

Feedback can take place in many forms, such as formative, summative, verbal and written. One model that may be used is Context, Example, Difference, Agree and Review (CEDAR), as it analyses what could be done differently next time and helps establish actions to improve practice

(Wildman, 2003). It can be very beneficial for the PS/PA to have a discussion with the student, as it provides an opportunity to interpret messages through observation of body language and voice tone, ask questions and clarify misunderstandings (Duers & Brown, 2009).

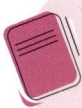

CASE STUDY: USING THE CEDAR MODEL

Emma is a second-year nursing student currently undertaking a clinical placement in a paediatric oncology ward. Emma's PS, Hetal, observes her interactions with patients and their families. Hetal recognises the importance of providing effective feedback to help Emma enhance her nursing practice.

Context

Hetal begins by contextualising the feedback within the specific tasks and situations Emma encounters during her clinical placement. For example, after witnessing Emma's communication with a distressed parent, Hetal provides feedback on her empathetic approach and effective communication skills.

Example

Hetal highlights specific examples of Emma's interactions, praising her for actively listening to the parent's concerns and offering reassurance.

Difference

Hetal focuses on highlighting the difference between Emma's performance and the desired standards of nursing practice. In this instance, Hetal explained that Emma could have taken the parent to a quiet space where there was privacy and confidentiality could be maintained. By identifying specific gaps in Emma's practice, Hetal helps her understand the standards expected of her as a nursing student and future registered nurse.

Agree

Both Hetal and Emma agree on the importance of aligning feedback with Emma's learning objectives and clinical experiences. They

Continued

CASE STUDY: USING THE CEDAR MODEL—cont'd

discuss Emma's goals for the placement, such as improving her nursing skills and enhancing her ability to communicate effectively with patients and families. Hetal ensures that the feedback provided resonates with Emma's aspirations and supports her professional development as a nurse.

Review

Throughout Emma's clinical placement, Hetal regularly reviews the feedback provided and evaluates Emma's progress. They meet periodically to discuss Emma's performance, reflect on her achievements and identify areas for further improvement. By reviewing Emma's reflections together, Hetal gains valuable insights into Emma's learning journey and adjusts the feedback accordingly to meet her evolving needs.

TIPS

Here are some tips from second and third year nursing students

- Believe in yourself.
- Speak up and ask questions.
- It's okay not to know something rather than pretend you do.
- Be organized.
- Build positive relationships with the staff on the placements.
- Get to know your patient group.
- It's ok to say you're unsure of completing a physical task if you're not feeling competent.

COACHING

Coaching is another type of support available to nursing students and is seen as an important contributor to the success of individuals, which is also evident in career planning and professional development (Narayanasamy & Penney, 2014).

Coaching can be defined as 'a collaborative solution-focused, results-orientated and systematic process in which the coach facilitates the enhancement of work performance, life experience, self-directed learning and personal growth of the coachee' (Association for Coaching, 2023).

This approach is important and valuable in practice learning environments, as it can provide significant changes in individuals in relation to achievement, fulfilment and joy (Narayanasamy & Penney, 2014).

Coaching plays a vital role in nursing students' journey by boosting their motivation and desire to learn. Sometimes this can be impacted by many contributing factors such as previous experiences, failures and self-efficacy, which can also have an impact on the student's confidence. The coach's role is to help students regain their drive and work towards their personal goals. Moreover, continuous learning and development are crucial for satisfaction and can enhance motivation positively. Through coaching, nursing students can recognise their significance in their field and witness results and achievements of goals. Ultimately, the process of learning, growing and accomplishing brings about a sense of joy. Without any of these elements, it's easy to feel drained and disheartened, viewing learning as dull and spirit dampening. Coaching addresses these challenges, ensuring students stay engaged, fulfilled and joyful in their educational journey. (Narayanasamy & Penney, 2014).

THE PRACTICE SPIRAL MODEL

There are many other coaching models available; however, this gives you an idea of how it can benefit your learning. Nursing students who have experienced coaching in the practice learning environment have identified many benefits such as increasing confidence, developing problem-solving and leadership skills, feeling more relaxed and overall contributing to the enjoyment of the placement (Underwood et al., 2019).

Stage 1

Explain and demonstrate
Your PS/PA will explain, describe and demonstrate a practical skill by breaking it down into a step-by-step process to allow you to understand what is involved and expected.

Stage 2

Reflect on learning
This gives you the opportunity to reflect, make notes and practice using relevant equipment.

Stage 3

Review progress
Reflect on the goal, assess if you are making positive progress towards achieving the goal. Positive feedback should be given regarding your progress and set the agenda for further sessions and input.

Stage 4

Plan to practice again
Further sessions should be arranged to allow further practice where you can demonstrate the skill you have learned and further sessions can be planned if required.

TIPS

Here are some tips from second and third year nursing students

- You'll have rough days at placement when you question whether nursing is actually for you. Don't give up; what you're feeling is valid.
- Placements and the course in general are like a rollercoaster with the ups and downs. It's worth it in the end when you're holding your degree.
- Remember, you're accountable for your actions at all times, even in the first year.
- Always try and take something from your placements—even if it's somewhere you aren't enjoying or know you aren't going to work in the future.
- BE KIND (To everyone. It can be a lonely and difficult time for others. Juggling studies and family life isn't easy.)
- Tea and coffee go a long way!
- Enjoy the experience.

CONCLUSION

Practice learning environments are an integral part of your nursing student journey. They should be supportive areas where you feel part of the team and your contribution is valued. There should also be a variety of learning opportunities and experiences available to help you develop your knowledge and skills. These learning environments will be challenging, and it won't be plain sailing; however, this will help develop your confidence and resilience and shape you into the nurse you want to become. As the nursing students who have been in your shoes have said, enjoy the experience!

Good luck on your journey.

TIPS

Useful online resources:

- **Think Positive about Student Mental Health**
  https://www.thinkpositive.scot/
- **Support in Mind Scotland**
  https://www.supportinmindscotland.org.uk/
- **National Wellbeing Hub**
  https://wellbeinghub.scot/

Space for reader's own reflection:

_____

_____

_____

_____

_____

_____

_____

_____

_____

_____

_____

_____

_____

_____

_____

_____

_____

_____

_____

REFERENCES

Association for Coaching. 2023. Coaching Defined. Association for Coaching. https://www.associationforcoaching.com/page/CoachingDefined

Burgess A, Mellis C. Feedback and assessment for clinical placements: achieving the right balance. Adv Med Educ Pract. 2015 May 19;6:373-81. doi: 10.2147/AMEP.S77890. PMID: 26056511; PMCID: PMC444531.

Cant, R., Ryan, C., Hughes, L., Luders, E., Cooper, S., 2021. What helps, what hinders? Undergraduate nursing students' perceptions of clinical placements based on a thematic synthesis of literature. SAGE Open Nurs. 7, 237796082110358. doi:10.1177/23779608211035845

Clynes, M., Raftery, S., 2008. Feedback: an essential element of student learning in clinical practice. Nurse Educ. Pract. 8 (6), 405–411.

Doyle, K., Sainsbury, K., Cleary, S., Parkinson, L., Vindigni, D., McGrath, I., Cruickshank, M., 2017. Happy to help/happy to be here: identifying components of successful clinical placements for undergraduate nursing students. Nurse Educ. Today 49, 27–32. doi:10.1016/j.nedt.2016.11.001

Duers, L., Brown, N., 2009. An exploration of student nurses' experiences of formative assessment. Nurse Educ. Today 29 (6), 654–659.

Fleming, N., 1987. VARK - A Guide to Learning Styles. https://vark-learn.com/

Hand, H., 2006. Assessment of learning in clinical practice. Nurs. Stand. 21 (4), 48–56.

Harris, C., 2018. Reasonable adjustments for everyone: exploring a paradigm change for nurse educators. Nurse Educ. Pract. 33, 178–180. doi:10.1016/j.nepr.2018.08.009

Hoy, G., George, S., 2018. New standards on the supervision and assessment of students in practice. Nursingtimes.net. https://cdn.ps.emap.com/wp-content/uploads/sites/3/2018/11/181114-New-standards-on-the-supervision-and-assessment-of-students-in-practice.pdf

Immonen, K., Oikarainen, A., Tomietto, M., Kaariainen, M., Tuomikoski, A.M., Kaucic, B.M., et al., 2019. Assessment of Nursing Students' competence in clinical practice: a systematic review of reviews. Int. J. Nurs. Stud. 100, 103414. doi:10.1016/j.ijnurstu.2019.103414

Narayanasamy, A., Penney, V., 2014. Coaching to promote professional development in nursing practice. Br. J. Nurs. 23 (11), 568–573. doi:10.12968/bjon.2014.23.11.568

NHS Education for Scotland. 2008. Quality Standards for Practice Placements (QSPP). NHS Education for Scotland, Edinburgh. https://www.nes.scot.nhs.uk/media/323817/qspp_leaflet_2008.pdf

NHS Education for Scotland. 2019. Practice Learning Handbook: For Practice Supervisors and Practice Assessors. Turas Learn. NHS Education for Scotland, Edinburgh. https://learn.nes.nhs.scot/54944

NHS Education for Scotland. 2020. Practice Education Facilitators (PEFS). NHS Education for Scotland, Edinburgh. https://www.nes.scot.nhs.uk/our-work/practice-education-facilitators-pefs/

NHS Education for Scotland. 2020. Preparation for Practice Supervisors and Practice Assessors, Supporting Effective Practice Learning. Turas Learn. NHS Education for Scotland, Edinburgh.

NHS Education for Scotland. 2024. Preparation for Practice Supervisors and Practice Assessors, Supporting Effective Practice Learning. Turas Learn. NHS Education for Scotland, Edinburgh.

Nursing and Midwifery Council. 2018a. Future Nurse Standards of Proficiency for Registered Nurses. Nursing and Midwifery Council, London. https://www.nmc.org.uk/standards/standards-for-nurses/standards-of-proficiency-for-registered-nurses/

Nursing and Midwifery Council. 2018b. Realising Professionalism: Standards Framework for Education and Training. Part 2: Standards for Student Supervision and Assessment. Nursing and Midwifery Council, London. https://www.nmc.org.uk/standards-for-education-and-training/standards-for-student-supervision-and-assessment/

Nursing and Midwifery Council. 2018c. Standards for Student Supervision and Assessment (Part 2). Nursing and Midwifery Council, London. https://www.nmc.org.uk/standards-for-education-and-training/standards-for-student-supervision-and-assessment/

Nursing and Midwifery Council. 2018d. Standards for Pre-Registration Nursing Programmes (Part 3). Nursing and Midwifery Council, London. https://www.nmc.org.uk/standards/standards-for-nurses/standards-for-pre-registration-nursing-programmes/

Posthuma-Coelho, A., 2016. Theoretical vs Practical Knowledge. Medium. https://medium.com/@amandaposthuma/theoretical-vs-practical-knowledge-86cab1113abd

Preparation for Practice Supervisors and Practice Assessors, Supporting Effective Practice Learning.

Prithishkumar, I., Michael, S., 2014. Understanding your student: Using the VARK model. J. Postgrad. Med. 60 (2), 183. doi:10.4103/0022-3859.132337

Royal College of Nurses. 2017. Guidance for Mentors of Nursing and Midwifery Students. Royal College of Nurses. https://placementhub.our.dmu.ac.uk/wp-content/uploads/sites/5/2016/08/RCN-mentor2017.pdf

Standards of proficiency for registered nurses. 2018a. https://www.nmc.org.uk/standards/standards-for-nurses/standards-of-proficiency-for-registered-nurses/

Tee, S.R., Owens, K., Plowright, S., Ramnath, P., Rourke, S., James, C., & Bayliss, J. (2010) Being reasonable: Supporting disabled nursing students in practice. Nurse Educ. Pract. 10 (4), 216–221. doi:10.1016/j.nepr.2009.11.006

Underwood, S., Green, J., Walton, R., Hackett, K., Cooke, J., Pegg, M., Armstrong, C., 2019. Evaluating the impact of a coaching pilot on students and staff. Br. J. Nurs., 28 (21), 1394–1398. doi:10.12968/bjon.2019.28.21.1394

Wildman, A., 2003. CEDAR Feedback Model. https://annawildman.com/cedar-feedback-model/

Willis Commission. 2012. Quality with Compassion: The Future Nurse Education. Report of the Willis Commission on Nurse Education. RCN, London.

Worrall, K., 2007. Orientation to student placements: needs and benefits. Paediatr. Nurs. 19 (1), 31–33.

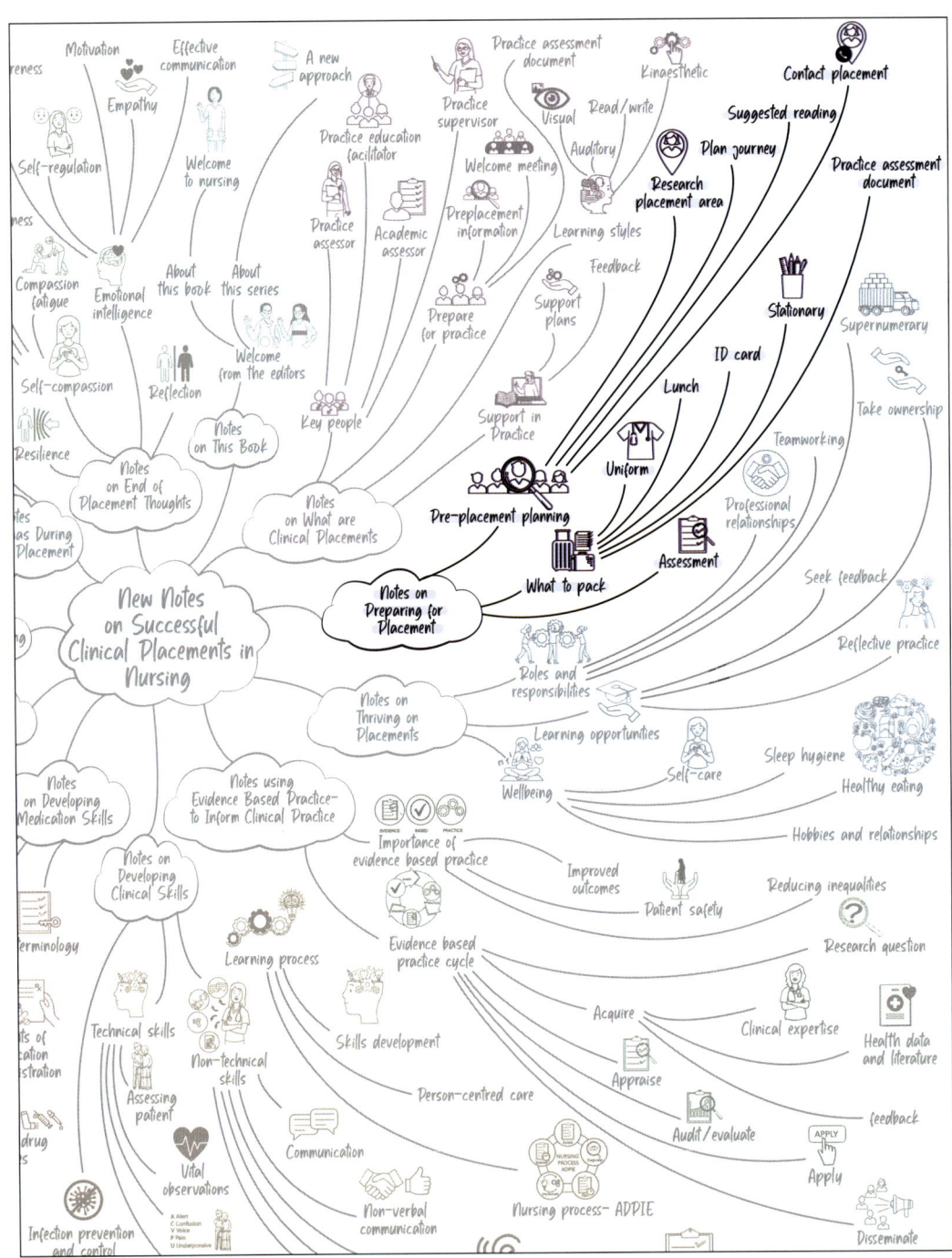

NOTES ON PREPARING FOR PLACEMENT

Katie Anderson (she/her) ■ **Cameron Smith (he/him)**

INTRODUCTION

You are about to embark on your first clinical placement. Congratulations and how exciting! Most nurses will remember their first placement: being full of excitement and nerves but also acknowledging the realisation of putting the theory into practice. You will have spent some time in university exploring key themes and undertaking preparation for placement. This chapter aims to build upon these themes and provide you with some helpful hints and tips to guide you in your preparation for placement.

As a nursing student, your experience is different from that of other university students, as you will spend 50% of your time in theory and 50% in clinical practice; therefore placements are a big deal. This is based upon the Nursing and Midwifery Council (NMC) preregistration standards (NMC, 2023), where you are required to undertake a minimum of 2300 practice learning hours. Your higher education institute (HEI) will work closely with practice partners to identify and provide students with a range of placements to enable you to experience environments to deliver holistic care to people of all ages.

You will have a variety of learning environments during your course, which will include primary, secondary and social care settings, which can further be defined into acute, community and specialist settings. Your placements will enable you to draw upon your theory and embed your knowledge within clinical placements while enabling you to demonstrate your skills relevant to your stage of practice. While undertaking your clinical placement, you will be supervised and assessed by practice supervisors and assessors. These registrants will support you to achieve the proficiencies relevant to your field of nursing practice. We shall explore supervision in our next chapter.

During your placement, you will also be provided with opportunities to attend alternative learning experiences related to your primary placement. This will enable you to gain a wider understanding of patient care, departments, specialities and organisations. This will also provide you with an opportunity to work with a multidisciplinary team and alongside professionals who may be able to sign off on skills you have undertaken with them.

Each setting will require specific preparation and consideration due to the differences in care provided. Hopefully, this chapter will help you organise and prepare yourself.

Before we start, it's important to take some time to think about how you are feeling and ask yourself what you are worried about. It may also be beneficial to think about your strengths and weaknesses as well as ask yourself what you would like to learn and what you hope to achieve while on your clinical placement.

What are your worries and hopes for your upcoming placement?

_____

_____

_____

_____

_____

_____

PRE-PLACEMENT PLANNING

Being notified of your first clinical placement is an exciting time; however, it can also leave you feeling nervous and overwhelmed.

Your university will usually notify you of your placement allocation a few weeks before your start date. If you have not received notification or if you experience challenges with your allocation, please reach out to your placement link plenty of time before your start date to enable the team to support you.

Once you have your allocation, we suggest you start finding out about the clinical area/specialty and consider the location of your placement. You may wish to begin by undertaking some research into what specific health needs/skills those within your care or placement area may require. For example, you may wish to revisit your anatomy and physiology, body systems or key clinical skills that you may be able to demonstrate during your time.

Your HEI may provide you with a profile of the area which will enable you to think about your placement in further detail. For example, it may identify what learning opportunities you can aim to achieve, what preparation work you may need to undertake as well as what the working shift pattern is for the area. This information is crucial to help inform your preparation, such as childcare and hobbies, or help structure study time to research the area.

Another useful link you may wish to explore prior to placement is care opinion. This is a national online platform where the public can share feedback about their experience of the health and care systems. You can review the latest patient stories at www.careopinion.org.uk.

You may also wish to connect with your student union, nursing society, wider university support networks or senior students. They may have already been to your clinical area and may be able to provide some top tips as well as offer recommendations or advice about accommodation and travel. Based on your clinical environment profile and term-time address, you may need to consider whether you need to find accommodation to stay close by or consider what transport you will need to get to placement on time. For example, your clinical placement shift

Placement Environment: Ward 1A Surgical Inverdeen General Hospital IV21 798 Inverdeen Contact: Charlie Wilson Telephone: 02535 452376 Contact Email: charlie.wilson@inverdeengeneral.com		
Speciality: General Surgical		
Learning Opportunities: Pre- and Postoperative Care, Medication Management, Pain Management, Wound Management, Essential Nursing Care, Intravenous Infusions and Therapies, Preoperative Assessment Department, Outpatient Department, Theatre.		
Interprofessional Learning Opportunities: Dietician, Pharmacist, Physiotherapist, Occupational Therapist, Specialist Nurses, Speech and Language Therapist.		
Preplacement reading: Elliott, N. and Girvin, J., eds., 2024. *How to be a successful nursing student*. Elsevier.		
Days: Monday to Sunday	Hours: 12-Hour Shift Pattern	Other Information: Day and Nightshift
Other information relevant to this placement		
Student lockers: Yes	Changing facilities: Yes	Catering: Yes
Reading materials: Yes	Library access: No	Study area: No

pattern may be from 07.00 to 19.30. You will be expected to be in the clinical environment ready to receive handover at 07.00. Your placement may be 1 hour 30 minutes away; therefore it will add an additional 3 hours to your working day with your commute to and from placement. You therefore may wish to consider staying in a bed and breakfast closer to the area to support your health and wellbeing.

Sleep, nutrition and downtime are all important aspects to consider as well as your personal safety. Driving 1 hour 30 minutes after a 12-hour shift could become challenging 3 or 4 days in a row. Depending on when your clinical placement is, you may experience finding accommodation challenging due to holiday times; therefore it is important to be organised well in advance. Through your union or nursing society, you may also be able to identify additional students who may be in the same area or clinical environment as you. This could mean you could consider renting accommodation together to reduce costs.

'I had one placement where I was Monday to Friday, 9 a.m. until 5 p.m. Normally the journey would have only taken 30 minutes by car, but because I was travelling during the peak times, it took me well over an hour'.

Natalie Elliott, RN

It's always a good idea for your first placement to do a trial run of how to get there and how long it will take. You could time your practice run with a preplacement visit to meet with your supervisor or assessor.

TIPS

In preparation for your practice run, you may wish to consider the following:

- Ensure you identify the correct public transport.
- What bus number/train times is it that you need? How long does each journey take, inclusive of stops?
- Is there a cycle route you could take instead? Are there bike lockers nearby or on site?
- What route would you take if driving? You may need to consider local traffic/roadworks to ensure you attend on time.
- Is there any parking at your clinical placement? Do you need a permit to park? Who do you need to contact to obtain a permit?
- How much will each journey cost you? Is there a weekly/monthly pass you could buy to reduce the costs?
- Could you car share with fellow students?
- Do you need to complete documentation, for example, preapproval forms/mileage forms/share insurance documents with your HEI prior to going out on placement?

'I had a placement where the parking was free, but it was a 10-minute walk to the hospital from the car park, so I had to factor this additional time into my travel time'.

Simon James, RN

Your university will have a link lecturer or placement team to offer advice and support regarding travel and accommodation, so please do reach out to them in advance of your clinical placement.

'Sometimes students might find it difficult to glean information from the area's profile, or perhaps you can't quite visualise where the service fits in relation to the patient experience. Your practice education link team is a useful point of contact to signpost you onto further information about the area or educational resources to be able to reference within your preplacement activities. They can also help you to identify with more depth and rationale what theoretical elements of your programme might be helpful to you during this placement. This can then all supplement a discussion to achieve proficiencies or identify gaps in your knowledge'.

Ciara Moloney, practice education link lecturer

Your education provider will notify you of your placement area's contact details; however, they may also be able to provide you with an audit or overview of the environment. This may include:

- Patient demographics and specific care needs to those within the environment
- Main learning opportunities
- Associated learning environments you may be able to visit
- Suggested preplacement reading
- Previous student feedback
- Interprofessional learning opportunities
- Student support networks
- Shift patterns/hours

All of these can help inform you of what to expect as well as prepare you prior to contacting your clinical area.

Reaching out to your placement area can be scary, as you want to set a good impression of yourself. Your university will provide you with guidance on when to contact your clinical area; this is normally 2 weeks before your start date. When contacting your clinical area, make sure to remain professional as per the (NMC, 2023).

NMC

THE NMC SAYS

20.10 Use all forms of spoken, written and digital communication (including social media and networking sites) responsibly, respecting the right to privacy of others at all times.

Whether contacting by email or telephone, make sure you introduce yourself and the university you are studying at as well as what stage/year of nursing you are in. Fig. 2.1 gives a useful example of how to do this.

Clinical areas may support healthcare students from several universities, so ensuring to clearly communicate who you are and where you

> Hello, my name is XXXX and I am a XX year nursing student from XXXX. Could I please speak with XXXX.
> I am very excited to start placement here on XXX and I'm wondering if now is convenient for me to ask some questions?
> I was wondering if you are able to give me my rota, along with the start and finish times. Will I be expected to work nightshift or weekends? I have children so it would be helpful to know so that I can arrange childcare.
> I have some commitments during my placement, and I was wondering if it would be possible not to rostered for XXXX.
> Will I be expected to wear my uniform?
> Do I have allocated practice assessor and supervisor?
> Can you tell me about the catering facilities, will I have access to a microwave, hot water, canteen?
> Is there anything you would like me to do to prepare for starting and do you have an induction booklet?
> Thank you very much for your time, I look forward to meeting you and the team on XXXX.

Fig. 2.1   Provides some useful ideas on how to approach this (Elliott N, 2024).

are from is important. If you are calling, we suggest contacting your clinical area outside of peak times such as at the beginning or at the end of a shift. Clinical environments can be very busy, and at times you may not be able to talk to the identified member of staff when you call due to workload or shift patterns. Therefore, be patient with the staff and environment; if they cannot answer you straight away, offer to call back, or leave a number that they can contact you on.

If contacting by email, ensure to use your university email address and not your personal account. Fig. 2.2 provides some helpful tips on email etiquette.

When contacting your clinical area for the first time, we suggest you have a notepad and pen handy to make any notes of advice or essential information that is shared with you. You may also wish to make a list of questions you have for the area, such as:

- Are there changing facilities available?
- Is there a locker for my personal items?

Email Etiquette
For students
Writing a professional email may not sound like a big deal, but it's actually a skill in itself

Greet your contact properly
- Include a greeting! It can be as simple as "Dear Dr. Smith," or "Hello, Mrs. Carter," Only use first names IF the person introduced themselves in such a manner. Otherwise use a FORMAL title like Dr., Mrs. or Ms.

Use real words
- Don't use text speak or lots of slang in your message – keep it professional.
- Txt spk mks ur msg hrd 2 read nd on look rly unprofesh!!!

Be polite
- Always remember to say "please" and "thank you" as necessary throughout the email. Instead of demanding be thoughtful and polite. If you are upset about something give yourself some time to calm down and relax so you don't say something you may not actually means to say. *You catch more flies with honey...*

Be brief, positive, and friendly
- Anyone you email may be busy, so make sure you aim for short and sweet. Portray a friendly tone and give options if necessary to show you are willing to work with the other person.

Proofread your email before sending it
- Look over your message for any grammar or spelling mistakes that stand out. Check for tone and make sure your concern is addressed correctly.

Fig. 2.2 Helpful tips on email etiquette.

- What kitchen facilities are available to me, such as a fridge and microwave?
- Who should I report to on my first day?

Have a think about some questions specific to you that you may wish to ask your clinical area prior to starting.

_____

_____

_____

_____

_____

_____

When contacting your clinical area, you may wish to request a preplacement visit, which is an opportunity for you to attend your clinical placement to familiarise yourself with the environment as well as meet key members of staff, such as your practice supervisor or assessor, before officially starting your placement. When engaging with your clinical area, ask what date and time would be suitable for you to visit. The clinical area will be able to inform you of dates and times that might be best dependent on clinical need. A preplacement visit will also enable you to familiarise yourself with travel arrangements, as previously discussed, and the route to take to your environment, so you are prepared on the first day of your placement.

Undertaking your first placement is exciting; however, it is natural to feel nervous too. Undertaking a preplacement visit will hopefully help alleviate any concerns you have, as you will be able to ask questions, for example, what learning opportunities are available, if there is a locker for your bag and if there is a fridge you can use for your meals. The member of staff showing you around may also be able to provide an insight into the skills and procedures you will be able to learn and demonstrate too.

SOCIAL MEDIA
@CYPSTNN

'Preplacement visits for nursing are an exciting opportunity to familiarise yourself with the setting, meet the team and ask questions. It's a change to get a feel for the environment and start building relationships'.

It is also a fantastic opportunity to ask questions you may have prior to your first day. It provides you with an opportunity to further explore the expectations or skills you may be required to demonstrate or provide to those in your care prior to your placement starting. Being proactive in your approach to your placement demonstrates initiative, organisational skills and enthusiasm, all of which are values you require in nursing.

SOCIAL MEDIA
@JamesWade1807

'1- be clear on what you need to achieve relation to your own proficiencies, skills and assessments you need to complete. 2- Have a weekly plan on what you aim to achieve 3- ensure orientation initial interview mid-way point and final assessment process is followed'.

'The benefit of a student attending a preplacement visit allows the student to know where they are going and get key information prior to starting their placement, which will assist them in their preplacement learning activities. It might give an opportunity to meet your practice assessor and practice supervisor prior to starting. It will help alleviate some anxieties about attending placement'.

Kirsty Lamond, practice educator

Gathering as much information prior to placement and being prepared will hopefully ease any anxiety you may experience and help you physically and mentally prepare for placement.

SOCIAL MEDIA

@CaridacClinic

'Do some pre reading about the area you are going to be working in. Take a packed lunch and plenty of fluids. Pens, little pocket notepad in tunic pocket. A positive attitude and a smile. And don't put too much pressure on yourself! You are there to learn'.

WHAT TO PACK FOR PLACEMENT?

So you know where you are going on placement, you've undertaken your preplacement visit and now it's time to get ready for your first shift. The first question many students ask is, 'What should I take to placement?' First, we advise you to invest in a suitable rucksack/bag to hold all your belongings that you will need to take to placement. We recommend a rucksack with two straps to enable you to carry your belongings with even distribution over both shoulders. You will be required to carry a lot of equipment, and we want you to protect the health of your back, as you have a long career ahead of you.

From our own personal experience and our role in supporting students in placement, we have formulated a checklist of key items to take with you to placement:

- Your uniform plus a spare: A spare uniform is always good to have in case you need to change. You never know what might happen on placement which may require you to change your uniform. A helpful hint also is to pack a carrier bag with you. This is for the uniform you change out of, as it may be dirty. Please also refer to your university/placement uniform policy to make sure you meet the standards as expected.
- Fob watch: Please ensure your watch is a wipeable one only and not a metal one, for example. The rationale for this is to ensure you meet infection control standards to reduce the potential risk of infection.
- Pencil case: A nurse can never have too many black pens. . .

- Lunch and snacks: Depending on how long your shift is, you may have to pack all your meals for 1 day. For example- Breakfast, snack, lunch, snack and dinner. Hence, you may need a large rucksack, or you may need to buy a lunch bag also. Meal preparation is key for nutritional value, cost and organization when on clinical placement. When you are undertaking multiple shifts together, you may have little time to go to the shops in between; therefore being organised and prepared with your food can save time, and it's one thing you can be prepared with during a busy period. When on shift, it can become hot, and at times you may feel dehydrated. The investment of a water bottle would be helpful, as you can have this with you at all times during your shift.
- Access to your clinical assessment documents: These are a vital piece of equipment, as you and your practice supervisor and assessor will start to utilise them from day 1. You may have a physical copy of your documents; therefore we suggest placing them into a protective sleeve, ensuring it is wipeable. This is to protect your documents; however, be mindful not to dismantle and reassemble them into another folder and that your original document is in its original state. This is to ensure your document remains legible for your academic assessor and future practice assessors to review your progress and eventually confirm you have met all the requirements of the programme. If you have an electronic copy of your documents, ensure you and your supervisors have access to them prior to starting placement. If you experience any challenges with this, please contact your university link lecturer for support.
- Notepad: When on placement, you may wish to make notes about a variety of things such as conditions, format of the ward and further suggested reading; therefore having a notebook on you can be a valuable tool. A helpful hint we were given as students was to buy two small address books. In one, you can write all the conditions you come across in alphabetical order. In the other, you can write commonly used drugs along with side effects and route of administration, again in alphabetical order. This means that in each clinical environment you attend, you can add to this 'bank' of knowledge as well as refer back to your book for guidance.

- ID card: When on clinical placement, it is vital you share who you are with others. This could be with those within your care or other members of staff. Therefore it is important to always have your ID on show. We would strongly suggest you don't use a lanyard due to safety challenges. The rationale for this is that a patient/member of the public may grab a hold of it around your neck, or it could get caught on a piece of equipment and therefore poses potential harm to you. Instead, we suggest using an ID badge holder that can clip onto your uniform. Again, please ensure it is wipeable to reduce the risk of infection.
- Personal belongings: We know that you will take personal items to placement with you, for example, your phone or purse/wallet. Where possible, try to take the minimum number of personal belongings. You are going to be busy on shift and therefore shouldn't need to always have personal items with you. However, to ensure the safety of your belongings, you may wish to ask about a locker at your preplacement visit and/or take a padlock and ask where you can store your personal belongings safely.
- Hair accessories: Try to limit the amount of hair accessories you use. At times, you may be asked to remove them due to safety concerns, for example, escorting a patient to a CT scan. Also, be mindful that a patient may pull them out, either intentionally or unintentionally.

GETTING THE BALANCE RIGHT

Clinical placements are exciting with all the opportunities available while also being able to link theory with practice; however, you can become consumed by placement. Therefore maintaining your wellbeing is a priority throughout your nursing career.

NMC

THE NMC SAYS

20.9 Maintain the level health you need to carry out your professional role.

As highlighted, your placement can become consuming. For example, you could be working 5 days a week or undertaking 12-hour shifts for multiple days, which may be a change to your routine. When starting university, you will begin to form relationships with fellow nursing students. This support network is great, as you are all experiencing and navigating your nursing journey together; however, it can also mean that a lot of conversations or meetings together can be based around nursing. It's important to try and get a balance so that you can 'switch off' from nursing while able to focus on your personal life too. The following are some key topics to consider in relation to your wellbeing.

Competing priorities

As you begin your placement, it's a ti when you need to consider how to balance study and work as well as personal commitments. Your focus should be your placement; however, we acknowledge that you may have external work in which to undertake also.

It's important to be mindful that although you are undertaking shifts within a clinical setting, this experience is linked to the university and will be embedded within a clinical module; therefore you will have module requirements to obtain. At times, students sometimes lose the link between the university and clinical practice and see them as two separate identities; however, this is not the case. See it almost as a long-distance module in which you have proficiencies and skills to demonstrate in order to achieve a passing grade for the placement.

We know many students will potentially have a part-time job to support them through their studies. Therefore, prior to undertaking your placement, you may wish to have a discussion with your employer to inform them of the shifts you may be about to embark on, the location of your placement as well as discuss flexibility in your role. For example, you may wish to consider reducing your hours while on placement.

There are many elements of your practice modules, for example, being organised, engaging with the public and undertaking shift work while also learning and demonstrating skills and proficiencies. All of these can take their toll or potentially lead to burnout if you're unable to manage the work/life balance. If you experience challenges in obtaining the right balance, we suggest you reach out to your practice supervisor or assessor in the first instance. This will enable you to discuss any flexibility with the clinical area; however, also reach out to your personal tutor or your link lecturer to discuss support mechanisms in place from the university.

Shift pattern

As mentioned, undertaking a preplacement visit and contacting your clinical area prior to starting will enable you to obtain your off duty for a few weeks in advance. Being proactive and obtaining your shifts will enable you to manage your personal life such as childcare and important life events such as weddings. Prior to starting placement, if you identify any key dates/challenges you may have, please let them know in advance. You can then facilitate an open and honest conversation with your practice supervisor and assessor about the challenges, and you can negotiate your shifts; however, bear in mind this would be for exceptional circumstances. However, it may also enable you to look ahead at your days off during which to rest, work or undertake activities and hobbies.

Wellbeing activities

When undertaking your placement, you can become consumed by it and feel you are living, breathing and talking about all things to do with nursing. However, it's important to try and maintain some normality in your routine such as your wellbeing activities. This is key to enabling you to have some downtime away from nursing as well as supporting your mental wellbeing. For example, you may already go swimming, go for a walk in the evening, meet friends or undertake mindful practices in your normal everyday life. However, when undertaking clinical placement, these practices may need to be adapted due to shift work. As highlighted, you may be able to obtain your off duty for a few weeks in advance, which will enable you to look at rescheduling your activities or even attending an alternative class.

Maintaining your wellbeing is vital when undertaking clinical placement, and we will explore this theme further in the next chapter.

ASSESSMENT PREPARATION

As identified, you will spend 50% of your time on clinical placement and will be assessed during your time throughout it as per the NMC education standards (2023). Just like a theory module, it is important to study and be proactive in your learning to demonstrate your skills and competence.

Prior to attending placement, you will be provided with your clinical assessment documentation. If you experience challenges in accessing, for example, an electronic copy or you haven't received your physical copy, please contact your link lecturer to resolve this prior to placement.

It is vitally important to spend time reading through your documentation to ensure you have full understanding of your assessment and to clarify any questions you have about it prior to your first shift. Initially, you will be asked to undertake preplacement activities; this is an opportunity for you to undertake research in your clinical area as well as identify learning opportunities you wish to achieve. Please ensure to undertake these activities, as this demonstrates professionalism and enthusiasm and aids in your learning when meeting with your practice supervisor or assessor for the first time.

As students, the ownership is upon you to lead and direct your learning, and your practice supervisors and assessors are there to support you. While on placement, you will have skills and procedures to undertake as well as demonstrate your knowledge and understanding of holistic care and conditions. Prior to your placement, we would suggest you consider identifying the skills and procedures you may be exposed to within your clinical area and ones where you may be able to get involved in and undertake depending upon your stage of education. It's important to take time to think carefully about your stage and scope of practice to ensure you set out realistic and achievable learning opportunities. During your initial meeting with your practice supervisor and assessor, you will have an opportunity to discuss your thoughts and objectives. Your supervisors may also be able to add additional comments and/or identify learning opportunities available to you that you were unaware of within the environment. In addition to your primary clinical placement, you may also identify or suggest additional learning opportunities. You may wish to think about alternative clinical areas you could visit your clinical placement, for example, outpatient clinical wards, operating theatres, high-dependency wards, community nurse and general practice nurse.

These additional opportunities may enable you to be exposed to further skills and procedures as well as help you to understand and formulate a patient's journey and the care that is provided during each stage.

SOCIAL MEDIA
@gailWil83708216

suggests to 'Ask lots of questions, take lots of notes, ask to follow a patients journey and to observe anything that's happening'.

TIPS

Once you have started placement, engage with a service user and ask what professionals or services they have been in contact with during their journey. This may help you identify additional learning opportunities.

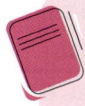

CASE STUDY

Supriya was on placement with a community nursing team; however, she identified that she wished to be an observer in operating theatres. She asked her practice supervisor, James, if this would be possible. James explained that while this would be interesting and Supriya may care for an individual following surgery,

Continued

CASE STUDY—cont'd

the link to immediate care is distanced as well as potentially distanced physically; that is, she may need to travel to an acute hospital setting. Instead, James suggested it may be more appropriate to spend time with a practice nurse, specialist community nurse, occupational therapist or pharmacist. These are professionals who are in direct contact with those who are seeking care from her primary practice placement. Her placement will be over a period of a few weeks, and therefore it's important to be organised and ensure she obtains the most out of the placement as she can.

Throughout your placement, you are continually assessed through key reviews. You will have an initial meeting with your practice supervisor and assessor, with a follow-up interim and final meeting. At your initial meeting, you may wish to highlight the dates when the following meeting will be undertaken. This enables you to remain focused as well as set out objectives to meet prior to these dates.

It's important to be organised when attending these meetings. You may wish to ensure you have key bullet points written down of aspects you wish to seek clarity about if you are unsure as well as share what you have done well and areas in which you feel you could enhance or gain confidence. These meetings should be supportive and an opportunity to share your thoughts and views with your practice assessor and/or your supervisor.

CONCLUSION

This chapter aimed to explore how to prepare you for your clinical placements. It's an exciting time to start your first placement and your nursing career, and we hope you enjoy your journey to becoming a registered nurse. Starting and adapting to a clinical placement can be challenging while maintaining your personal life; throughout this chapter, we have explored ways to make your transition to placement easier as well as ways to look after yourself. We wish you all the best as you embark on your clinical placements.

Space for reader's own reflection:

_____

_____

_____

_____

_____

_____

_____

_____

_____

_____

_____

_____

_____

_____

_____

_____

REFERENCE

Elliott N. 2024. How to be a Successful Nursing Student. Elsevier.

Nursing and Midwifery Council. 2023. Standards framework for nursing and midwifery education. https://www.nmc.org.uk/globalassets/sitedocuments/standards/2024/standards-framework-for-nursing-and-midwifery-education.pdf

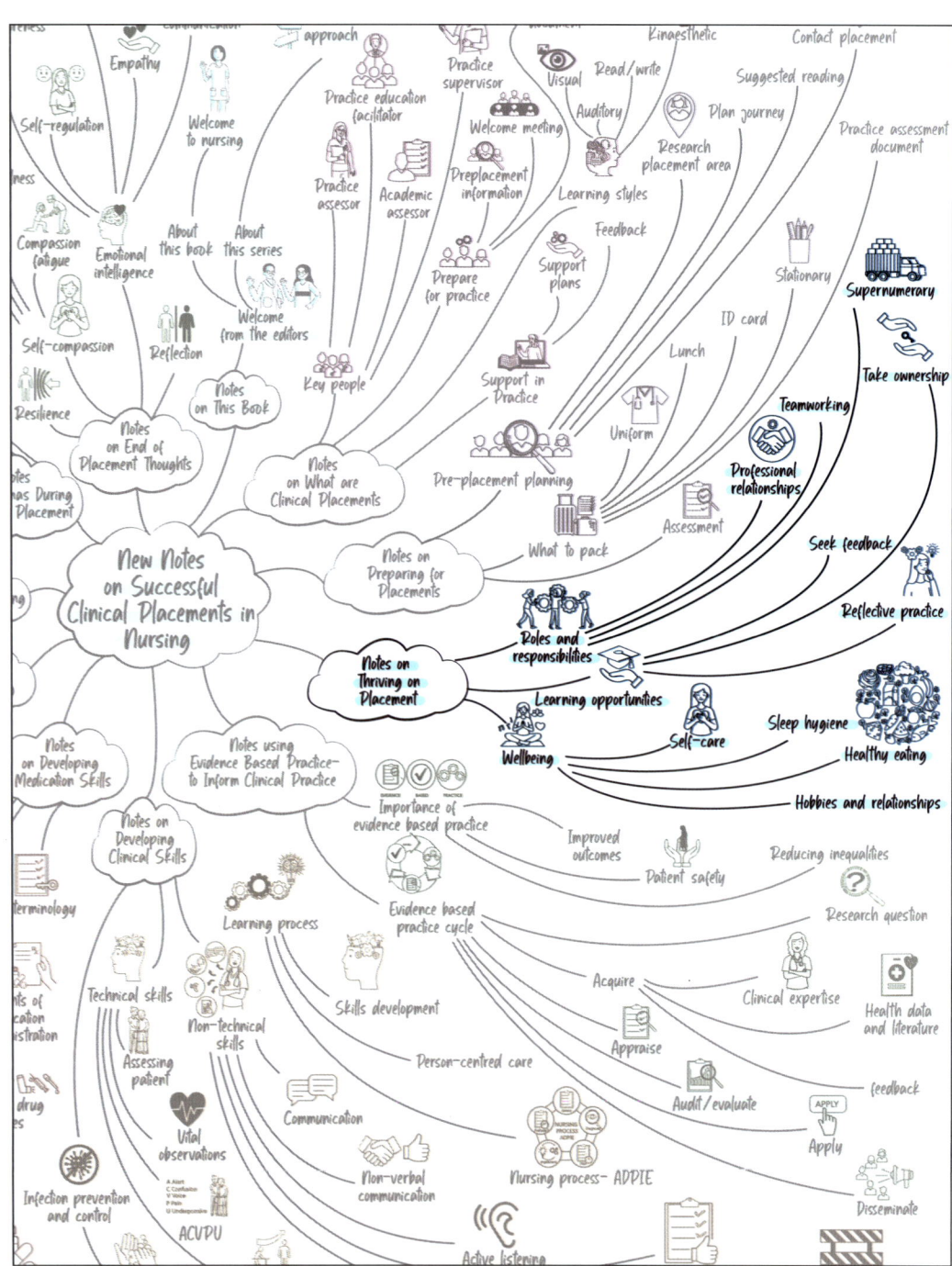

New Notes on Successful Clinical Placements in Nursing

NOTES ON THRIVING ON PLACEMENT

Cameron Smith (he/him)   ■   **Katie Anderson (she/her)**

INTRODUCTION

Within the last chapter, we explored how best to prepare for placement; within this chapter, we aim to consider how to get the best out of your placement and thrive.

It's an exciting time to start your placement for the first time; you may begin to think about the care you will provide and what learning opportunities you will be exposed to while also demonstrating the knowledge and skills you have learnt during your time at university. That said, it can be an anxious and daunting time, as you are entering a new and unfamiliar environment with multidisciplinary team members you don't know, as well as engaging with the public and demonstrating the values of a nursing student.

This chapter aims to explore ways in which you can thrive during your placement by providing you with helpful hints and tips.

Thriving on placement is a skill which you may need time to develop as a first-year student. You may need to reflect upon your wellbeing and consider whether you have met your personal needs to thrive on placement. As mentioned in the previous chapter, you may need time to think of ways in which to manage your priorities as well as consider if you need support from others in order to be the best version of you. Nursing is a challenging yet rewarding job; therefore ensuring you are fit to undertake placement will enable you to do the best you can.

During your first few days, you will spend time familiarising yourself with the physical environment, for example, knowing where key consumables or equipment are stored as well as understanding the routine of the clinical environment. This can take time and may differ each day; therefore don't put too much pressure on yourself to know everything within the first few days. While navigating the physical environment, you will also spend time getting to know key individuals who will play a part in your progress as well as patient journeys, for example, your practice supervisor and assessor. Depending on your environment, the multidisciplinary team you work with may change regularly due to shift work; therefore you may be required to introduce yourself to others multiple times and vice versa. We understand this can be repetitive; however, once you have settled into your clinical area over a period of a few weeks, this should lessen. As highlighted, you will have key professionals who will help guide your learning through the placement; these will be your practice supervisor and assessor. These registered professionals will support you in achieving your proficiencies and requirements for your clinical module. We shall further explore the themes of supervision, learning opportunities, support networks and wellbeing to enable you to thrive on placement.

Take a moment to think about what would support you in being able to thrive on placement. What could you do to ensure you're prepared and fit to flourish on placement? What do you need from others to help you grow and develop on placement?

_____

_____

_____

_____

_____

_____

ROLES AND RESPONSIBILITIES

In 2016, the Nursing and Midwifery Council (NMC) looked to review and update their educational standards. The NMC consulted with nurses, midwives, health and social care partners as well as education providers within the United Kingdom. The NMC also sought feedback from patients, carers and the public regarding the future of nurses and midwives and education and practice learning experiences that would be needed to prepare them. The NMC professional standards for education and training standards were published in 2023 and consist of three parts:

- Part 1: Standards framework for nursing and midwifery education
- Part 2: Standards for student supervision and assessment
- Part 3: standards for preregistration nursing programmes

During placement, you will have identified members of staff undertaking supervision. You will work with several healthcare professionals who will provide guidance, support and feedback to enhance your knowledge and skills.

Fig. 3.1 identifies the connection between roles ensuring the student is at the centre of supervision.

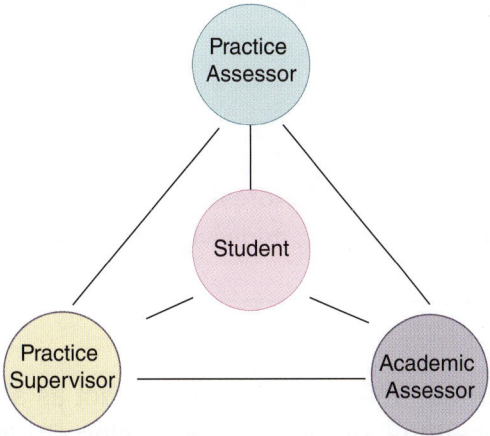

Fig 3.1 **Regulatory roles for the supervision and assessment of nursing students (NES, 2019).**

Professional relationships

Starting a new clinical area can be daunting and exciting. You might be wondering what skills or procedures you might undertake while also considering how the team you're joining works and how you will fit into this team. Developing relationships with the multidisciplinary team is vital to help you settle into the area as well as enable you to seek support from those around you. These individuals will be key to supporting your growth and development both personally and professionally; this may in turn also increase in your confidence.

SOCIAL MEDIA

@justacarehomegirl

'make it your mission to learn, stay open minded, speak to as many people as possible'.

Your practice supervisor and assessor are the key to supporting your transition to the clinical environment as well as your journey through your placement. Developing a professional relationship with your supervisors is vital to enable you to obtain your learning outcomes and develop your confidence in the care you provide. Your practice supervisor and assessor will be registered nurses with the NMC. As registered professionals, they will uphold the NMC (2018) in which they are required to:

NMC

THE NMC SAYS

20.8 Act as a role model of professional behaviour for student and newly qualified nurses, midwives and nursing associates to aspire to.

Therefore they must uphold their values and act as a role model to you and also your educational provider. As a nursing student, you must also reflect these values to demonstrate the NMC code of conduct (2018). Having a good working relationship with others can have a positive impact upon you and can make a difference in your experience and engagement. When developing professional relationships, you must consider your professional role and boundaries.

It is generally not the expectation that nursing students engage with their supervisors like they are best friends. In addition to this, it is also not expected that you would contact/engage with your supervisor via social media. These actions could blur professional boundaries and potentially cause conflict.

NMC

THE NMC SAYS

20.6 Stay objective and have clear professional boundaries at all times with people in your care (including those who have been in your care in the past), their families and carers.

To help you develop your professional relationships with your supervisors, you may wish to demonstrate and develop key attributes such as:

- Active listening: This means actively attending to what is being said and how it is being said. It is listening without making judgements or letting your own perceptions act as a barrier to what is being said by the other person. Active listening indicates that you are working hard to understand the other person and enables trusting relationships, rapport, mutual interest and understanding (Grant and Goodman, 2019).
- Working as a team: As a nursing student, teamwork will be one of the key components of the role. Teamwork links directly to meeting the NMC code (2023) by prioritising people, practising effectively, preserving safety and promoting professionalism and trust. The team you work with may be inclusive of many different roles, for example, registered and nonregistered staff members. Effectively engaging with others to meet the same outcome creates a successful working environment, which ultimately leads to better person- or family-centred care.

SOCIAL MEDIA
@PUNC20_michelle

'I thrive by taking every opportunity the team give me, being practice and having a team who love to encourage and support me.'

NMC

THE NMC SAYS

8.2 Maintain effective communication with colleagues.

8.4 Work with colleagues to evaluate the quality of your work and that of the team.

8.5 Work with colleagues to preserve the safety of those receiving care.

7.3 Use a range of verbal and non-verbal communication methods, and consider cultural sensitivities, to better understand and respond to people's personal and health needs.

As we have mentioned, it's important to nurture and develop professional relationships with others; however, at times, these relationships may not be formed as easily or may break down over time. Should you experience any challenges with your practice supervisor or practice assessor, you should seek support from the practice education team and the practice education lecturer/link lecturers. It is important to address any challenges at the earliest opportunity, and the education teams can support you in doing this. You will not get into trouble, and these teams are there to support you through the challenges you are experiencing. You may, however, wish to raise concerns in relation to care, supervision and professionalism as examples; again, we would signpost you to contact your link lecturers to discuss, as you will be able to undertake internal or external raising concerns processes.

Supernumerary status

Prior to or during your clinical placement, you may hear the term 'supernumerary status' as a student; however, you may be unclear as to what this means.

The NMC (2023) states: 'Students in practice or work placed learning must be supported to learn without being counted as part of the staffing required for safe and effective care in that setting. Placements should enable students to learn to provide safe and effective care, not merely to observe; students can and should add real value to care. The contribution students make will increase over time as they gain proficiency, and they will continue to benefit from ongoing guidance and feedback. Once a student has demonstrated that they are proficient, they should be able to fulfil tasks without direct oversight. The level of supervision a student needs is based on the professional judgement of their supervisors, taking into account any associated risks and the students' knowledge, proficiency and confidence'.

Therefore, as a student, you are supported to undertake your learning without the challenge or conflict being accounted for in staffing numbers. This enables students to focus on their learning needs and consolidate their practice while being supported by practice supervisors and assessors.

SOCIAL MEDIA
@rsheridan2390

'To any new students about to go out into practise one bit of advice would be to use your supernumerary status to your advantage, spoke out to other teams for a day, learn as much as possible or my personal favourite sit and talk to your patients'.

LEARNING OPPORTUNITIES

Starting a new placement is exciting, but it can also create some level of anxiety, which is normal. Every placement will provide you with various learning opportunities and support you in developing your knowledge and skills. Before you start placement, it is important to familiarise yourself with the module learning outcomes, platforms and proficiencies, and skills annexes. Before you start, think about what your objectives are, what you hope to achieve in each placement learning experience and what learning opportunities might your placement offer that will help you in achieving these objectives.

Being proactive and take ownership of learning

THE NMC SAYS

6.2 Maintain the knowledge and skills you need for safe and effective practice.

As a nursing student, you will be supported by several professionals before, during and after your clinical placement; this could be practice supervisor, practice assessor or link lecturer. However, you are accountable for your own learning, and your learning needs are your responsibility (Practice Assessment Document [PAD] Scotland, 2023).

SOCIAL MEDIA
@slaterbooth1

'Be proactive. Speak with your supervisor and let them know what skills you need to learn and gain experience on. Listen at handover and speak to other members of staff (along with your supervisor) if they are doing things you need to learn'.

TIPS

To help you make a positive start to each of your placements, you should complete your preplacement activities. These activities could be:

1. Contacting your clinical placement and ascertaining your shift pattern as well as arranging a preplacement visit.
2. Reading the clinical environments profile as provided by your higher education institute.

3. Writing notes or a summary on what care the practice learning environment provides.
4. Identifying a condition or situation you may come across within your clinical area and providing a literature search of these.
5. Identifying learning from your theory modules that would support your learning within the clinical environment.
6. Identifying learning from clinical skills that would support your learning within the clinical environment.

These activities will give you the chance to think about what learning opportunities will be available for you in each of the placement areas. When you are thinking about what learning opportunities there might be, it might be good to refer to the proficiencies and skills annexes in your practice assessment documents. You may wish to think about how the learning opportunities will help you in achieving these. It is good to go into each placement with an understanding of what that area does; thinking about the learning opportunities before you start placement will help you to discuss your learning needs and set your objectives when you have your initial meeting with your practice supervisor and assessor.

SOCIAL MEDIA
@SuzieParryJohn

'students... its ok to be proactive and strategic with saying out what competences and skills you want to focus on. Take the driving seat don't be a passenger'.

SOCIAL MEDIA
@ed_nurse_uk

'Be prepared, know exactly what you need to achieve for the year/placement and what you personally want to know/observe practice and I will do my best to make sure the opportunities if they arise my student will get what they need'.

The initial meeting with your practice supervisor and assessor will give you an opportunity to work collaboratively with them to discuss the learning experiences you may be exposed to while on placement and how these will link to the skills and procedures you will need to achieve over the duration of your undergraduate programme. It also provides an opportunity to explore what to expect from the environment and each other's expectations in your roles/stage. This initial meeting also marks the start of your ongoing assessment. At your initial meeting, you should also plan provisional dates for your midway and final assessments.

You will need to be proactive when you are on placement and may need to seek out additional learning experiences.

SOCIAL MEDIA
@Ujala935523512

'Lastly I believe I taking initiative and being proactive in volunteering for opportunities to observe or participate in patient care activities, procedures and clinical simulations'.

Some placement areas will have rotational programmes around various additional learning experiences that directly link into their area; in some cases, this will be planned before you start placement, and in other cases, you may need to plan these additional learning experiences yourself. This is an opportunity for you to demonstrate your leadership skills by taking responsibility for your own learning needs.

SOCIAL MEDIA
@Mattgordon83

'Embrace everything, even if it isn't your passion, it might change. See everything, get involved, you never know you might see a different perspective. Use your initiative, no questions are silly questions. Lastly make sure you do your pre placement visit'.

When you are on placement, it is important that you seek regular feedback on your performance and how you are progressing towards meeting your objectives. Your practice supervisors and assessors are responsible for providing you with regular formative feedback, support and guidance. However, you should also be proactive in seeking feedback. Throughout your placement, you will have the opportunity to work with various members of the multidisciplinary and multiagency teams. This will help you achieve your proficiencies and skill annexes while also helping you develop your knowledge. It is important to seek feedback from any member of the team you work with, as you can use the additional notes pages in your practice assessment documents to have this feedback recorded. This will help you to reflect and will support your practice supervisor and assessor develop an understanding of how you are progressing when you are not working directly with them. Seeking regular feedback will help your practice assessor when they come to complete your midway and your final assessment, as they can draw upon a range of feedback.

> 'This may seem like a lot to remember, but my main point to take away from all of this is to be proactive and engage with your placement area as much as you can'.
>
> **Doreen Dube, nursing student**

Reflective practice

Reflective practice is a necessary skill of nursing to ensure continuous learning and improvement. Reflection fosters the development of self-awareness while fostering evaluation and learning from a situation (Toews et al., 2021). This may enable individuals to understand actions and emotions which may result in changes to your own or others' future practice, both personally and professionally (NMC, 2024).

NMC

THE NMC SAYS

9.2 Gather and reflect on feedback from a variety of sources, using it to improve your practice and performance.

There are many ways in which you can undertake reflection, some of which can be undertaken by yourself and/or with others, such as your practice supervisor or assessor. Some ways in which you can undertake reflection are:

- Written reflective accounts: These can be undertaken individually and either shared with others or kept to yourself.
- Journaling/blogs: These can be undertaken individually or with others. Again, you may wish to keep these accounts to yourself or share with others, such as publishing a blog.
- Group reflection sessions: These will be undertaken as part of a group discussion. Usually, you will have a facilitator to help navigate the conversation and ensure support is provided during and after the session.
- Schwartz rounds: These sessions are often undertaken on a monthly basis with a time frame identified, for example, up to 1 hour. All members of staff from all disciplines are invited to a session where challenging emotional issues are discussed related to patient care (The Kings Fund, 2024).
- Clinical supervision: Clinical supervision is the term used to describe support provided to professionals to explore practice and restorative and professional reflection. You will be assigned a professional with whom to critically reflect upon your professional practice and development as well as your wellbeing. These sessions are protected with dedicated time assigned to provide you with a safe space to reflect.

One common way in which you can undertake reflection is through debriefing. A debrief is a moment in which to pause with those involved with a situation or care provided and reflect. A clinical debrief enables you to reflect upon your shift or a specific event that has happened while you have been on placement. An opportunity to debrief at the end of each shift can help you develop your decision making, clinical judgement and critical thinking; it will also provide you with an opportunity to reflect on what you have achieved during a shift, what you have learned from it and how you could enhance your clinical practice in the future. Some placement areas will have team debriefs; these often happen following an incident, and it is important for you as a student nurse to be invited to these debrief sessions and to attend.

SOCIAL MEDIA
@JamieJMMcNab

'Seize every opportunity, reflect at the end of each shift, Appreciate the value in delivering "basic" care'.

Support networks

We hope that your placement learning experiences are all very positive for you; however, there may be occasions where you will require additional support. As student nurses, you will have a range of support available to you if you do come up against challenges when you are on placement. Prior to starting your placement, familiarise yourself with the various support networks that you can turn to in the placement area as well as the support offered by your education provider.

As well as formal support networks, you may wish to also consider peer support groups. Peer groups can enhance professional and personal development. They can be found in a variety of environments such as universities/placement areas/social media/external university services or additional university services. It's an opportunity for individuals from a range of backgrounds to come together to offer practical help, advice, a listening ear or feedback to benefit the needs of a group. Although you may all come from a varied background, you all have on key theme in common: nursing. Peer support can bring individuals together to one space to help enhance your learning environment and student experience.

Advantages of peer support networks can be:

- Increase in self esteem
- Increase in mental health support
- Developing positive and diverse professional relationships
- Sense of belonging and community

Fig. 3.2 shows the importance of peer support networks available to nursing students whilst studying nursing at university.

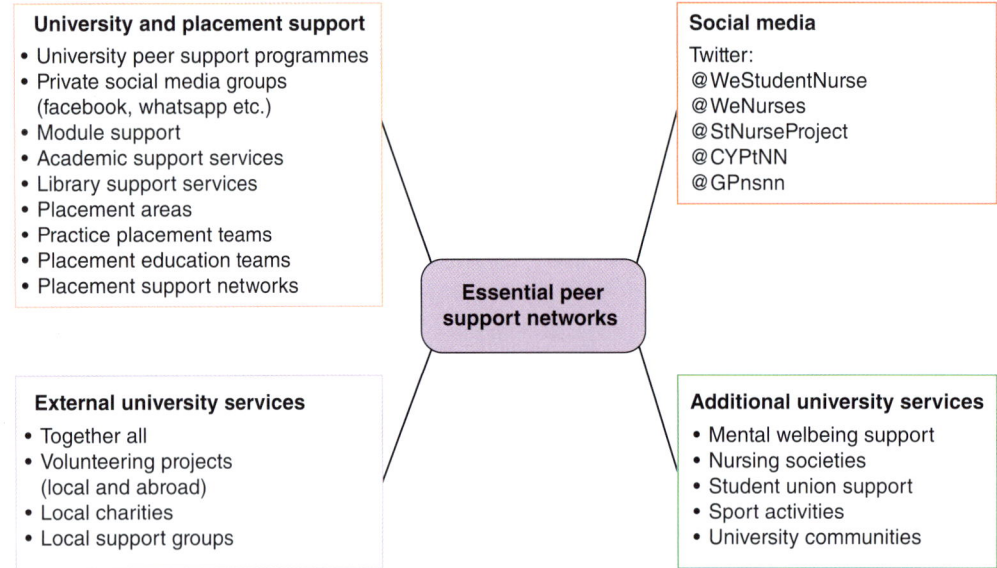

University and placement support
- University peer support programmes
- Private social media groups (facebook, whatsapp etc.)
- Module support
- Academic support services
- Library support services
- Placement areas
- Practice placement teams
- Placement education teams
- Placement support networks

Social media
Twitter:
@WeStudentNurse
@WeNurses
@StNurseProject
@CYPtNN
@GPnsnn

Essential peer support networks

External university services
- Together all
- Volunteering projects (local and abroad)
- Local charities
- Local support groups

Additional university services
- Mental welbeing support
- Nursing societies
- Student union support
- Sport activities
- University communities

Fig 3.2.   Benefits of peer support networks. From How to be a Successful Nursing Student, Fig 1.1, Oxford, Elsevier Ltd, 2024.

WELLBEING

NMC

THE NMC SAYS

3.1 Pay special attention to promoting wellbeing, preventing ill health and meeting the changing health and care needs of people during all life stages.

Wellbeing is a term that is used often within everyday society; however, each individual has a different perception of the term, and these can be used interchangeably.

Abraham Maslow (1954) proposed that as humans, we have several basic needs to thrive socially and emotionally and develop growth. All of these are vital as you embark on and throughout your nursing career. However, the World Health Organisation (WHO, 2021) has identified the foundations of wellbeing in broader terms, and these are inclusive of physical, mental, spiritual and social wellbeing.

Maslow (1954)'s basic needs included (Fig. 3.3):

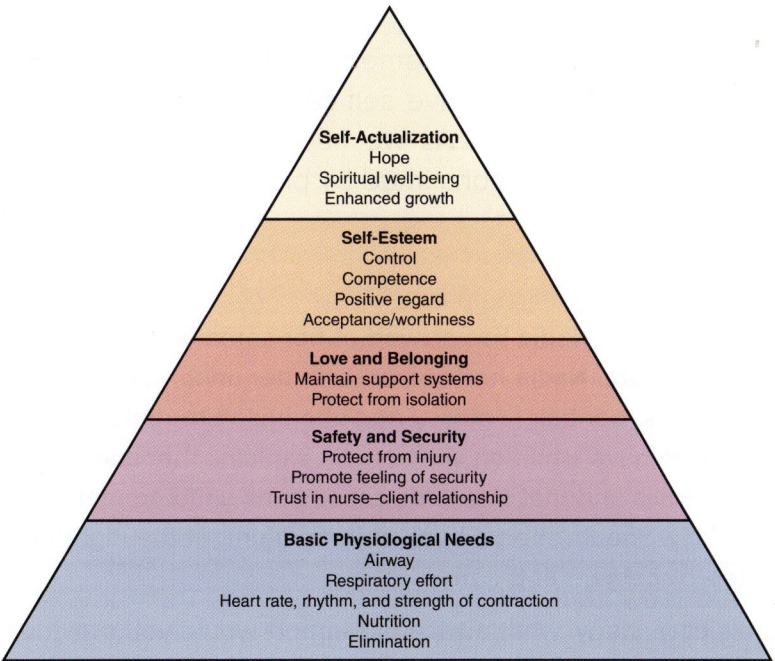

Fig 3.3 Maslow's hierarchy of needs. From Harkreader H, Hogan MA, Thobaben M: Fundamentals of Nursing: Caring and Clinical Judgment, ed 3, Philadelphia, 2007, Saunders.

As a nursing student, you are in a unique position where you will undertake many clinical placements in a variety of settings. This means your mental and physical health will be challenged due to the environments, and you may need to adapt the care you provide to individuals and families in these settings. It's important to be able to pause and recognise your own wellbeing needs in order to develop supportive and coping mechanisms. Being able to recognise and nurture your own needs early in your career will enable you to deliver safe, effective and high-quality care while also promoting lifelong professional wellbeing.

NMC

THE NMC SAYS

20.9 As nurses you must maintain the level of health you need to carry out your professional role.

Your time during and out of placement will become precious; therefore it's vital that you embed positive self-care needs into your lifestyle to maintain a healthy balance. As we have mentioned in the previous chapter, you can become consumed by placement.

CASE STUDY

Stage 1 student Nadia has arrived at her community placement 10 minutes late. Nadia has arrived with her uniform underneath her own clothes, her hair is messy and she hasn't brought any breakfast or lunch to have while on shift. Nadia explains that she stays in student halls and that she undertakes bank shifts to make ends meet financially. She finished a bank shift at midnight the night before and started placement at 8 a.m.

In this case study, what advice or support would you provide to Nadia?

Please pause for a moment and consider what are your self-care needs.

_____

_____

_____

_____

_____

_____

As mentioned in the previous chapter, you may have to make adaptations to your personal life and routine due to placement routine, for example, shift work. However, to support you being able to thrive in placement, we should, where possible, try to maintain key elements that reflect Maslow's hierarchy of needs.

The following are some key themes in which to consider in aiding your wellbeing during placement.

Sleep hygiene

It's important to consider your normal sleep hygiene. Adopting a healthy bedtime routine, no matter the time of day/night, is vital for your wellbeing. Key aspects include ensuring to obtain a minimum of 8 hours sleep, facilitating a calm and peaceful bedtime environment and considering a darkened room using blackout curtains/blinds or an eye mask. You may also experience sleeping during the day for the first time; you may not be used to the noise created during the day, so you may wish to consider earplugs also. These are all positive steps to support your sleep hygiene. The Royal College of Anaesthetists' Fight Fatigue Campaign (2019) identified that 84% of anaesthetic trainees felt too tired to drive home safely after a night shift, with 57% further sharing they experienced an accident or a near miss when driving home. Therefore good sleep hygiene is vital to your safety and wellbeing (Fig. 3.4).

Travel time

Travel to and from placement can be challenging and may impact your wellbeing if not considered. Initially, you may wish to consider whether there is an option to stay closer to your clinical placement. If staying closer is not an option, then you will need to consider which mode of travel will get you to placement on time. Some questions worth considering are:

- Is public transport an option, or can you drive?
- Do you need a parking permit?
- Will you be travelling between a multitude of clinical areas or individuals' homes?
- Can you car share?

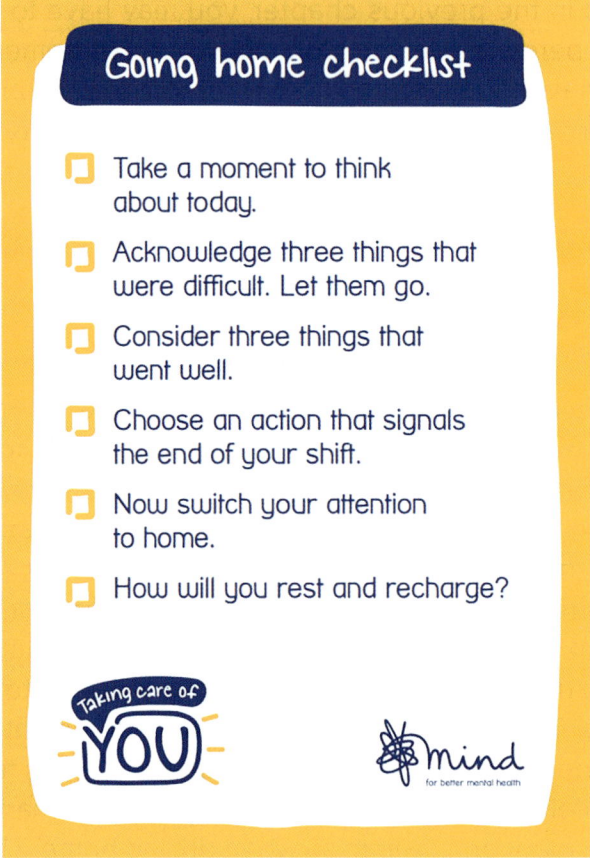

Fig 3.4   Going home checklist. Mind (2024)

- Will you have to take more than one mode of transport?
- Can you claim expenses prior to your placement?

 'I had one placement where I was Monday to Friday, 9 a.m. until 5 p.m. Normally the journey would have only taken me 30 minutes by car, but because I was travelling during the peak times, it took me well over an hour'.

Natalie Elliott, RN

Although the practical aspect of travelling needs consideration, the commute to placement can be a valuable breathing space. The commute to and from placements can give you some protected space to think and unwind. It is often the buffer between clinical placement and home life, thus helping not to blur the boundaries and/or helping to leave 'work' at work.

Some areas may also adopt a 'going home checklist' for yourself and colleagues.

Healthy eating

During clinical placement, you may be working several shift patterns; these can range from Monday to Friday, working 12-hour day/night shifts or even long days. Being proactive and organised in relation to your eating habits is vital and a key area of your health which should not be overlooked. You may underestimate the amount of energy a shift can consume, physically and mentally. Ensuring your body is supported by a nutritious meal throughout the day can help to overcome this and ensure that you remain in the best health during your working pattern.

It's easy to choose unhealthy meals/ snacks, as they are easy to grab and eat on the go; however, if you are undertaking this behaviour over 5 days or a long period of time, this will have an impact on your energy skills as well as overall health. Try to be mindful of this, and consider small, subtle, healthier choices you can make.

> *'Some of the barriers that nurses have identified in relation to these unhealthy habits are: inadequate working conditions, such as shift work or nursing workload; poor eating habits among fellow nurses (peer nurses); and limited availability of healthy food options at work'.*
>
> **–Forcada-Parrilla et al., (2022)**

Ensuring you have all your meals for the day can take time and organisation. If on a 12-hour shift, you may have to consider the following meals:

- breakfast
- morning snack

- lunch
- afternoon snack
- evening meal

This takes time to prepare as well as consideration of how you will carry all your food and where you will store it. As mentioned in the previous chapter, you may need to think about your rucksack size and or a separate lunch bag in which to carry it all. When contacting your clinical area for the first time, you may wish to ask about what storage facilities they have for your food.

Often at times, you may be on shift for possibly 3/4 days together, or you may work 5 days in a row. Being organised and being prepared with your meals can enable you to have that downtime after shift to process what you have seen or been involved in rather than considering having to cook. By batch cooking meals, you can cook a large proportion of food at one time, therefore reducing the amount of time spent cooking, reducing food wastage and reducing the amount of electricity or gas you are using, which is both good with respect to being organised and for your finances.

When considering your food choices, think of easy and simple recipes that may help you feel fuller for longer, for example, bananas and porridge. Having a nutritious meal that can see you through a little longer will help with those busy shifts when breaks can get delayed.

In the following, some suggestions have been given below by students to support nutrition.

SOCIAL MEDIA
@mozzaedwards

'Baked potatoes done in a microwave look different to oven baked, but split filled with cheese, scrambled egg, houmous or beans are cheap and fill'.

SOCIAL MEDIA
@SarahLouiseJ

'This is literally fresh pasta (can use dry I do when I'm short on money), turkey breast (I use chicken if it's cheaper and free what's left), crème fresh, parmesan and Italian spices. Its such a cheap meal and if you have stuff left can make something else'.

SOCIAL MEDIA
@SarahSt51234485

'I lived on pasta, chopped up ham and pesto on placements! Can be eaten hot or cold'.

SOCIAL MEDIA
@SarahLouiseJ

'Soup as well. My god what a life saver. If you ever have any spare money get a soup maker. I throw everything in the fridge in it so nothing goes to waste'.

SOCIAL MEDIA
SimonJa39523855

'grains/noodles and cold meat with some sauce over the top'.

SOCIAL MEDIA
@Stew77Laura

'Big batch of any veg roasted then added to pasta, cous cous, wraps, top with grated cheese, cottage cheese, sweet chilli sauce, pesto, delicious hot or cold and make enough for 3 x 12 hour shifts'.

SOCIAL MEDIA

@kayleighmmanley

'Anything that can be batch cooked! Pasta bakes, chilli, curries, soups (butternut squash and sage is a personal fav), paella's, jambalaya. And apart from pasta bakes, these can be frozen so I have a selection of meals to choose from'.

SOCIAL MEDIA

@BrianWebster18

'I like to make an omelette (so a few eggs and then any choice of extras such as onions, tomatoes, anything really) and then pop the whole omelette onto a wrap. It's an amazing, cheap, quick breakfast (or any time meal) and feels like a fakeaway McDonalds Breakfast wrap'.

SOCIAL MEDIA

@sarah16107480

'Batch cook at weekend. Satay noodles- pack of dried noodles, cooked. Stir fry onion carrot, cabbage, mushrooms, $+/-$ tofu. Make sauce with peanut butter and chilli sauce, with a little water to thin it out. Divide into 5 portions and keep in the fridge. Or couscous with roast veg and chicken or halloumi- can do a jar of roast veg or cook alongside something else. Cook chicken or other protein and divide up and mix with grated carrot/ cabbage/ apples and vinaigrette as a salad'.

Often, nursing students don't pack enough food for a shift; therefore it's better to have more than not enough; there is no worse feeling than feeling hungry on shift, and you are only halfway through the day. Take some time to write out some meal ideas for when you're on placement.

_____

_____

_____

_____

_____

_____

Hobbies and relationships

Clinical placements can easily become your whole life, and it is easy to become consumed by them. Often, nursing students (and, indeed, nurses) can find themselves rescheduling seeing friends and family, cancelling gym sessions, putting off going to clubs or not being as social as they once were. This is often because by the end of the working day, nursing students are tired and mentally preparing for the next day; however, maintaining a 'normal' schedule is vital to meeting basic health and wellbeing.

As nursing students, you are keen to impress and demonstrate all that you can while on placement; however, this can take its toll. As mentioned, you can be overwhelmed by it and find yourself only talking about nursing or placement. While this is exciting and demonstrates your passion, you need to be able to switch off from the role. Therefore ensuring the connections with friends/family and undertaking the things you enjoy are vital. Sticking to your normal schedule can also support your mental wellbeing, as there may be challenges on placement. A walk in the park, journalling, knitting, meeting a friend for a coffee or going to the gym may enable you to have some downtime and gain a different perspective. As mentioned, it can be difficult to maintain some normality; therefore you may wish to discuss with family and friends and arrange to see them on alternative days and times. It can take a bit of reworking, but the benefits far outweigh the inconvenience of rescheduling.

What things do you think will help you to maintain a good work/life balance?

_____

_____

_____

_____

_____

_____

CONCLUSION

This chapter aimed to explore how to thrive while on clinical placement. We have explored roles and responsibilities, professional relationships, learning opportunities and wellbeing, all key themes to help aid you to thrive on placement. It is an exciting time to start your nursing journey, especially when you undertake your first clinical placement. However, entering and settling into a new clinical environment other than university can be challenging and overwhelming.

We have provided you with hints and tips as well as an opportunity to pause and consider how you may implement or manage some of these themes when on placement. We have also provided you with support networks or individuals with which to connect to aid your success.

We hope, as you transition through your nursing journey, that you will be able to implement and develop some of these strategies to thrive on future placements.

Space for reader's own reflection:

_____

_____

_____

_____

_____

_____

_____

_____

_____

_____

_____

_____

_____

_____

_____

_____

_____

REFERENCES

Dube, D., 2021. Engage with your placement area as much as you can. Nurs. Times. https://www.nursingtimes.net/students/engage-with-your-placement-area-as-much-as-you-can-20-07-2021/

Forcada-Parrilla, I., et al., 2022. The influence of doing shift work on the lifestyle habits of primary care nurses. Nurs. Rep. 12 (2), 291–303.

Grant, A., Goodman B., 2019. Communication and interpersonal skills in nursing, fourth ed. Sage Publishing, London, p. 97.

Maslow, A.H., 1954. Motivation and personality, Harpers.

Mind. 2024. Going home checklist. https://www.mind.org.uk/media-a/4577/tcoy_leaving_work_cl_poster_stg1_v3.pdf

National Health Service Education for Scotland. 2019. A national framework for practice supervisors, practice assessors and academic assessors in Scotland. https://www.nes.scot.nhs.uk/media/fxdd4d01/scottish_approach_to_student_supervision_and_assessment_interactive.pdf

Practice Assessment Document (PAD) Scotland. 2023. https://learn.nes.nhs.scot/65764

Royal College of Anaesthetists. 2022. Fight fatigue resources. https://anaesthetists.org/Home/Wellbeing-support/Fatigue/-Fight-Fatigue-download-our-information-packs

The Kings Fund. 2024. Schwartz center rounds. https://www.kingsfund.org.uk/insight-and-analysis/projects/schwartz-center-rounds

The Nursing and Midwifery Council. 2018 https://www.nmc.org.uk/standards/code/read-the-code-online/

The Nursing and Midwifery Council. 2023. https://www.nmc.org.uk/globalassets/sitedocuments/qa-link/quality-assurance-handbook.pdf

The Nursing and Midwifery Council. 2023. Our role in education. https://www.nmc.org.uk/education/our-role-in-education/

The Nursing and Midwifery Council. 2023. Standards framework for nursing and midwifery education. https://www.nmc.org.uk/globalassets/sitedocuments/standards/2024/standards-framework-for-nursing-and-midwifery-education.pdf

The Nursing and Midwifery Council. 2024. Supporting information for reflection in nursing and midwifery practice. https://www.nmc.org.uk/globalassets/sitedocuments/standards/supporting-information-for-reflection-in-nursing-and-midwifery-practice.pdf

Toews, A., Martin, D., Chernomas, W., 2021. Clinical debriefing: A concept analysis. J. Clin. Nurs. 30 (11), 1491–1501.

World Health Organization. 2021. The Geneva charter for well-being, World Health Organization, Geneva. https://www.who.int/publications/m/item/the-geneva-charter-for-well-being

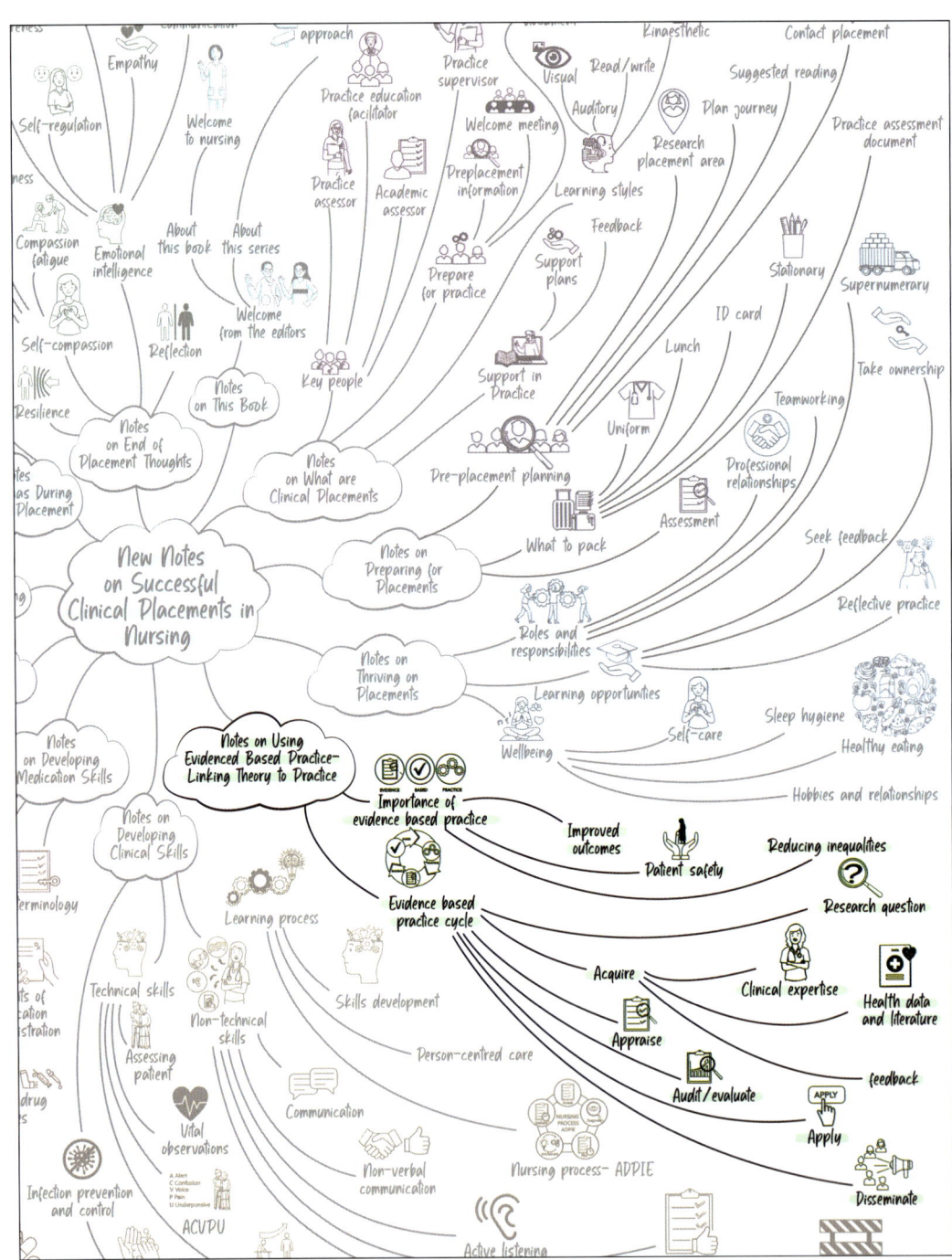

NOTES ON USING EVIDENCED BASED PRACTICE–LINKING THEORY TO PRACTICE

Jessica Lister (she/her) ■ Steffi Ward (she/her) ■
Emily Mycock (she/her) Megan Kirk (she/her) ■
Sarudzai Makaza (she/her)

INTRODUCTION

This chapter aims to dispel the myths of perceived complexity surrounding evidence-based practice (EBP) and enable nursing students to quickly realise that EBP is a skill they will soon excel in and use daily throughout their student and postregistration career to meet the requirements of the Nursing and Midwifery Council (NMC) (2018) code.

NMC

THE NMC SAYS

6 Always practise in line with the best available evidence.

The chapter aims to provide practical information to support nursing students to become evidence-based registered nurses, guiding them through sourcing and critiquing different types of evidence and applying and disseminating this into practice to ensure the highest standards of care for their patients.

The possibility that nursing care may look and feel different from what is taught in simulation or guided by best practice is explored, and students are guided as to what they can and should do.

The chapter ends with valuable tips on being creative to ensure that you maximise learning opportunities.

But first, what is research, and why is it important in nursing? Research is the creation of new knowledge to establish facts and reach new conclusions. In nursing, it allows us to develop EBPs that improve patient care, enhance clinical outcomes and ensure safety. Research fosters a culture of continuous improvement, critical thinking and professional development, ultimately leading to better healthcare systems and patient satisfaction.

The evidence of hierarchy

There are many different sources of evidence available. The evidence of hierarchy, as presented by DiCenso et al. (2009) (adapted by De Brun, 2013), offers a useful summary of how the evidence can vary in hierarchy, based upon the strength of their research methods, and guides you to first search for a recent systemic review or National Institute for Health and Care Excellence (NICE) guidance, and if that is not available, to then move down the hierarchy to the next level available.

WHAT IS EVIDENCE-BASED PRACTICE, AND WHY IS IT IMPORTANT TO NURSING CARE?

As a nursing student and later as a registered nurse, you must deliver care, treatment and advice based on the best available evidence or best practice (NMC, 2018).

EBP refers to registered nurses obtaining and using the best available evidence to inform clinical decision making and improve patient health outcomes. EBP guides the achievement of the best outcomes for individuals and supports the efficient use of resources. It helps registered nurses develop a knowledge base and confidence, have awareness of

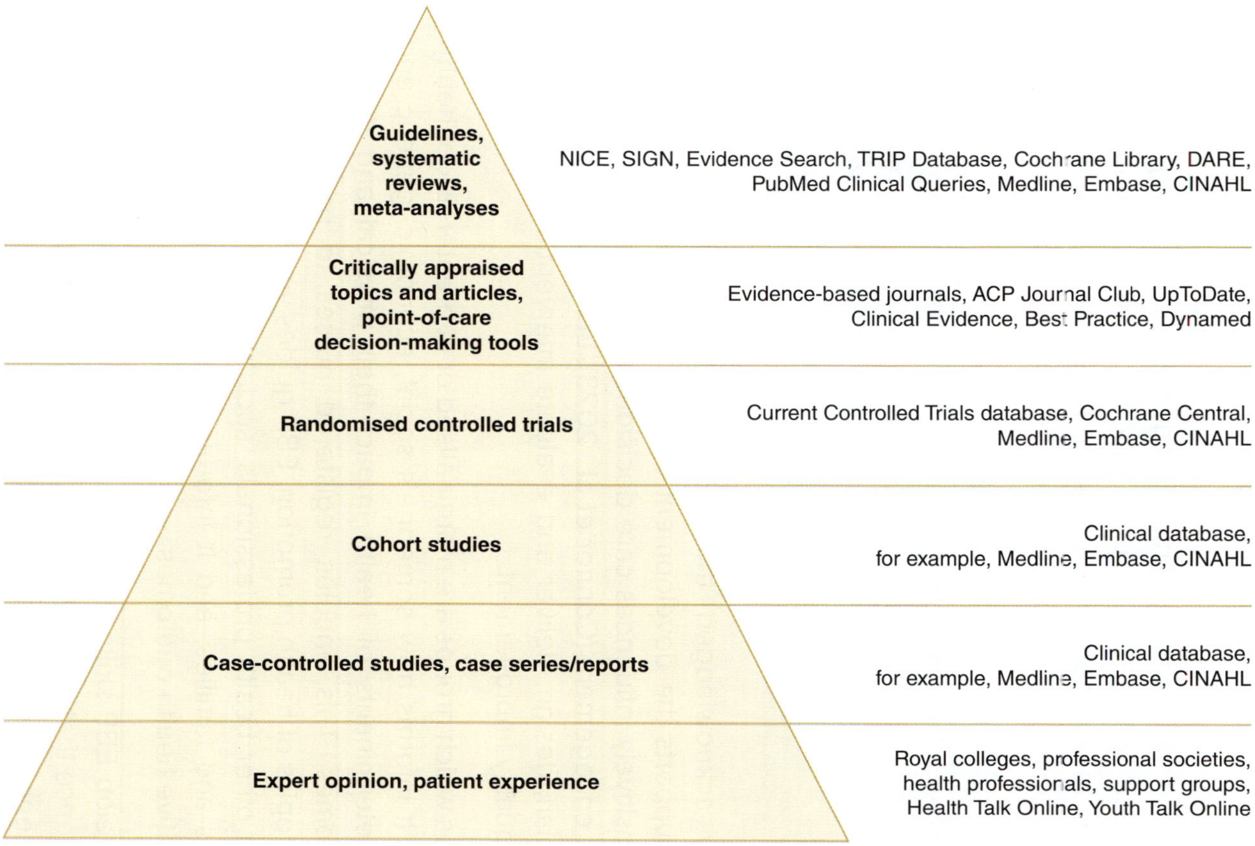

Fig. 4.1 The Evidence of Hierarchy. *DARE*, Database of Abstracts of Reviews of Effect; *NICE*, National Institute for Health and Care Excellence; *SIGN*, Scottish Intercollegiate Guidelines Network; *TRIP*, Turning Research Into Practice. From DiCenso A, Bayley L, Haynes RB. (2009) Accessing pre-appraised evidence: fine-tuning the 5S model into a 6S model. Evidence-Based Nursing, 12(4):99-101.

Guidelines, systematic reviews, meta-analyses — NICE, SIGN, Evidence Search, TRIP Database, Cochrane Library, DARE, PubMed Clinical Queries, Medline, Embase, CINAHL

Critically appraised topics and articles, point-of-care decision-making tools — Evidence-based journals, ACP Journal Club, UpToDate, Clinical Evidence, Best Practice, Dynamed

Randomised controlled trials — Current Controlled Trials database, Cochrane Central, Medline, Embase, CINAHL

Cohort studies — Clinical database, for example, Medline, Embase, CINAHL

Case-controlled studies, case series/reports — Clinical database, for example, Medline, Embase, CINAHL

Expert opinion, patient experience — Royal colleges, professional societies, health professionals, support groups, Health Talk Online, Youth Talk Online alternative options and thus make informed clinical decisions based on the needs, situations and the legal frameworks and evidence presented to them.

EBP permeates everything you do as a nursing student, from your academic work to understanding clinical guidelines and nursing skills on placement. There will be times during placement when you may have academic work to complete, or you want to research the evidence base and practical application of clinical guidelines or processes.

 'Using evidence and reading the newest guidelines allows me to provide patients with the best care possible. It means that during placements I am able to practice confidently as I have the knowledge to do so'.

Willow Ajibode, student learning disability nurse

It is widely acknowledged that EBP significantly improves care outcomes, supports the development of nursing leadership and team cohesion, positively influences care decisions and improves safety, inclusivity and engagement (Connor et al., 2023). EBP enables nurses to effectively plan, design, deliver and evaluate interventions to support continuous quality improvement.

EBP identifies which groups are marginalised or at greater risk of health inequalities. It informs how someone's social, economic, genetic and biological determinants of health impact their physical and mental health outcomes. This enables registered nurses to prioritise risk factors and topics of health promotion. EBP guides you to work in partnership with other health professionals, social care agencies, service users, carers and families, and it informs person-centred thinking to achieve positive health outcomes.

You will develop EBP skills that support you in identifying robust and reliable evidence that aligns with the person you care for, empowering them and keeping them at the heart of decision making. EBP will guide you to think critically, be inquisitive and continuously learn from reflection and evaluation while also being a catalyst to support continuous improvement.

How do you feel about seeking out evidence to support your practice?

_____

_____

_____

_____

_____

EVIDENCE−BASED PRACTICE AND THE NMC CODE

As you become more familiar with the NMC code, you will gain an appreciation for its dependency upon EBP across the four themes of prioritising people, practising effectively, ensuring safety and promoting professionalism and trust (Fig. 4.2). This requires a commitment to embed evidence-based thinking into all aspects of decision making and should be seen as central to daily practice to ensure public protection.

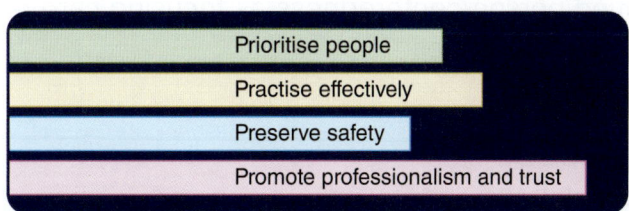

Fig. 4.2   The four themes of the code (NMC, 2018).

Prioritise people

NMC

THE NMC SAYS

1 Put the interests of people using or needing nursing or midwifery services first. You make their care and safety your main concern and make sure that their dignity is preserved, and their needs are recognised, assessed, and responded to. You make sure that those receiving care are treated with respect, that their rights are upheld and that any discriminatory attitudes and behaviours towards those receiving care are challenged.

The evidence shows that working in partnership with individuals results in improved engagement, improved concordance, people being committed to their care plan, increased knowledge and, unsurprisingly, improved health outcomes. It takes less time and costs less compared to those who are not engaged.

It is therefore essential that nurses undertake holistic assessment, advocate for their patients where needed and devise person-centred care plans. This duty extends beyond the therapeutic relationship and includes challenging any discriminatory attitudes or behaviours others may present and making reasonable adjustments to meet person-centred care needs.

Personalised, person-centred care is a key element of the NHS Long-Term Plan (NHS England (NHSE), 2019). The Personalised Care Institute (2024) identified person-centeredness as focusing care on the individual's needs and preferences.

SOCIAL MEDIA
@chris_dlamini

'The nurse's role in person centred planning is to ensure that the patient remains the focal point of the planning through supporting their views to be heard and their needs met. It is not about the wishes of the professional and services'.

SOCIAL MEDIA
@EmmaLyle6

'The patient is the main focus of person-centred care, and it enables positive relationships and holistic care between nurses, the patient and their careers and families'.

NHS England (NHSE) (2024) further highlights that using these principles to guide clinical decisions ensures that care is respectful and responsive to the individual. Person-centred approaches rely upon EBP. Only through the nurse collating information about the person—their support system, their baseline, their usual activities, hopes and dreams, likes and dislikes—are they then able to work with the individual to develop person-centred care and support plans.

SOCIAL MEDIA
@sweetleaf3001

'To be truly person centred starts with following human rights principles and affording people choice and control'.

SOCIAL MEDIA
@RuwaniHysinth

'Person centred approaches is necessary in order to provide support that reflects the lived experience of the individual including identifying their strengths and aspirations'.

To obtain the needed evidence, the nurse will need to review the person's notes, speak to the individual and/or their carers/family, and use their observation skills to tailor their interactions and interventions to meet the person's requirements.

Being person centred therefore requires you to understand available treatment options to meet the person's needs and agree on the right solution for the individual problem presented. For example, there is little point in suggesting a treatment option which is not available in the United Kingdom or presenting a treatment information leaflet in a communication style the person cannot understand.

Being person centred also requires you to be aware of how cultural, religious or any personal individual factors may influence a person's ability or desire to engage with a treatment plan or how past experiences of care may influence a person's ability to build a therapeutic relationship with you. In practice, this may therefore require you to research an individual's needs that you are not familiar with.

Prioritising people, researching, observing, asking, collaborating and sharing (ROACS) can be used to help to remember the steps needed to deliver person-centred care and achieve the principle of ROACS (Fig. 4.3).

It is essential to be familiar with the research and best practice guidance to meet the person's needs and consider how this can be achieved

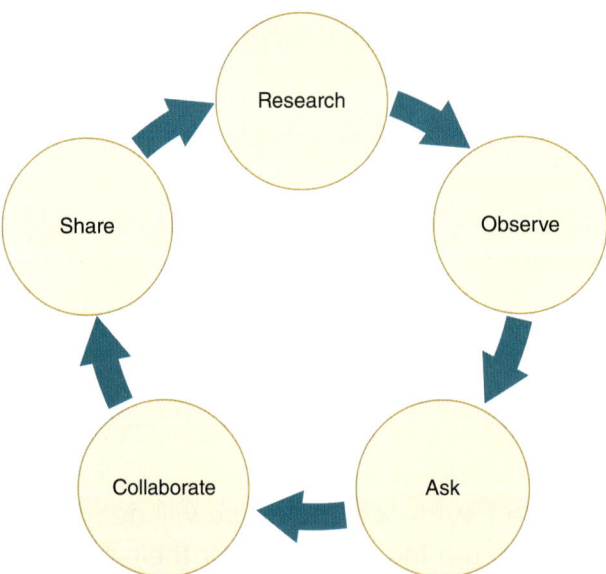

Fig. 4.3   Researching, observing, asking, collaborating and sharing (ROACS) model.

in a person-centred way. Listen to your gut instinct and take note of your observations; what seems to work for the individual? Is the health assessment or intervention accessible to them? If not, why? What can you do to support access? Listen to what is and is not said. Collaborate with the person and the multidisciplinary team to agree on the plan of care and, finally, check that any adjustments needed are highlighted on their notes and share the valuable evidence you collate to enable consistently high-quality care, enable the development of others and reduce health inequalities people face.

TIPS

- If the person cannot tell you their preferences, ask someone who knows them well. Find out what they are interested in, and use this as a topic of conversation to gain their interest and attention and enable the development of a therapeutic relationship. This will not only transform the person's experience of care; it will also enable collaborative working and adherence.
- Pay attention to what the child, nonverbal adult or person who struggles to self-advocate doesn't say. Silence can speak volumes if you listen!

How will you ensure that the evidence you use to inform your decisions is documented and shared?

_____

_____

_____

_____

_____

_____

Practise effectively

NMC

THE NMC SAYS

6 Nurses must assess need and deliver or advise on treatment or give help (including preventative or rehabilitative care) without too much delay and to the best of your abilities, based on the best evidence available and best practice. You communicate effectively, keeping clear and accurate records and sharing skills, knowledge, and experience where appropriate. You reflect and act on any feedback you receive to improve your practice.

As nurses, we all start our careers with a low baseline of skills and knowledge, yet students often report feeling 'out of their depth'. If you feel a task is beyond your current level of competence, you are expected to say so. We recommend that you take opportunities to research the needs of those who you are caring for and to ensure you are familiar with best practice guidance, sharing your knowledge and reflections to support the development of others where appropriate. It is always a good idea to observe the activity several times if it is a complex task; assist if you can and reflect throughout these learning opportunities. When you are ready to perform a clinical task, always do so under supervision until you are confident with how to perform and, importantly, know what to do if there are any complications.

That said, you should be confident in your transferable skills. As long as you ask for help when needed, remain curious, consider the evidence and practice in a person-centred way. You really can't go wrong!

TIPS

Tap into various social media outlets, or there may already be a best practice group or communication network designed for sharing new ideas/innovations that you can join. If not, you could consider starting one. Virtual chat groups are easily accessible to most people.

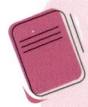

CASE STUDY

A community nursing team observed a significant improvement in patient outcomes by applying EBP. During visits to patients for wound care, the nurses used the latest research on aseptic techniques, resulting in faster healing and reduced infection rates. By following NICE and Scottish Intercollegiate Guidelines Network (SIGN) guidelines, along with the most up-to-date evidence, Emma ensured her practice was current, effective and safe. This adherence not only enhanced patient care but also built trust with patients and colleagues.

Preserve safety

NMC

THE NMC SAYS

13 You make sure that patient and public safety is not affected. You work within the limits of your competence, exercising your professional 'duty of candour' and raising concerns immediately whenever you come across situations that put patients or public safety at risk. You take necessary action to deal with any concerns where appropriate.

If you have seen something in clinical practice that you are unsure about, it is important to discuss this as early as possible. The NMC code clearly states, even as a nursing student, that you must raise your concerns immediately, especially if you are being asked to practise beyond your role, experience or training (NMC, 2018). Your observations provide an important source of evidence to support lessons being learned and improvements to be made. Having this conversation will also support your own reflection and development.

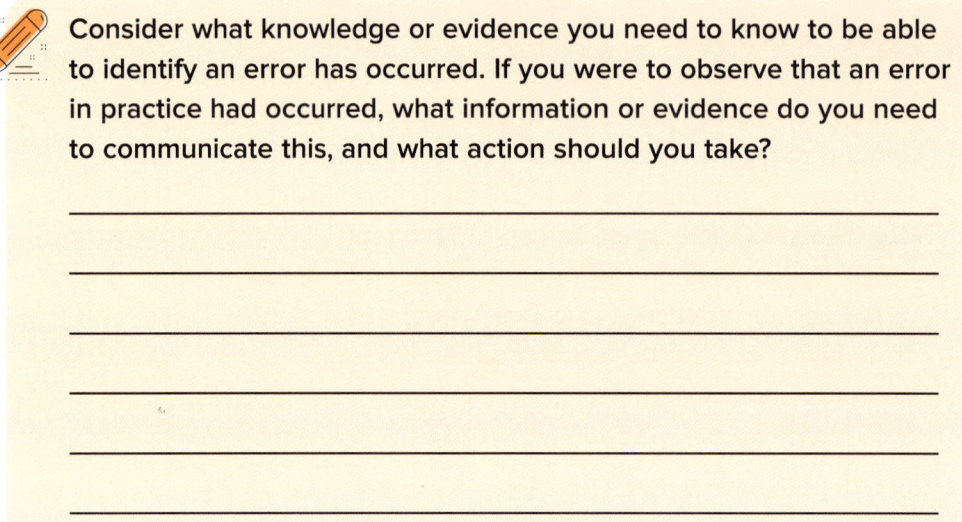

Consider what knowledge or evidence you need to know to be able to identify an error has occurred. If you were to observe that an error in practice had occurred, what information or evidence do you need to communicate this, and what action should you take?

_____

_____

_____

_____

_____

_____

Ideally, you will discuss it with the person involved or who was leading the shift at the time. If you do not feel comfortable with this, speaking to your supervisor, practice accessor (PA) or university will enable you to get the right support and ensure the issue is addressed.

Using your communication and EBP skills, you will be able to share concerns in a professional manner, engage support and develop collaboration, enthusiasm and motivation to generate change.

Most often, a conversation with the right people at the right time will help clarify any questions and catalyst continuous improvement. The communication skills you employ for these conversations will impact on the outcomes you achieve. We like to use 'TAPPS' to help guide our response to any concerns we may have:

TAPPS considerations

Time: Find an appropriate time to ask your question. What is the urgency? How long is needed for the discussion?

Appropriate: Is it relevant to what is happening? Are you maintaining the confidentiality, respect and dignity of the patient/staff member? Are you using the right reporting process?

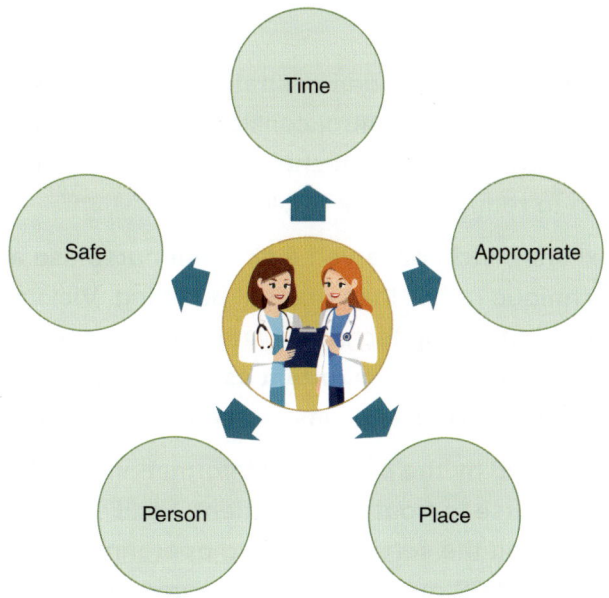

Fig. 4.4   TAPPS model.

Place: Do you need to find somewhere appropriate to have the discussion?

Person: Have you found the right person to discuss your question with? This could be your supervisor, PA, ward manager or personal tutor at the university.

Safe: Is it safe to disclose the information? Is the patient/staff member safe, and do you need to use other safeguarding or risk assessments in the situation?

University teaches EBP as identified within the relevant NICE, SIGN, national frameworks and standard operating procedures (SOP). There may be times, however, where practice looks and feels different depending on the environment, staffing and resources available within the clinical setting.

CASE STUDY

Vicki, a nursing student on placement in a gastroenterology unit, had recently completed nasal gastric (NG) feeding simulation at university and was looking forward to building her clinical experience in

Continued

CASE STUDY—cont'd

practice. Vicki's supervisor demonstrated and explained how to set up an **NG** feed, infection control considerations and how to use a gradual pumping saline flush technique to create a swirling motion in the stomach to reduce the risk of blockages.

On her next shift, Vicki observed a different nurse use a continuous flushing technique rather than gradual pumping. Vicki asked about the difference in flushing technique and was advised that the technique chosen was not important as long as it was aseptic, completed every 4 hours and was correctly documented.

Vicki felt confused by the conflicting information but didn't want to challenge the nurse in front of the patient. Vicki searched for the evidence and read the service standard operating procedure for **NG** feeding and the **NICE** guidelines, and she completed a literature review on different flush techniques. Vicki then arranged to meet with her **PA**, where she discussed what she had seen, reflected upon how she felt in the situation and considered the evidence she had reviewed.

Throughout the process, Vicki used her professional curiosity to compare and question the evidence supporting safe nursing practices and used this to help her reflect and discuss it with her supervisor.

What did Vicki do well, how could she have done it differently and what might you have done in her place?

_____

_____

_____

_____

_____

_____

If you do not feel this conversation has been resolved and you are concerned about patient care, you have several options, depending on the urgency of the situation. The first step should, wherever possible, be to speak to your supervisor, the shift manager or the team manager. Depending upon the concern, you may also want to speak to your placement link lecturer or student services, who can support you.

Promote professionalism and trust

NMC

THE NMC SAYS

20 We must always uphold the reputation of your profession. You should display a personal commitment to the standards of practice and behaviour set out in the Code. You should be a model of integrity and leadership for others to aspire to. This should lead to trust and confidence in the profession from patients, people receiving care, other health and care professionals and the public.

Nursing students and registered nurses must maintain clear professional boundaries, demonstrate a commitment to honesty and integrity, and inspire trust and confidence in the profession. Building trust with those you care for and with your colleagues is an essential component of the nurse's responsibility. Sharing the current evidence base with patients impacts their experience of care as well as their adherence to any treatment decisions. Indeed, one of the leading causes of nonadherence results from a lack of trust in the prescribing or administering clinician, with patients not having their concerns alleviated or being given the required information to make an informed choice. As students and registered nurses, our patients look to us for guidance and answers, and we have a responsibility to provide an honest appraisal of the evidence. This provides an opportunity for the nurse to understand and respond to a patient's concern and enables them to make informed decisions based on the evidence presented to them, building trusting relationships which promote professionalism and trust with those we care for and other health and care professionals and the public.

Consider how you can share the evidence with patients to enable them to make informed decisions. How will you deliver this, and what resources, if any, will you use?

_____

_____

_____

_____

_____

_____

CASE STUDY

Emma, a first-year nursing student, demonstrated the importance of promoting professionalism and trust through EBP. When discussing treatment options with a patient with diabetes, she provided clear, jargon-free explanations and used printed brochures from reputable sources such as the NHS. Emma also used a tablet to show an informative video on diabetes management. By scheduling follow-up sessions to address any concerns and using decision aids, she empowered the patient to make informed decisions. This approach not only enhanced the patient's understanding and trust but also highlighted Emma's commitment to professional, evidence-based care as per the NMC code.

_____

_____

_____

_____

_____

AN INTRODUCTION TO THE EVIDENCE−BASED PRACTICE CYCLE

Throughout this chapter, we have talked about using the 'best available evidence', but how do you know what is the best available, and where is it available? How can you determine what is fact and what is fiction, what is bias and what is applicable to your practice?

Utilising EBP involves a series of steps that guide you through asking, acquiring, appraising, applying, evaluating and sharing evidence in practice.

Fig. 4.5 is an have adapted version of the Sackett et al. (1997) "5 Steps of Evidenced-Based Medicine" model, which includes sharing to help ensure your practice is aligned with all four themes of the code (NMC, 2018).

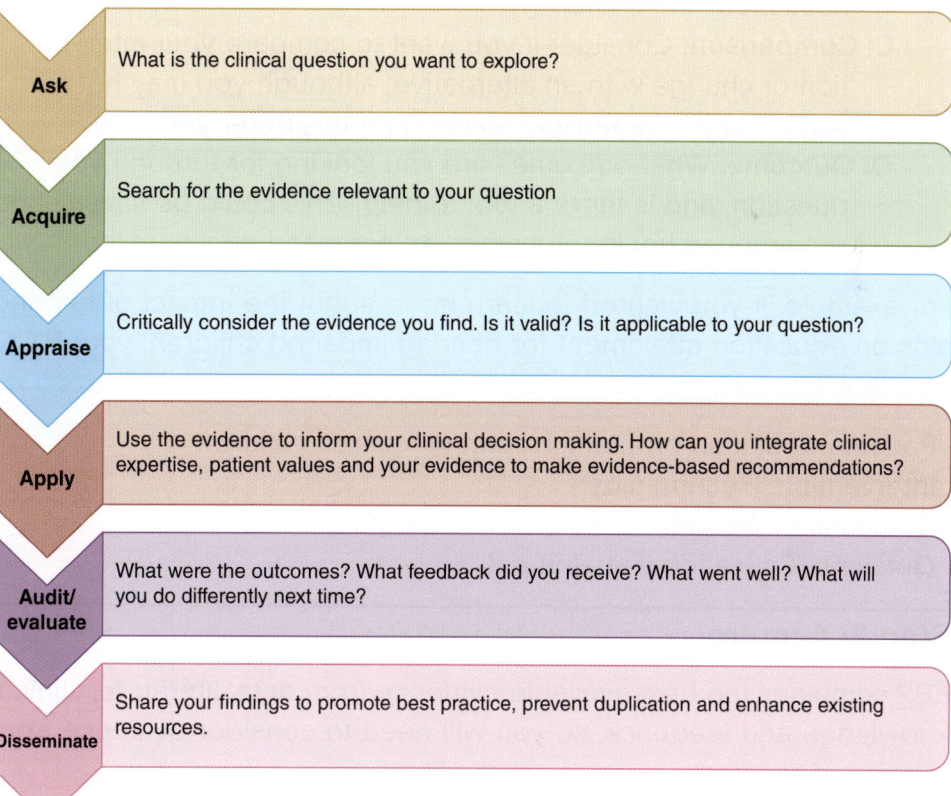

Ask — What is the clinical question you want to explore?

Acquire — Search for the evidence relevant to your question

Appraise — Critically consider the evidence you find. Is it valid? Is it applicable to your question?

Apply — Use the evidence to inform your clinical decision making. How can you integrate clinical expertise, patient values and your evidence to make evidence-based recommendations?

Audit/ evaluate — What were the outcomes? What feedback did you receive? What went well? What will you do differently next time?

Disseminate — Share your findings to promote best practice, prevent duplication and enhance existing resources.

Fig. 4.5   Steps of evidence-based practice.

Step 1: Ask

It is important that you are clear on what it is that you want to ask. While this may seem obvious, you'll be surprised by how many hours can be lost by being too broad, resulting in poor quality of subsequent search results not relevant to your target topic.

PICO is a helpful framework to help you clarify your topic question and make sure you search for relevant evidence:

PICO search framework.
P: Patient/population/problem: What patient group, population or specific problem are you focusing on for your research? Consider patient characteristics such as *age* or *gender* or if they have a medical condition.
I: Intervention: What is the intervention or the change you want to know more about? This may be a treatment option or diagnostic tool.
C: Comparison: Consider if you want to compare your intervention or change with an alternative, although you may not always find a comparison, so don't let this deter you.
O: Outcome: What outcomes are you looking for through your question, and is there a tool to help? This could be satisfaction or improved health outcomes or increased quality of life.

For example, if you wanted to learn more about the impact of hearing aids on education attainment for hearing-impaired children, your PICO may look like this:

Patient/population/problem: Hearing-impaired children
Intervention: Hearing aids
Comparison: No aids
Outcome: Educational attainment

Step 2: Acquire

EBP combines the best available evidence from data, literature, clinical knowledge and feedback, so you will need to consider evidence from a range of sources.

- Health data and literature: What do the available text and data sets tell you?

- Clinical expertise: What do the experts say? What do your own clinical experiences tell you?
- Feedback: What was the patient's experience of care? What do their family or advocates say?

Fig. 4.6 introduces the variety of evidence sources available (can you think of others?). Choosing which evidence to consult will depend on your question and the detail you need. For example, in evaluating the effectiveness of treatment, it's essential to gather feedback from patients, consult with clinicians and review relevant literature. As you progress in your career, you may also need to collect local data such as DNA rates and patient feedback. This can include both compliments and complaints. By taking a comprehensive approach, you'll be able to make informed decisions and provide the best care for your patients.

Where to obtain data

Health data and literature. NICE provides evidenced-based guidance and quality standards for treating and caring for those with specific diseases or conditions in England and Wales. NICE is funded by the Department of Health and Social Care, and its guidelines are considered to be best practice and aims to reduce inconsistencies in care and treatment. While care and treatment decisions will be based upon clinical

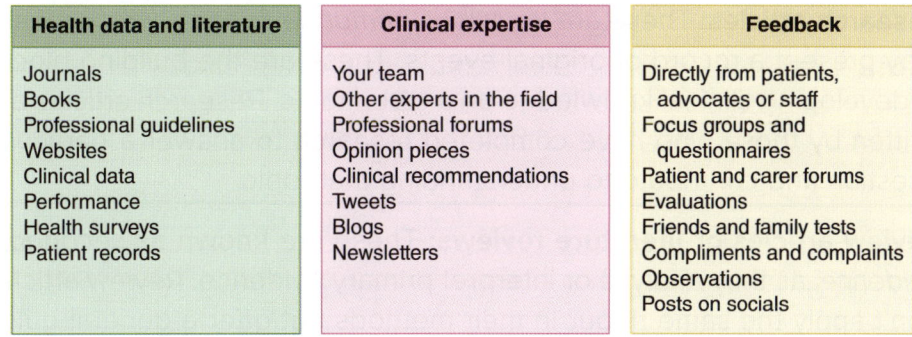

Health data and literature	Clinical expertise	Feedback

Journals
Books
Professional guidelines
Websites
Clinical data
Performance
Health surveys
Patient records
	Your team
	Other experts in the field
	Professional forums
	Opinion pieces
	Clinical recommendations
	Tweets
	Blogs
	Newsletters
		Directly from patients,
		    advocates or staff
		Focus groups and
		    questionnaires
		Patient and carer forums
		Evaluations
		Friends and family tests
		Compliments and complaints
		Observations
		Posts on socials

Fig. 4.6   Sources of evidence for evidence-based practice. From DiCenso et al. (2009) by De Brun (2013).

judgement, patient presentation and preferences and available re-sources, NICE recommendations should inform decisions made.

Health journals

Journals will be your main go-to for information throughout your training and professional career, as they offer up-to-date information, often written by experts for academic researchers and contain a variety of different styles of articles concerning new research or practice developments. The best place to find journal articles will be from an online database such as CINAHL or Cochrane Library through your university library.

Journals often offer the benefit of being peer reviewed by experts before publication, supporting the credibility of the information provided. Where books offer a broad overview, journal articles tend to provide a more specific focus and, given their target audience, may be more challenging to read while you become familiar with academic terminology.

Systematic reviews: Finding a systematic review on your topic can be like finding gold! They offer a rigorous, comprehensive, nonbiased summary of all the published and grey literature that meets defined eligibility criteria. They aim to answer a clinical question and will often use the PICO framework to offer recommendations for practice. Their reference list enables you to identify publications you want to read in full. These reviews also help increase your understanding of how to analyse research critically.

Research articles: These are known as *primary evidence*, which means they present a record of original events. These are the building blocks of developing clinical knowledge on a given topic. Research articles are written by those who have completed research to answer a particular question and contribute to understanding that topic.

Review articles or literature reviews: These are known as *secondary evidence*, as they analyse or interpret primary evidence. Review articles don't apply the same rigour in their methods but offer a general guide to what is already known about the topic and may suggest areas for further research.

Case studies: Case studies offer a detailed study of a particular case or group of cases, topic or person and are mostly used in clinical or social research. Case study research can include qualitative and/or quantitative methods. They are good at describing and evaluating a subject or problem and may offer a different outlook on a subject or challenge existing theories.

Opinion pieces: These offer informed articles written by professionals who want to share their opinions on a topic or subject. While most opinion pieces are written by experts on the topic, such as clinicians, academics, researchers or policymakers, the evidence base used to form these opinions can vary.

Books

All universities will have an academic library where you can obtain hard copies and, more frequently, electronic copies of academic books. Books offer a great starting point with easy-to-access information that tends to provide a broad overview and explanations of a field or different models of practice.

However, be aware that books can quickly become outdated and can be time consuming to scan. Generally, books go through a less rigorous review process than journals. You want to use books published within the last 5 years, especially if they are about clinical practices or medication, as these topics are subject to frequent updates and changes.

Websites

The internet is probably the most convenient method of sourcing up-to-date evidence. It offers instant access to professional standards and guidance, including NICE guidance and other valuable information about health and social care, including health literature, services available, population statistics, patient feedback and signposting to online communities and charities. However, be cautious when using basic search engines. You need to ensure the websites you are browsing are safe, accurate and up to date. We recommend using professional or government-endorsed websites where possible; our favourites are in the recommended resources at the end of this chapter.

TIPS

- Make friends with the librarian at the university library. They are a great source of information, have advanced library search skills and often run helpful workshops.
- Get an Open Athens account. This will give you access to online research databases and allow you to search more extensively. The librarian can help you set up an Open Athens account.

Clinical expertise

You will have access to an abundance of care staff who offer a wealth of information and experience. Many will have a special interest in a particular area of practice and will have undertaken enhanced training and further study.

For example, if you want to explore suitable therapies for stroke patients, speak to or arrange to shadow the clinical nurse specialist attached to the stroke ward. The ward clerk will be able to give you advice on welcoming family, the healthcare support worker will have valuable information about engaging and motivating patients, and the occupational therapist will give you useful information about the impact upon a person's daily life, expected recovery and longer-term treatment plans.

While this can feel intimidating, most people love to be asked for their views on something, especially when they have a particular interest or have dedicated their careers to that topic. Consider the perspectives of a range of people to support your depth and breadth of knowledge.

Luckily for you, contacting experts and obtaining their thoughts have never been easier. Search for social media posts, blogs, presentations and discussion forums, or even reach out through good old-fashioned emails!

TIPS

Don't be afraid to ask if you can book time with a person to talk about your topic. This has several benefits, as it enables the person to offer a time when they are less busy and think about what information they want to share. They may even signpost you to useful information or other experts to consult.

Feedback

Obtaining and giving feedback is an essential part of developing your nursing practice, and the NMC has identified it as an important element of continued professional development.

Patient feedback is a valuable source of information to help assess and evaluate individual and wider population treatment delivery, outcomes and experience of care. This provides vital evidence that will identify areas and priorities for improvements.

It is good practice for students and nurses to ask individuals about their experience of care and any areas they think we can improve. This will also identify any areas of the person's care plan that need adapting.

Consider asking the patient if they think treatment is working well or if they are likely to stop adherence on discharge. Are the person-centred outcomes being achieved? Has there been an improvement or a decline? What contributed to this? Consider also if there are any common themes that may give an indication of more generalised patient experience. For example, one person complaining of poor sleep may lead you to question pain management or an individual's stress or positioning, whereas several people saying they hadn't slept well may lead you to ask questions about the ward environment at night.

It is also just as important to listen to what those who struggle to communicate say. Does a child appear scared and need reassurance? Does a person with learning disabilities seem confused and need information adapted? Is an interpreter or signer needed? Is an older person disorientated and needing information repeated more frequently? Does a surgical patient seem happy and relaxed, or do they appear to be in pain or overly anxious?

Don't forget, however, that one person's experience may be very different from another's, so avoid making generalisations unless there is sufficient evidence to support this claim. You will also be able to gain feedback from several nondirect sources, such as compliments and complaints, thank you cards and social media.

For a well-rounded understanding of how others view your performance, make the most of the team and ask them to share their thoughts rather than just relying upon your mentor's feedback. This information will be invaluable to enhance your reflections and continuous development.

TIPS

Remember that giving feedback is important to others' development. Consider in advance how you can offer this in a constructive, polite manner that uses a coaching approach to support continuous development. This approach will support your leadership skills development and encourage others to use the same supportive approach as you.

Undertaking a literature search

A literature search is the most effective way to 'acquire' published evidence on the question you want to explore. It offers a structured approach with several steps to help make it more manageable.
You have already decided on the clinical question or topic you want to explore and have used PICO to identify your key terms/concepts.

Synonyms. Next, consider using synonyms alongside your key concepts. A synonym is a word or phrase that means nearly or the same as another word. For example, if you are researching 'hearing loss', you could also use the terms 'hearing impairment' or 'deafness'.

Your P in PICO may therefore be:

P: Hearing impaired children/deaf children/children with hearing loss.

Consider using limiters. Limiters offer a great way to help sift out articles that are not relevant to your search. For example, you may wish to exclude papers over 10 years old, not in English or from countries with very different healthcare options from the United Kingdom. Therefore knowledge cannot be transferred to your population.

Run your search. You should now be ready to run your search. If you receive an extensive number of search results or 'hits', review your search strategy and consider combining some of your search terms using Boolean operators to reduce irrelevant papers further.

Boolean operators. Boolean operators are simple words (AND, OR, NOT, AND) that focus your search and help increase the number of positive results, or hits, and reduce inappropriate hits. They save you time by focusing on useful results and eliminating hits that would otherwise need to be reviewed before being discarded.

AND: This helps to narrow the search, as both terms must be returned. If one of the terms is absent, the item will not be included in the resulting hits.

OR: This broadens your search, as either or both of the terms will be included.

NOT or AND NOT (depending on the search engine you use): This will narrow your search to discount searches that include the NOT term.

Using '*' searches for plurals or word variations. For example, using nurs* in your search might find articles that include words such as nurse, nurse or nursing.

Using inverted commas, "", can help with multiple words next to each other such as 'differential diagnosis'.

Using parentheses, (), gives priority to the keywords within; for example, (hearing loss OR deaf) and child* will give hits containing hearing loss and children and deaf and children, but it will not return hearing loss or deaf where children are not included.

An example of all those operators working together in our search example might look like:

P: "Hearing impaired" OR deaf OR "hearing loss" AND Child* OR paediatric NOT adult*
I: Hearing aid*
C: no aid*
O: educational OR academic AND attainment OR achievement

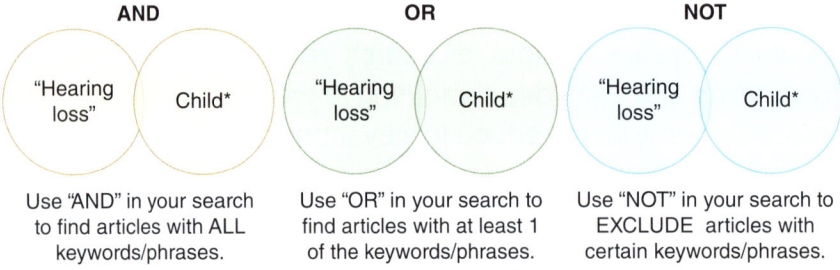

AND	OR	NOT
Use "AND" in your search to find articles with ALL keywords/phrases.	Use "OR" in your search to find articles with at least 1 of the keywords/phrases.	Use "NOT" in your search to EXCLUDE articles with certain keywords/phrases.

TIPS

Search for both full and abbreviated words, for example, BP and blood pressure—this will increase your search results, as not all article titles include abbreviations alone.

Step 3: Appraise

Appraising the evidence is vital to achieving EBP, ensuring that you do not use false or unreliable information in your decision making. While this may initially seem daunting, as you take these steps, you will quickly grow in your confidence as an EB practitioner who utilises critical knowledge and problem-solving skills to coordinate complex care for individuals.

Using critical appraisal tools will guide you through the wealth of information available, pointing you towards papers that are relevant, reliable and of value to your nursing practice and quickly identifying those that may be biased or unreliable.

The first step in appraising your results is evaluating the sources of your hits. Using this process, you can further focus your time by discounting inappropriate results despite including them in your Boolean operators hits list.

A useful tool to help you determine your hits' credibility would be the "CRAAP test" devised by Sarah Blakeslee at the University of Chicago (2004) (Fig. 4.7), which guides you to review the credibility of the paper's currency, relevance, authority, accuracy and purpose, helping you to identify those which are more trustworthy and, importantly, those which you may wish to discount.

The credibility spectrum shown further enables the identification of the variability in credibility for each CRAAP domain. The higher the credibility in each domain, the more reliable the paper.

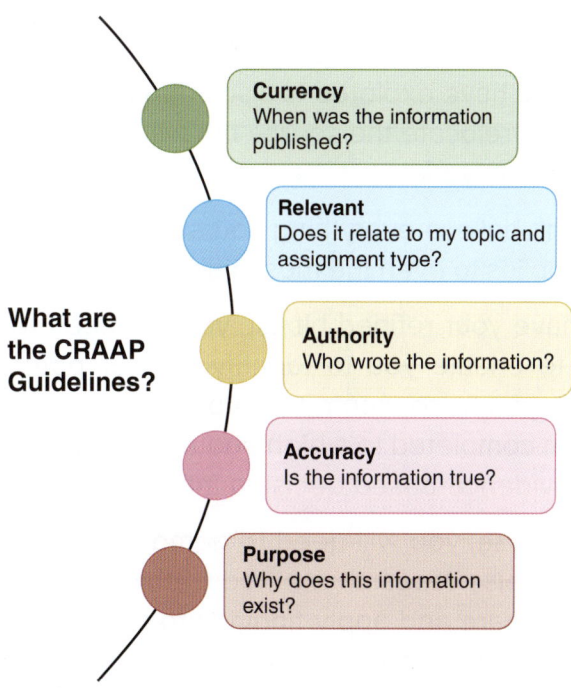

Fig. 4.7 The CRAAP test. Blakeslee S. (2004) LOEX Quarterly 31(3):4. Available at https://commons.emich.edu/loexquarterly/vol31/iss3/4.

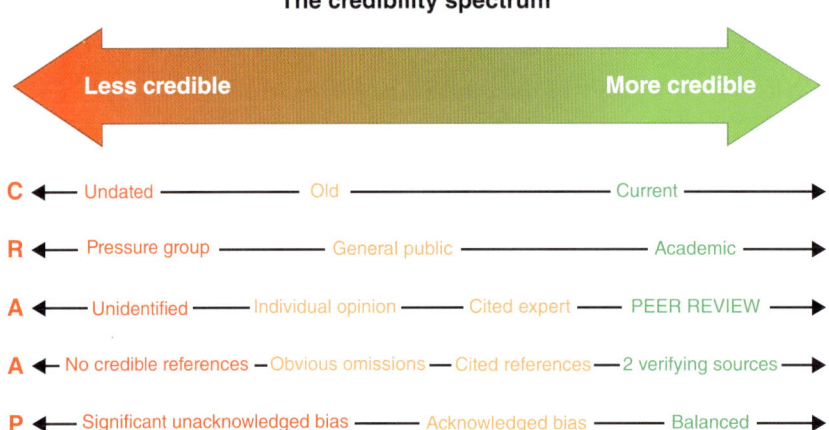

The credibility spectrum

Used with permission from Charles Darwin University. https://libguides.cdu.edu.au/findinginformationsources/evaluatingsources.

Once you have completed your search and are satisfied with the results you have found using the steps given, it is important that you save your hits list and search strategy. Keeping a record of the databases or evidence sources you have explored is also important. This not only saves time if you need to relocate the source but will also help you with referencing your piece of work.

Just like you can't believe everything you see on Facebook or read online, the same applies to even the most highly regarded medical journals.

Now that you have your refined hit list, you will need to appraise each of the papers to enable you to identify bias or potential fake news quickly, allowing you to concentrate on papers which are of value and which have been completed to a high enough standard for you to utilise to inform your evidence-based decision making.

As a registered nurse, you will need to demonstrate an understanding and ability to appraise research methods, ethics and governance critically and to use, share and apply findings to inform and promote best nursing practices, which are drawn from the knowledge, skills and abilities you have built through experience (NMC, 2023).

A critical appraisal will guide you through a series of questions, such as how old the paper is, what the credentials of the authors are, how big or small the study was and whether its findings are transferable to your clinical setting. Does the design match the research question? Has the paper been peer reviewed, and are there any biases or conflicts of interest you need to consider?

The most critical appraisal tools often offer a video guide for beginners online. It's well worth taking time to watch these while you are learning the roles! The most used tools are:

There are many ways of collating and presenting the information you find in your searches. Keeping a log is a very useful strategy to ensure you can quickly refer to your findings and make comparisons between papers. Here is a case study of appraising evidence to help guide you.

CASE STUDY

Getting to grips with the evidence you find

Steffi needed to appraise various pieces of research to support their next assignment. They used recommended databases such as Library Plus, CINHAL and ProQuest to find the evidence and CASP to appraise the evidence collected. Steffi created a spreadsheet with the main points from each piece of research on to offer a quick reference to their findings.

'There was so much information in each piece of research, I was becoming confused, so I put the most important information from each piece into a spreadsheet; then I could find what I needed quickly and make comparisons easily. This made it much easier to find what I needed when I was writing my assignment'.

This is what Steffi's evidence log looked like:

JBI	CASP	STROBE
Can be used to assess qualitative/quantative research Easy to use Can be used to assess the reliability of evidence that underpins guidelines used in clinical practice	Tools are similar to JBI Can be used to assess qualitative/quantative research Can be used to assess rigour in research Often recommended by universities	This tool is used to assess quantitive research Can help demonstrate a more rigorous research process and meet publication requirements

Fig. 4.8 Critical appraisal tools. *CASP*, Critical Appraisal Skills Programme; JBI, Joanna Briggs Institute; *STROBE*, Strengthening the Reporting of Observational Studies in Epidemiology.

Author (year of publication)	Country of origin	Title	Is there an abstract?	Ethics approval indicated?	Study type, e.g., RCT, qualititive	Methods used	Inclusion/ exclusion criteria	Sampling, e.g., snowball, purposive	Most important discussion points	Findings (transferab-ility, generisab-ility)	Is there evidence of bias/ conflict of interest?
Smith et al. (2019)	United Kingdom	An exploration of student nurse experiences of clinical placement and development of their understanding of evidence-based practice	Yes	Yes, full ethics, including Helsinki Declaration, local board and written consent from participants	Qualititive	Semi-structured interviews, thematic analysis	Final year nursing students, aged 18–55 years	Snowball sampling	Clinical placement enables practical development of EBP. Students feel they need more time in practice	Students consolidate their understanding of EBP clinical practice.	No conflict of interest declared in the study

Fig. 4.9   Evidence log example. *EBP*, Evidence-based practice, *RCT*, randomized controlled trial.

Step 4: Apply

Once you have searched for and critiqued the evidence you have found, you need to consider how best to apply it in practice. It is important to consider the evidence, the recommended solution to the problem and, more importantly, the system and individuals you are working with. Beyond this, as a registered nurse, you are expected to prioritise the best interests of the people you care for when providing person-centred, safe and compassionate evidence-based care (NMC, 2023).

Mathieson et al. (2019) identified several barriers to implementing EBP, including time, lack of statistical understanding and lack of academic confidence. Recognising these will enhance your opportunity to overcome any barriers you or your colleagues may face. Those who are not confident searching or critiquing evidence will benefit from support, guidance and an effective role model.

If you identify a new piece of evidence or practice guidance, it is quite likely that your placement area will have a clinical governance process to support the application to practice and amendment of care pathways. Leaders will also need to consider the workforce's capabilities and competencies and available resources and arrange for any training or amendments to SOP that may be required to ensure consistency and effective evaluation.

As a student, we recommend that you use team meetings and supervision to consider how to best apply evidence which is new to you and the process required to update and amend care pathways where required.

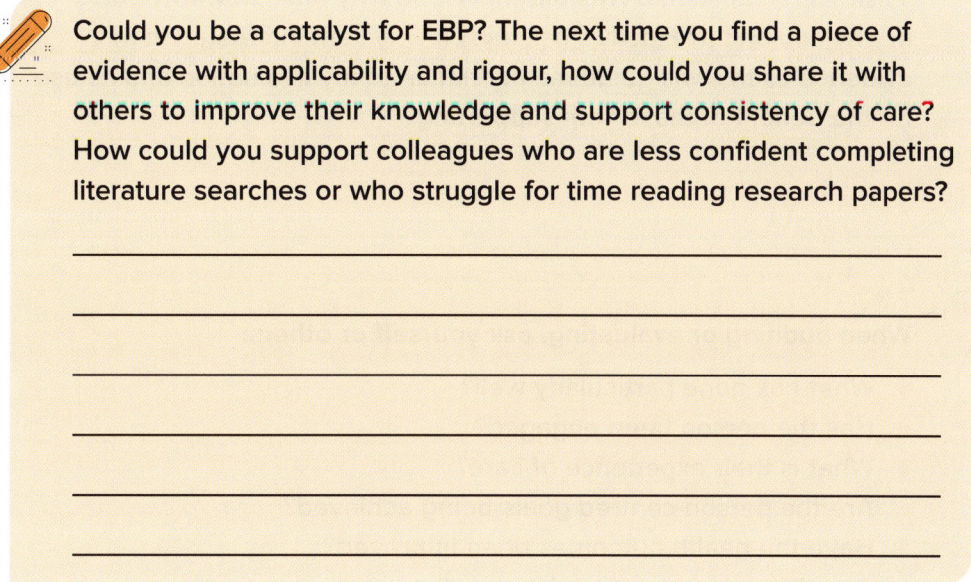

Could you be a catalyst for EBP? The next time you find a piece of evidence with applicability and rigour, how could you share it with others to improve their knowledge and support consistency of care? How could you support colleagues who are less confident completing literature searches or who struggle for time reading research papers?

_____

_____

_____

_____

_____

_____

Step 5: Audit/evaluate

Audit and evaluation are essential to EBP and practising safely and effectively.

THE NMC SAYS

9.2 You must gather and reflect on feedback from a variety of sources, using it to improve your practice and performance.

This includes actively seeking feedback if your practice is clinically safe and effective and if your patient would agree. Adopting this line of thinking to your practice as a nursing student will help shape your learning and the value base you bring to your decision making while accelerating your decision-making expertise and, ultimately, the quality of care you deliver.

SOCIAL MEDIA

@JimmyJimrid

'I ask WHY questions. Why did this work, why did it not, why could it, why couldn't it? Finally, I ask myself why I am interested in this evidence as this will guide me in relation to my evaluation and its use for the benefit of those I am supporting'.

TIPS

When auditing or evaluating, ask yourself or others:

- What has gone particularly well?
- Has the person been engaged?
- What is their experience of care?
- Are the person-centred goals being achieved?
- Have the health outcomes been improved?
- Are all services required involved?
- Did the intervention have the desired outcome? Would everyone agree?
- What do the data say?
- Has there been a change in performance, outcomes or satisfaction? If so, why?
- Is this aligned with the lived experience?
- How could things be improved?
- What is needed to sustain and embed improvement?
- How can you share best practices locally or further afield?

TIPS

Explore opportunities to spend time with the research and development teams. They are likely to have several clinical evaluations being undertaken which you may be able to support.

Step 6: Disseminate

NMC

THE NMC SAYS

9.4 Support students' and colleagues' learning to help them develop their professional competence and confidence.

Nursing students can influence care delivery and play an important role in supporting a culture which shares and appreciates the value of evidence and can be a catalyst to influence its wider dissemination. Consider to whom the evidence topic is most relevant and who can influence and support change. Target your audience, and consider their learning needs. Do you need to share with clinicians, managers, or quality and governance leads?

While it's not common practice for nursing staff to put direct quotations from NICE guidance or research into care plans, this can help to make it clear what the theory is behind the planned practice.

'It's so important that nurses review and incorporate evidence into their clinical practice. As the care plan is the basis of this, including the under-pinning evidence in the care plan documentation will help to clarify the theory supporting interventions, ensure a consistent approach and help the nurse to measure and evaluate clinical effectiveness and outcomes'.

Gwen Moulster OBE, consultant nurse

Sharing your knowledge with others is also a great way to remember key information and help you to develop confidence. This could be on a 1:1 basis or a group. It may be informal, such as showing another student how to use the ward's communication book or sharing a piece of evidence in a team meeting. As you develop through your programme, your abilities to support others' development will continue to grow, and this can then progress to teaching clinical skills in which you have gained competence.

MAXIMISE LEARNING OPPORTUNITIES

How often have you thought, 'I know I saved that evidence somewhere!' From the start of your course, there will be pieces of legislation, SOP, NICE guidelines and so on that you will use repeatedly. We suggest you create a 'most useful documents' folder on your PC or laptop to store these in one place so they're easy to find. Don't underestimate how much time you will spend searching for frequently used documents over the 3 years!

TIPS

Collate evidence using a little pocketbook:

It is impossible to remember all the activities you complete and the information you are given. However, having an account can be very useful to guide reflections and support continued learning. We recommend using the 'little pocketbook' strategy. Invest in a small pocket-sized book that will fit into your tunic pocket. Use this to make notes of to-do lists, useful contacts, dates of activities you've undertaken or meetings you have been to. You can keep bullet-point notes to support later, more in-depth reflections.

Use the front cover to note useful information you may wish to refer to regularly, such as baseline readings for clinical observations, SEPSIS 6, the Bristol Stool Chart, maximum doses of regular drugs or sections of the Mental Health Act.

Remember: don't keep confidential or patient-identifiable information in your pocket, and always dispose of any confidential waste per the local data protection policy.

CONCLUSION

This chapter aimed to introduce nursing students to the realisation that they already use a range of evidence to inform their practice and that EBP is central to adhering to the code.

We have introduced different types of evidence and considered the reliability of this and its application to practice. We discussed how students can ensure person-centred care, practice according to professional and legal framework and how they can be catalysts for implementing EBP.

We hope students feel confident about their abilities to source, interpret and apply a range of evidence, depending upon the individual and clinical needs presented. Just as nurses are lifelong learners, we, too, need to be lifelong evidence-based practitioners to meet the ever-changing needs of our populations, learn from development in practice and consistently deliver high standards of personalised nursing care.

TIPS
Recommended Resources

- Nursing and Midwifery Council (NMC): www.nmc.org.uk
- National Institute for Health and Care Excellence (NICE): www.nice.org.uk/guidance
- SIGN: www.sign.ac.uk/our-guidelines/
- NHS Education for Scotland: www.nes.scot.nhs.uk/our-work/
- Research matters: What excellence looks like in NHS Wales: www.healthandcareresearchwales.org
- Evidence - Public Health Wales (nhs.wales)
- Health and Care Research Wales Evidence Centre: www.researchwalesevidencecentre.co.uk/
- Royal College of Nursing (RCN): www.rcn.org.uk
- NHS Library & Information Hub: www.library.NHS.uk
- Office for National Statistics: www.nomisweb.co.uk
- NHS website: www.nhs.uk/live-well/
- NHS Digital Staff Passport: https://beta.staffpassports.nhs.uk

Space for reader's own reflection:

_____

_____

_____

_____

_____

_____

_____

_____

_____

_____

_____

_____

_____

_____

_____

_____

_____

_____

_____

_____

REFERENCES

Accessing pre-appraised evidence: fine-tuning the 5S model into a 6S model. Evidence-Based Nursing, 12(4):99-101 Cited in De Brun, C (2013) Finding the Evidence. A key step in the information production process. The Information Standard Accessed on 30.4.23 Accessed at: www.england.nhs.uk/tis/wp-content/uploads/sites/17/2014/09/tis-guide-finding-the-evidence-07nov.pdf

Blakeslee, S. 2004. The CRAPP Test. LOEX Quarterly. 31 (3), Article 4. Accessed April 16, 2024. www.commons.emich.edu/do/search/?q=author_lname%3A"Blakeslee"%20author_fname%3A"Sarah"&start=0&context=913693&facet=

Connor, L., Dean, J., McNett, M., et al. 2023. Evidence-based practice improves patient outcomes and healthcare system return on investment: findings from a scoping review. Worldviews Evid. Based Nurs. 20, 6–15. https://doi.org/10.1111/wvn.12621

David L. Sackett, Evidence-based medicine, Seminars in Perinatology, Volume 21, Issue 1, 1997, Pages 3-5, ISSN 0146-0005, https://doi.org/10.1016/S0146-0005(97)80013-4

DiCenso, A., Bayley, L., Haynes, R., 2009. Accessing pre-appraised evidence: fine-tuning the 5S model into a 6S model. Evid. Based Nurs. 12 (4), 99–101 in NHSE. 2013. The Information Standards Guide. Finding the evidence. Accessed April 15, 2024. www.england.nhs.uk/tis/wp-content/uploads/sites/17/2014/09/tis-guide-finding-the-evidence-07nov.pdf

Goleniowska, H., Griffiths, T., Laverty, H., Smith, E., Russ, M., Turner, D., et al., 2019. The Moulster and Griffiths Learning Disability Nursing Model: A Framework for Practice. Jessica Kingsley Publishers.

Mathieson, A., Grande, G., Luker, K., 2019. Strategies, facilitators, and barriers to implementation of evidence-based practice in community nursing: a systematic mixed-studies review and qualitative synthesis. Prim Health Care Res. Dev. 20, e6.

NHS England (NHSE). 2019. NHS Long Term Plan. https://www.longtermplan.nhs.uk/wp-content/uploads/2019/08/nhs-long-term-plan-version-1.2.pdf. Accessed April 4, 2024.

NHS England (NHSE). 2024. Universal Personalised Care: Implementing the Comprehensive Model. https://www.england.nhs.uk/publication/universal-personalised-care-implementing-the-comprehensive-model/. Accessed April 4, 2024.

Nursing and Midwifery Council (NMC). 2018. The Code. https://www.nmc.org.uk/globalassets/sitedocuments/nmc-publications/nmc-code.pdf. Accessed April 3, 2024.

Nursing and Midwifery Council (NMC). 2023. Future Nurse: Standards of Proficiency for Registered Nurses. https://www.nmc.org.uk/globalassets/sitedocuments/standards-of-proficiency/nurses/future-nurse-proficiencies.pdf. Accessed April 3, 2024.

Personalised Care Institute. 2024. https://www.personalisedcareinstitute.org.uk/what-is-personalised-care-2/

Sackett, D., Rosenberg, W., Gray, J., et al. 1996. Evidence based medicine: what it is and what it isn't: it's about integrating individual clinical expertise and the best external evidence. BMJ. 312, 71–72. http://dx.doi.org/10.1136/bmj.312.7023.71

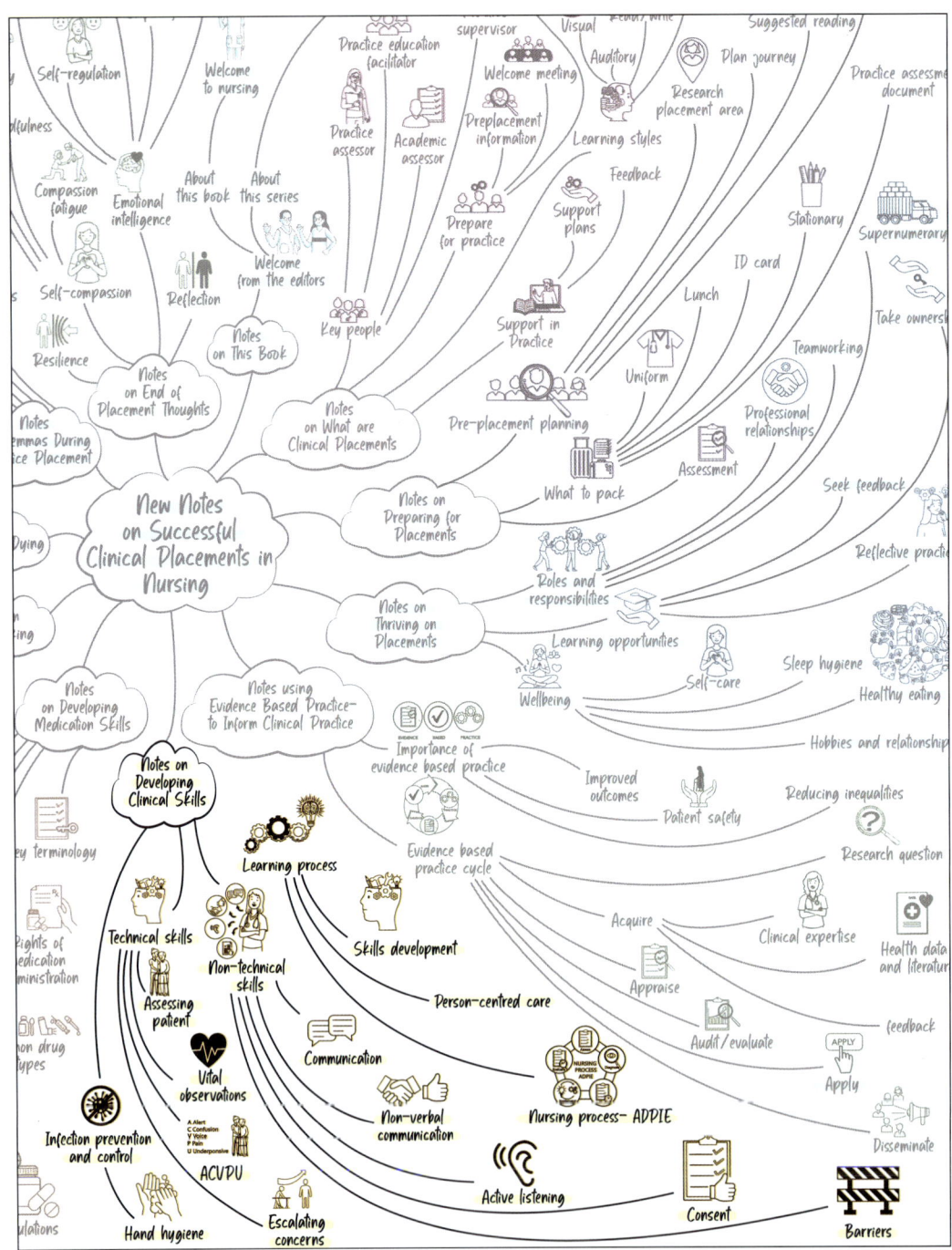

New Notes on Successful Clinical Placements in Nursing

Self-regulation
Welcome to nursing
Practice education facilitator
supervisor
Welcome meeting
Visual
Auditory
Plan journey
Suggested reading
Practice assessment document
Research placement area
mindfulness
Compassion fatigue
Emotional intelligence
About this book
About this series
Practice assessor
Academic assessor
Preplacement information
Learning styles
Feedback
Stationary
Supernumerary
Self-compassion
Reflection
Welcome from the editors
Prepare for practice
Support plans
ID card
Take ownership
Lunch
Resilience
Key people
Support in Practice
Uniform
Teamworking
Notes on This Book
Notes on End of Placement Thoughts
Notes on What are Clinical Placements
Pre-placement planning
What to pack
Assessment
Professional relationships
Notes Dilemmas During Practice Placement
New Notes on Successful Clinical Placements in Nursing
Notes on Preparing for Placements
Seek feedback
Reflective practice
Dying
Notes on Thriving on Placements
Roles and responsibilities
Learning opportunities
Self-care
Sleep hygiene
Healthy eating
Wellbeing
Notes on Developing Medication Skills
Notes using Evidence Based Practice to Inform Clinical Practice
Importance of evidence based practice
Hobbies and relationship
Improved outcomes
Patient safety
Reducing inequalities
Key terminology
Notes on Developing Clinical Skills
Learning process
Evidence based practice cycle
Research question
Rights of medication administration
Technical skills
Non-technical skills
Skills development
Acquire
Appraise
Clinical expertise
Health data and literature
Common drug types
Assessing patient
Person-centred care
Audit/evaluate
feedback
Vital observations
Communication
Apply
Infection prevention and control
A: Alert
C: Confusion
V: Voice
P: Pain
U: Unresponsive
ACVPU
Non-verbal communication
Nursing process- ADPIE
Disseminate
Regulations
Hand hygiene
Escalating concerns
Active listening
Consent
Barriers

NOTES ON DEVELOPING CLINICAL SKILLS

Kelvin McMillan (he/him)   ■   Hannah Nicholls (she/her)
■   Richard Greensmith (he/him)   ■   Matt Fallon

INTRODUCTION

Clinical skills are an essential part of the daily roles and responsibilities that make up the activities of a nurse, with a specific focus on the person-facing, hands-on and clinical procedures when maintaining welfare- and person-centred care. It can be difficult to define clinical skills in a sufficient way that would encompass and give justice to everything that a nurse would do in relation to the clinically related activities, especially across the four fields of nursing: adult, children's and young person's, learning disabilities and mental health nursing.

Generally, clinical skills are the daily deeds, delivery and dissemination of therapeutic interventions to support the welfare of a person or persons. These clinical skills are based on a combination of requirements from governance, the profession and the employer and are developed through experience. Within this chapter, the use of the terms 'person' and 'patient' will identify age ranges of all people across the lifespan, including babies, infants, children, adolescents, adults and elderly, and those with any physical, psychological or developmental condition that could affect health and wellbeing, such as medical, surgical or mental health conditions or specific learning difficulties/neurodiverse conditions.

This chapter will explore a variety of essential non-technical and technical clinical skills that you may encounter while learning within clinical placement environments. As you progress as nursing students, you will notice overlaps when using both nontechnical and technical clinical skills, for example, the need for communication when concerned about a patient's condition following a clinical assessment.

Examples of clinical skills being covered in this chapter include:

Non-technical skills:
- Communication skills
- How teams interact with each other
- Recordkeeping
- Planning patient care

Technical skills
- Infection prevention and control (IPC), including personal care
- Assessment skills
- Measuring clinical observations
- Procedural skills

THE LEARNING PROCESS

When you start attending your placements, you are required to show evidence of procedures you have learnt at the university. We refer to these skills as proficiencies. Your practice assessor or supervisor is responsible for ensuring you have confidence in demonstrating the skills you are required. Examples of skills you may learn in your first placement include:

- Basic assessment skills: checking a pulse, correctly measuring a patient's blood pressure, etc.
- Personal care: washing patients, oral care, assisting a patient to the toilet, etc.
- Communication: introducing yourself, gaining consent for procedures, etc.
- Medicine management: administering medication safely and under direct supervision of your practice supervisor/assessor.

To be proficient in providing care, you must first ensure that you have learned about providing care within the university (the theory element). Only by learning the theory, which incorporates an evidence-based approach, can we truly deliver care to a high degree standard required by the Nursing and Midwifery Council (NMC) and local health settings. Your practice assessor and/or supervisor is there to help bridge the theory into practice by providing you opportunities to practise skills and discuss how to develop your skills. You will also be supported by your academic assessor, who can provide guidance on how you develop certain skills if required.

Skill development and ability

Within health and social care, there are other complexities when trying to understand nursing terminology whereby you will learn the standardised language and common terms that are utilised within the nurse's role and also when working with the multidisciplinary team and interprofessionally. DeKeyser discussed the skill acquisition theory, which identifies that repeated exposure to certain skills will enhance your ability and capability so that you become proficient. Therefore this skill acquisition theory highlights five levels of development when utilising the skills, including novice, advanced beginner, competent, proficient and expert. Within your nursing programme, each of these will relate to your clinical skills from the start of your first year, that is, novice, to the end of your programme, that is, proficient and/or expert. Anderson's skills acquisition theory as adaptive control of thought highlights that skills are often based on two core elements (Fig. 5.1).

Knowledge type	Concept	Detail below any communication and interpersonal skills you use based in the two core elements
Declarative	When we begin to understand the concepts, theories and philosophies	For example, verbal skills
Procedural	When we begin to understand how to actively take part in/perform a procedure	For example, gaining consent and explaining the procedure to a new patient

Fig. 5.1   Skills acquisition theory, practice and activity.

Clinical placements

Clinical placements can take place in a variety of areas (Fig. 5.2). Each placement area will offer unique opportunities to learn skills, and you are encouraged as nursing students to take ownership of your own learning. Therefore it is important to highlight the importance of initial interviews/communication with practice supervisors/assessors regarding placement opportunities, as this is your opportunity to raise any learning needs you have.

As an adult learner, you take a key role in planning and negotiating your learning so that you gain the most from your time learning in clinical practice, but where to begin?

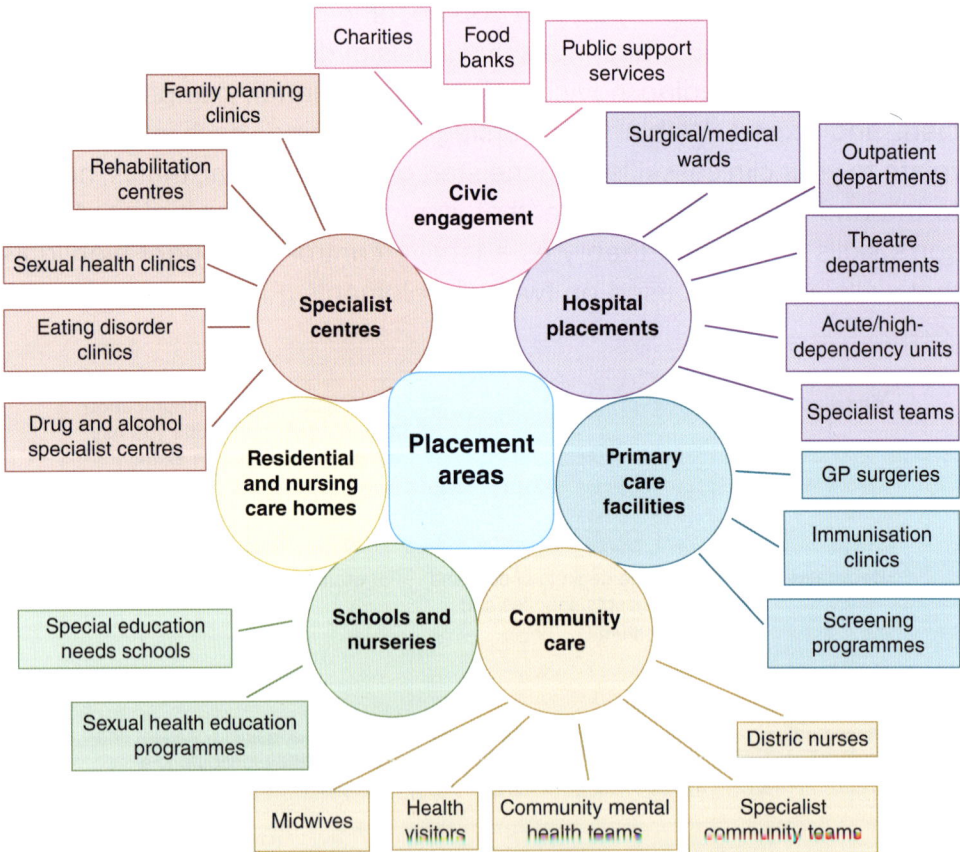

Fig. 5.2   Potential placement areas.

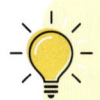

TIPS

- Find out where you are going and communicate with them.
- Talk to your practice assessors and supervisors about what they think you may be able to learn and what is realistic for you at this point of your course and placement area.
- Explore university resources about placement areas, with a list of potential learning opportunities.
- Speak to an education link nurse/team coordinating student placements, who may offer a student pack full of useful information for you.

Often there is a focus on the fundamental nursing skills for students in the first year of their course. Even if you have had prior experience of these in previous roles such as a healthcare support worker, it is important to think about applying these skills and delivering care in the context of a nursing student. For example, helping deliver personal hygiene evolves into assessing skin integrity, mood and nutritional status; recording clinical observations becomes a more detailed assessment of a patient's health by you talking to them and looking for any potential signs of deterioration alongside the measurements you are taking.

It goes without saying that a lot of the environments where nurses work are extremely busy. It's been in the media, and at the time of writing, there seems to be no sign of this changing. When negotiating learning opportunities, it is important that this is taken into consideration. While as a student nurse, you are supernumerary and shouldn't be counted in the staffing numbers, it can be very worthwhile for your learning and development to support the team you are placed with at busy times. This can be a good way to gain experience in the broad range of things you will be expected to do when you are a registered nurse (NMC, 2018).

Personal care:
- Washing/dressing/toileting and elimination.
- Patient positioning and assisting with mobilisation.
- Wound care and skin integrity assessment.
- Nutrition and hydration.
- Shaving.
- Maintenance of oral hygiene.
- Nail care.
- Bed making.

Communication skills:
- Person-/client-/family-centred communication.
- Strengths-based approaches to care.
- Holistic care.
- Individualised care.
- Ensuring the use of informed consent.
- Communication with the multidisciplinary team.
- Maintaining confidentiality.
- Maintaining safety.

Patient assessment:
- Assessment of activities of daily living.
- Basic A-E assessment.
- Pain assessment.

Assessment of the following health and social needs:
- Physical
- Emotional
- Social
- Cultural
- Sexual

Fundamental nursing skills:
- Medicine management.
- Documentation of care provision.
- Promoting sleep hygiene.
- Promoting independence.
- Infection control.
- Working collaboratively with patients and other healthcare professionals.
- Identification of own limitations.
- Knowledge of evidence-based practice.
- Knowledge of correct policies and procedures.

Fig. 5.3   Illustration showing the diversity of placements offered in major healthcare sectors, along with all fundamental skills that can be learned within all placement environments.

CASE STUDY

James, an adult field-of-practice nursing student, has been assigned to a placement at a residential care village. James is worried because he still has quite a lot of proficiencies to complete while he is on this placement and wonders about whether the opportunities available will help him to complete these.

Following discussion with one of the nurses at the residential village, James starts to spend time with some of the residents there. He notices that quite a few residents don't leave their private rooms and don't spend much time in the communal areas with other residents. From his other placements, James has learnt a lot about mental health conditions and wonders whether some of his learning may apply to some of the members of the residential village. James is curious and, with the permission of his practice assessor, decides to

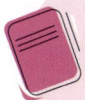

CASE STUDY—cont'd

organise a questionnaire for the residents, aiming to identify whether they feel supported and integrated within the residential home community. On receiving the results of this questionnaire, James identifies that several residents feel lonely, especially those who opt to stay in their private rooms a lot. James discusses this with the mental health enabler for the village, and they discuss organising coffee mornings where residents can meet each other, with a specific focus on those residents who have stated that they feel lonely. The mental health enabler also plans to attend these in case residents may need further emotional support.

In the case study, what skills do you feel James would have used?

_____

_____

_____

_____

_____

_____

Patient-centred care

The diversity of healthcare provisions has evolved due to increasing complexity of health needs within communities. As seen in the case study, while multiple residents live within the same residential area, variation in needs must be recognised by health and social care staff. As nurses, our patients should be at the heart of everything we do, and an approach we use is patient-centred care in which the individuals' own needs and outcomes are the focus of care. For this reason, nurses and other healthcare professionals are encouraged to develop thera-peutic relationships with patients, which is described as a connection

Six Elements of Person-Centred Care
1. Active listening. 2. Open-ended questions and reflective conversations. 3. Involvement of family and friends (with consent of the patient). 4. Understanding of individual preferences. 5. Empathy. 6. Shared goal setting and decision making.

Fig. 5.4   Six elements of person-centred care.

between a practitioner and a service user built on trust, mutual respect and a sense of hope.

There are alternative approaches to patient-centred care; however, all these models still place emphasis on ensuring the patient is at the centre of our care. These include:

- Person-centred care (Fig. 5.4): predominantly in adult nursing.
- Family-centred care: used in children's nursing.
- Client-centred care: used in mental health nursing.
- Welfare-centred care: aligned to all fields of nursing as a holistic review.

TIPS

As you will be looking after a diversity of patients, having cultural competence is critical to deliver compassionate care to all patients. Many cultures require very different needs to access healthcare services, so be aware of cultural stereotypes and stigmas that may act as barriers.

NURSING PROCESS: ADPIE

As a nursing student, you will have many opportunities to contribute to the delivery of patient-centred care. When assessing your patients, using the nursing process model by Ida Orlando is advised. This is a patient-centred, goal-oriented tool to support patient care based on the stages of:

- Assess: making a subjective and objective assessment. What is the current complaint? Medical History? Vital signs?

- Diagnose: your clinical judgement about actual or potential health problems to help prioritise your care.
- Plan: making personalised goals and outcomes that centre around the individual's unique needs.
- Implement: carrying out interventions as planned.
- Evaluate: reviewing the implementation to test whether the outcome has been achieved—consider reassessment.

Using the ADPIE approach can help you advocate for your patients, promote safety and increase critical thinking skills. The (NMC, 2018) identifies that:

Effective communication is central to the provision of safe and compassionate person-centred care. Registered nurses in all fields of nursing practice must be able to demonstrate the ability to communicate and manage relationships with people of all ages with a range of mental, physical, cognitive and behavioural health challenges.

NON—TECHNICAL SKILLS

While technical proficiency is crucial for nursing practice, developing non-technical skills is equally important in providing holistic and effective patient care. Non-technical skills, often referred to as soft skills, encompass a range of interpersonal, cognitive and emotional abilities that enhance communication, teamwork and clinical judgement. These skills are fundamental in building therapeutic relationships with patients, collaborating with healthcare colleagues and making sound clinical decisions under pressure. For nursing students, honing non-technical skills such as effective communication, teamworking, leadership and reflection not only improves patient outcomes but also contributes to a more supportive and efficient working environment.

Communication

As a nurse, you can bring healing to injury, ease to *dis*-ease, relief from suffering, coping from despair and laughter from tears through communication skills and interpersonal skills. You may know that you already have good communication skills, but there are many different traits of communication to consider. Communication skills include:

- Listening: Especially active listening, which requires you to listen to the speaker, understand what they are saying and respond while reflecting on what they said. You will also need to retain information for later on.
- Empathy: This is the ability to understand and share feelings with others. In other words, think in their shoes about how they might react to the information you are communicating, and then adapt communication appropriately.
- Verbal skills: Verbalising information requires the seven Cs to be effective:
  - Clear
  - Concise
  - Concrete
  - Correct
  - Coherent
  - Complete
  - Courteous
- Non-verbal skills: Thinking about how approachable you are to others and how you appear when communicating.

As a nursing student, you will offer therapeutic interventions whereby your skills will help to put the patient at ease, letting them feel relaxed and cared for while receiving treatment. Building therapeutic relationships with your patients is dependent on communication and also on interpersonal skills, which are based on a combination of personal abilities, insights and intuition from your own learning and experiences. These include the use of social skills, people skills, social intelligence and attachment skills among others that can support our interactions with other people.

Non-verbal communication

Communication and interpersonal skills also encompass various other methods such as non-verbal/non-linguistic, signs, symbols and images. Mehrabian (1972) considered this approach to communication in the 'communication theory' that considers nonlinguistic communication as the application of non-verbal cues. These are based on seven aspects that include:

- Facial expressions (such as a smile or rolling the eyes)
- Gestures (such as those of kinesics when waving hands around, coughing to get attention)
- Posture (the way we sit, stand, folding of the arms)
- Eye contact (regularly meeting the other person's gaze)
- Physiological changes (often those out of our control such as blushing, tearing up, laughter)
- Paralanguage (the intonation or tone of voice, pace and volume).
- Proxemics (the physical gap between individuals when either standing or sitting)

However, it is important to recognise that for all seven aspects, different cultural, societal, diversity, and community expectations would need to be considered as an essential clinical skill for communication as detailed by the (NMC, 2018):

NMC

THE NMC SAYS

At the point of registration, the registered nurse will be able to safely demonstrate:

1.3 Use appropriate non-verbal communication including touch, eye contact and personal space.

Active listening

Additionally, a core non-verbal skill is that of active listening in which you, as the recipient of what is being said (spoken language), will engage with intent to hear cues, for example, as a nursing student listening to what the patients say and don't say to you. With active listening, there is the 3R approach to support you in your practice

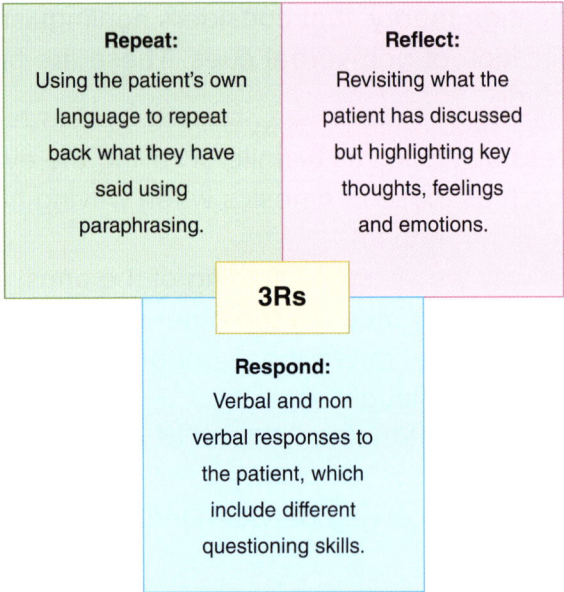

Repeat:
Using the patient's own language to repeat back what they have said using paraphrasing.

Reflect:
Revisiting what the patient has discussed but highlighting key thoughts, feelings and emotions.

3Rs

Respond:
Verbal and non verbal responses to the patient, which include different questioning skills.

Fig. 5.5   The 3R approach.

learning placement (Fig. 5.5). These skills will be essential for you as a nurse, as identified by the NMC (2018):

NMC

THE NMC SAYS

1.1   Actively listen, recognise, and respond to verbal and non-verbal cues and practice communication skills.

4.2.2 Active listening when dealing with team members' concerns and anxieties.

Gaining consent

To establish competency when performing clinical skills, you will be expected to practise clinical skills on your patients. It is normal to feel nervous when practising for the first time, but remember, your practice assessor/supervisor will supervise and support you when you practise. But before you do practise clinical skills on patients/service users, you must establish whether a patient gives consent for you to proceed. To help you, follow the above advice when introducing yourself, and ensure you explain clearly what the clinical skill will entail to the patient/service user.

Consent is a legal process that must be undertaken by all healthcare professionals, as stated within the NMC code:

NMC

THE NMC SAYS

4.1 Balance the need to act in the best interests of people at all times with the requirement to respect a person's right to accept or refuse treatment.

4.2 Make sure that you get properly informed consent and document it before carrying out any action.

If a patient or family member does not allow you to perform care, please do not take this personally. Put yourself in your patient's shoes; they will be feeling vulnerable and anxious, which can influence their way of thinking. If a patient does not consent to you practising clinical skills on them, acknowledge this, return to your practice supervisor/accessor and let them know.

Introducing yourself

A good introduction might open an opportunity for effective communication between you and your patients. You are training to be a patient's advocate, and an introduction can be the basis for developing trust between you and the patient/service user. With trust, a patient/service user may feel safe to approach you with questions or concerns.

The 'Hello, my name is' campaign was inspired by the experiences of Dr Kate Grainger, MBE, who, sadly, died from cancer in 2016. Dr Grainger started the campaign based on her experiences as a patient, where many staff failed to introduce themselves when interacting with her. Her campaign was initially promoted on social media using the hashtag #hellomynameis and has been widely adopted throughout the NHS in the United Kingdom. The following are some top tips for

TABLE 5.1 TOP TIPS FOR AN EFFECTIVE INTRODUCTION TO PATIENTS, INSPIRED BY THE 'HELLO, MY NAME IS' CAMPAIGN

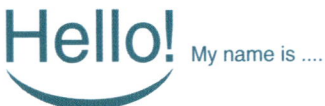

Assess communication needs	It is critical to prepare for any communication barriers and consider methods of overcoming these. Never assume how an individual communicates.
Introduce yourself	Ensure you gain the patient's eye contact and smile. Then introduce yourself by your chosen name and your role. For example, 'Hello, my name is _____, and I am a nursing student working with "the practice assessor/supervisor's name" to help look after you today'. Ensure you also acknowledge other family members/friends with the patient.
Acknowledge how they want to be addressed.	After introducing yourself, ask how the patient would like to be addressed. For example, would they like to be addressed by their title (Mr, Mrs, etc.), or by their first name or preferred way of saying their name. Ensure you ask for their preferred pronoun too.

introducing yourself which are inspired by the 'Hello, my name is' campaign (Table 5.1):

Handovers

These communication, interpersonal, social and people skills will all be important during your clinical placement experience, as you will be engaging with multiple members of the multidisciplinary team as well as relevant individuals surrounding your patients' care. However, an essential component of nursing is the handover: the periods before, during and after a placement shift where staff members provide a report about the people in their care, which often includes personal identifiers (e.g., name, age, gender), physical and mental conditions, treatment, and the health and social care needs to be managed based on their health and wellbeing status. During handover, it will be important to consider how you communicate the details about the patients you will be caring for, as this can influence how others communicate and interact with those patients.

Barriers to communication

It is evident that communication and interpersonal skills can be challenging when you consider all the expectations for getting the basics right when caring for our patients. As healthcare professionals, we may also identify potential barriers to effective communication with our patients. The reasons for this could vary widely and could include examples such as:

- The environment we are working in being noisy or very busy.
- Our patients' health status may affect their communication, such as if they have a neurological condition or are experiencing high levels of pain.
- There could be a language barrier.

It is our responsibility to assess and identify potential adaptations to minimise barriers, thus ensuring that all patients can communicate their needs and receive the care they require. Look at the following case study:

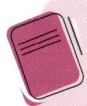

CASE STUDY: MILDRED

During a shift handover, you hear about a 75-year-old female who has been admitted to the clinical area after a fall in the street on a wet and rainy evening. It is reported that she appears to have been knocked unconscious and has dried blood in her hair. An access card was found on her, which helped to identify her name as Mildred.

Continued

CASE STUDY—cont'd

During the handover, it is reported that she seems quite disoriented, confused and a little agitated, as she keeps pushing staff away and appears to be waving her hands around when they try to help her. As a student nurse in your first year, you are asked to help Mildred to have a wash, get her changed out of the clothes she arrived in and see if she has a head wound.

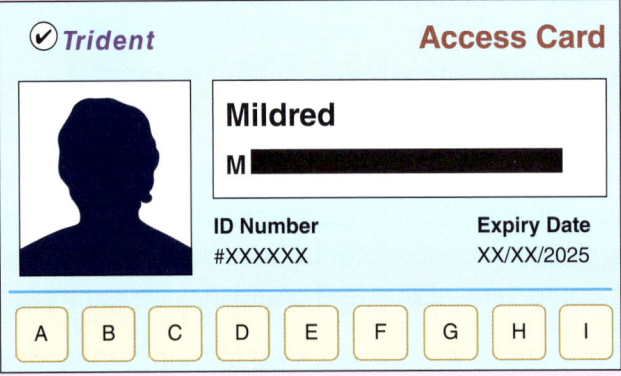

What do you think could be happening with Mildred? What do we know and not know about her? Can you think of any communication skills that could be used in this situation?

_____

_____

_____

_____

_____

_____

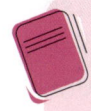

CASE STUDY

Mildred was attributed with being disorientated, confused and agitated, which can be common signs of the stress response. However, Mildred may also have a head injury such as concussion because she was knocked unconscious. Nursing requires the use of therapeutic communication, which utilises techniques that can assist with providing holistic patient care to support physical, emotional and mental health needs (e.g., person-centred care). Therapeutic communication involves observation and listening skills, specifically, active listening in which your focus is attentive to cues, be they spoken or demonstrated (you are 'switched on') so that you can respond to those cues appropriately. As Mildred arrived with an access card, this highlighted she has a disability, and in this case, it's detailed she was waving her hands around, but it is apparent Mildred is deaf, as she is using British sign language but with no response. (N.B. capital D suggests deaf from birth, and a small d suggests developmental deafness or hard of hearing).

Augmented communication and artificial intelligence

While there are barriers to communication, we are rapidly developing advancements in communication via the use of augmentative communication aids and artificial intelligence, which are often used to support or replace the spoken word (e.g., signs, symbols, images and technological devices), and as nurses in the 21st century, digital literacy is a key component to your communication skills as identified by the NMC (2018):

NMC

THE NMC SAYS

1 Underpinning communication skills

1.11 Provide clear verbal, digital or written information and instructions when delegating or handing over responsibility for care.

The Royal College of Nursing (RCN, 2018) considered that every nurse should be an e-nurse while being able to use technology to maximise care for patients, service users and carers. Information and communication technologies, telehealth, telecommunication technologies and health information technologies are driving healthcare forward and aiding communication, while technological devices can enhance our assessments of patients. These elements will support you in your practice; however, looking, listening, feeling, use of intuition and communication skills are all essential when managing the care of patients. It is also important to consider this when caring for patients with disabilities and specific learning difficulties to ensure that we offer the appropriate level of support to manage healthcare needs as detailed in the NMC (2018):

> *Where people have special communication needs or a disability, it is essential that reasonable adjustments are made to communicate, provide and share information in a manner that promotes optimum understanding and engagement and facilitates equal access to high quality care.*

For example, a patient may have a language barrier, which, if not addressed, could lead to difficulties in assessing somebody's neurology or gaining consent for assessments. Within the NHS, all service providers should have access to translation services, and when you go onto placement, one question you could ask is how you would book an interpreter should your patient benefit from one. As an example, NHS 111 can provide a confidential interpreter for telephone enquiries, and this is essential in ensuring that you address all your patients' needs and provide continuity of care by gaining the necessary information.

TECHNICAL SKILLS

Stepping out into placements to practise clinical skills is an exciting time. However, we must take care with how we approach patients and service users. You will be looking after patients who will be feeling vulnerable and scared and might have no certainty on how their health will be. Therefore taking into account key considerations when approaching a patient or service user is important.

Infection prevention and control (IPC)

A hospital should not be a place to do harm to patients. Unintentional harm to patients can be caused by a healthcare-associated infection, commonly caused by poor IPC practice. It is therefore critical to apply key principles of IPC when you deliver a clinical skill to a patient/service user.

For any microbe to multiply and survive, they must have certain conditions for this to occur. The main conditions are highlighted in the following image (Fig. 5.6). As health professionals, our commitment to IPC is to eliminate one or more conditions to prevent microbes from multiplying.

The principle of IPC is to remove conditions for microbes to survive or multiply or to prevent any chance of cross contamination. Microbes can be transmitted from person to person via:

- Direct contact: contact with lesions or a person with an infection.
- Indirect contact: environmental contamination such as touching a contaminated surface.
- Airbourne: water droplets spread through the air.
- Faecal-oral transmission: eating contaminated food with faecal matter on it, for example, if it's been near a contaminated water supply.

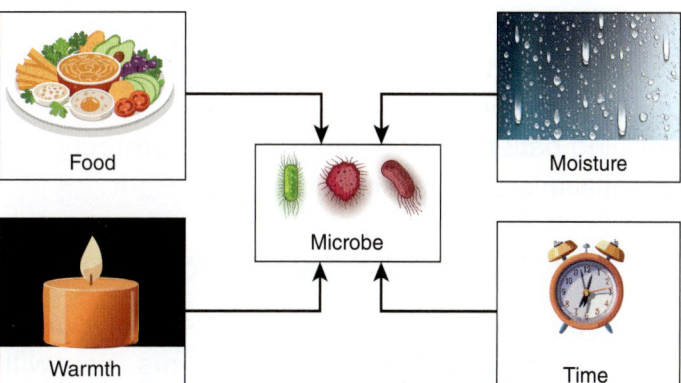

Fig. 5.6   The image shows four conditions that microbes require to survive and multiply.

Hand hygiene

A fundamental IPC practice you must do before performing any clinical skill is effective hand hygiene to reduce the possibility of cross contamination or/and remove one or more conditions to prevent microbes from surviving.

Look at the resource on how to perform effective handwashing by the World Health Organization (WHO).

Commonly missed areas include:

- the thumb and surrounding area at the base of the thumb
- in between the fingers
- under the nails
- the fingertips
- the palm of the hands
- the wrists

Handwashing must be performed at key moments within patient care. The five following key moments identify when you should be washing your hands effectively (WHO, 2009):

- Before patient contact: to eliminate any microbes on your hands before patient contact.
- Before a clean/aseptic procedure: to reduce risk of cross contamination during procedures.
- After body fluid exposure risk: to help protect you and others from potential microbe transmission.
- After patient contact: to help protect you and others from potential microbe transmission.
- After touching patient surroundings: to help protect you and others from potential microbe transmission.

Assessing your patient and escalating concerns

A key part of incorporating your clinical skills into your clinical practice is through completing patient assessments. You will learn and be involved in the many different types of assessments that healthcare professionals complete as you progress through the course, but high-quality patient assessments will consider their individual health and care needs to identify appropriate care plans. While you develop these skills, it is important that you involve your practice assessors and supervisors and are curious and ask questions when you are unsure of how to proceed. As you develop your skills, you will draw together your increasing knowledge of healthcare, anatomy and physiology, understanding of rationales for care and learning gained through experience to start understanding the decision-making processes. However, in the initial stages, you need to work within your limitations, as described by the NMC future nurse proficiencies (NMC, 2018). Some of the proficiencies which relate to assessment and documentation are listed in Fig. 5.7.

During your initial placements, one of your aims will be to master the basics of care provision. In the busy healthcare environment, every interaction with patients is valuable. It enables practitioners to gain insight into their patients, and their holistic care requirements. For example, in all care environments (both within hospitals and in non-acute care in the community) we care for patients' personal hygiene needs. For example, we may assist patients to have a wash. This enables a variety of assessments to take place, including assessing patients' skin integrity, mobility and limb strength and temperature, as well as elements such as assisting someone to the toilet.

Furthermore, having time to dedicate to a patient during personal hygiene can unlock more information about them, enabling you to gain a greater awareness of their history, such as their current health percep-

> 1.8 Write accurate, clear, legible records and documentation.
> 1.10 Analyse and clearly record and share digital information and data.
> 1.11 Provide clear verbal, digital or written information and instructions when delegating or handing over responsibility for care.
> 2.7 Undertake a whole body systems assessment including respiratory, circulatory, neurological, musculoskeletal, cardiovascular and skin status.

Fig. 5.7. Nursing and Midwifery Council (NMC) future nurse proficiencies.

Caring for patients' hygiene needs	Assessing for deterioration	Anything else?
• Monitoring patients' mobility and independence with completing their activities of daily living • Ensuring good patient positioning in bed to reduce development of a chest infection and reduce risk of muscle wastage • Completing skin assessments and utilising pressure ulcer risk assessments to consider whether patients' mattress/pressure-relieving equipment is appropriate • Monitoring and managing oral hygiene	• Utilising track and trigger scoring systems such as NEWS2 and PEWS to complete vital observations • Recognising the need for a structured assessment, including an A-E assessment • Monitoring fluid balance, hydration and nutrition • Consideration of mood and recognising when patients' mental and emotional health may require further attention • Using communication strategies to assess for changes	• Monitoring effect of medications for effectiveness/side effects • Considering other tools available to assist with recognising patients' needs, e.g., Bristol stool chart to monitor for constipation/diarrhoea and woundcare management

Fig. 5.8.   Examples of patient assessments. *NEWS2,* National Early Warning Score 2; *PEWS,* Paediatric Early Warning Score.

tions, mood and concerns, to identify their specific health needs. Patient- and family-centred communication is an essential skill that you will use in completing patient assessments. Fig. 5.8 provides further detail about some of the assessments that you may participate in when completing your clinical placements:

Recordkeeping

An important part of your patient assessments also entails learning how to accurately document your findings to ensure that other members of the multidisciplinary team can review these and act accordingly. You may also need to refer to multidisciplinary team members who haven't yet been involved with your patients' care. During your clinical placements, you will be guided by your supervisors to plan care in accordance with your assessment findings and identify when these referrals are appropriate.

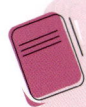

CASE STUDY

Ami, a nursing student, has been asked to complete a strict fluid balance for a patient who is not eating and drinking well after a surgery on their abdomen. This monitors the total intake and output that a patient has and works out the following calculation:

Total intake — total output = total fluid balance (the total fluid balance could be either a positive or negative number)

This may inform us about many aspects of a patient's condition, including whether they could be dehydrated or if their kidneys are functioning properly.

When completing the fluid balance chart, Ami needs to consider recording the following:

Intake:

- Drinks, for example, water, squash and juice
- Intravenous medications (given through a line such as a cannula), which could include drugs, bags of fluid and feed (called total parenteral feed)
- Nasogastric feed and/or water (this may be given through a tube in the nose or through the stomach)

Output:

- Urine, blood, vomit or stool (diarrhoea)
- Fluid draining from drains, such as surgical drains, chest drains

Providing individualised care

When completing patient assessments, we must ensure that we are approaching this in an individualised way, considering and drawing together some of our communication techniques discussed earlier in the chapter, specifically, using a person- and/or family-centred approach to care. To find out significant information about your patient, you may need to take a patient history and ask them questions about their care. Some things that you might want to ask your patient about include:

- Past medical history, including any medications that your patient normally takes, information regarding previous hospital admissions or surgeries
- Presenting condition and normal baseline: What led the patient to present to you today? Have they been to see any other health professionals in the lead up to requiring your care?
- Family: What support does the patient have? Does the patient have any children or people who are dependent on them? Do they have any significant family medical history which may need to be investigated further?
- Social history: Consideration of their activities of daily living and how they have been impacted by their illness is significant. Other elements to query could include asking whether the patient smokes or drinks, if they have carers to support them at home or if they have any cultural or religious factors that may influence their care requirements.

It is also important to consider that within societies, we are now looking after a higher range of patients with increasing complexity or variation in health. We need to be mindful of this, as it can influence variability in how a patient presents with a certain disease. For example, patients with scoliosis, a condition that causes twisting and curvature of the spine, may present with different forms of this. Some patients may experience minimal impact from the disease, and other patients may present with high levels of pain, have respiratory difficulties and require respiratory support.

If your patient has lived with a condition for a long period of time, they (or their family members) might be experts in these conditions, and they will be able to recognise when things have changed and provide you with some insight into how they normally feel or what their normal observations are. This will assist you in the care you provide, including implementing clinical skills and assisting your completion of concise, detailed and relevant assessments. This will enable you to recognise whether there have been any changes or deterioration and what you may need to escalate further.

Examples of factors that can influence variations in health include:

- Age
- Ethnicity
- Environmental factors
- Gender
- Development
- Upbringing
- Genetic factors.
- Congenital factors

Vital observations and track and trigger scores (NEWS2 and PEWS)

One main role that you may be asked to take on when on clinical placement is undertaking vital observations of your patients. You may start to hear clinicians and your supervisors refer to terminology such as 'NEWS' or 'PEWS'. This is a system called track-and-trigger scoring, which is used to assess patients' clinical observations to identify signs of deterioration to help determine when a patient's condition needs escalating to the medical team and other support services. NEWS stands for National Early Warning Score and PEWS for Paediatric Early Warning Score. Versions of these scoring systems are used across the United Kingdom, with the latest version of NEWS scoring being NEWS2, published by the Royal College of Physicians (2017). A national approach to PEWS was recently published by NHS England (2023) with the aim to standardise an escalation procedure for use within children's care.

 TIPS

Look at the NEWS2 and PEWS charts available on the Royal College of Physicians (NEWS2) and NHS England (PEWS) websites and familiarise yourself with the parameters for normal and abnormal observations for both children and adults.

Continued

TIPS—cont'd

Note: There are different **PEWS** charts for children depending upon their age!

It's important to have an awareness and understanding of the different needs of patients across the lifespan (from conception to death), as this is a requirement set by the NMC as part of the standards of proficiency for registered nurses.

You may notice that the scoring parameters differ greatly between the **PEWS** and **NEWS2** charts. This is because children undergo rapid development and growth within the first 3 years of their life. For example, infants and children tend to have a higher respiratory rate than adults due to reduced lung capacity, lung immaturity and increasing metabolism to fuel growth and development. The same principles apply to heart rate and blood pressure, too, except blood pressure is lower in infants and children due to having shorter circulatory pathways than adults.

These systems were implemented following several pieces of work in the late 1990s and early 2000s, leading to the publication of a report by the National Confidential Enquiry into Patient Outcome and Death (NCE-POD, 2005). This report looked at patients who either suffered inpatient (in hospital or while in a care facility in which they were admitted) cardiac arrests or had unplanned admissions to critical care. They found that many unwell patients had a period of instability, which usually started at least 12 hours preceding their admission to critical care or cardiac arrest. The National Patient Safety Agency (2007) conducted further research on this and found several themes relating to why deterioration was missed or not escalated appropriately, as detailed in Fig. 5.9.

These studies on deterioration led to the development of the National Institute of Clinical Excellence (NICE) Guidance CG50 (2007): 'The

> **Missed deterioration: common themes**
> Observations not being recorded;
> Deterioration not being recognised;
> Concerns not being communicated or escalated
> NPSA (2007)

Fig. 5.9   Common themes of missed deterioration.

Acutely Ill Adult in Hospital: Recognising and Responding to Deterioration'. This guidance outlines how we should monitor our patients in an acute hospital environment, how we should escalate concerns and the level of response required. One key recommendation from this was that physiological track-and-trigger scoring systems are used for all adult patients in acute settings.

Through utilising systems such as NEWS2 and PEWS, the aim is to improve safety by providing a common language that all practitioners in the NHS should be familiar with. A scoring system is assigned to each of the vital observations conducted. A normal observation scores 0, while an observation deviating outside of normal parameters could score up to 3. The score from each specific observation is then cumulatively totalled to provide a NEWS2 or PEWS score: the higher the score, the more unwell the patient potentially is.

Fig. 5.10 shows the vital observations typically measured in adult patients. All of these measurements result in a score that contributes to the cumulative NEWS2 score. The PEWS charts contain the same as the adult NEWS2 but also include measurements such as the capillary refill time (a measurement of how well perfused the patient is) and whether the patient is in respiratory distress (making a lot of effort with their breathing, such as using additional muscles to take deeper breaths). Temperature is generally not included within the scoring for the PEWS, and this is because an elevated temperature can be very normal for children who do not have an acute illness (children do not have the same mechanisms to regulate their temperature as adults do

Respiratory rate	The number of breaths that a patient takes over the course of 1 minute
Oxygen saturations	A device called a pulse oximeter measures the amount of oxygen in the blood as a percentage. Patients will also score if they are receiving oxygen therapy to maintain their oxygen levels.
Blood pressure	It is measured by a cuff that is typically placed around a limb. The cuff inflates and then deflates and calculates a measurement containing a high number (systolic) and low number (diastolic), e.g., 120/80 mmHg. The systolic measures the pressure in your arteries when the heart beats (contracts), and the diastolic measures the pressure in the arteries in between beats (at rest).
Heart rate	The number of times that the heart beats per minute. There are various pulses that can be felt around the body; generally the radial (wrist) pulse is chosen when calculating this.
Assessment of conscious levels	This involves identifying whether the pain is alert (and orientated to time, person and place), confused, responsive to either voice or pain, or unconscious. Anything other than a patient being alert needs to be escalated as a concern.
Temperature	Measures the patient's temperature through a probe, normally placed under the armpit or in the mouth.

Fig. 5.10   Measuring vital observations.

and therefore can easily have a high [>38 degrees] or low [<36 degrees] temperature), but there is a screening process for sepsis, a severe systemic infection whereby the body has an extreme response to infection (World Health Organization, n.d.) if patients' temperatures are outside of normal parameters.

TIPS

Look at the Royal College of Physicians (2017) NEWS2 resources again, and identify whether the following individual observations scores as a 0, 1, 2 or 3:

Respiratory rate: 20 breaths per minute
Oxygen saturations: 96% on room air
Heart rate: 104 beats per minute
Blood pressure: 128/88 mmHg
ACVPU status: alert
Temperature: 37.2°C

Calculate the cumulative NEWS2 score based upon these observations.

_____

_____

_____

_____

_____

_____

The answer is a NEWS2 Score of 1

This patient is scoring at present due to a heart rate of 104 bpm. However, while their respiratory rate is still scoring as with 'normal range', if it rises any further, then this will also contribute towards the cumulative NEWS2 score.

TIPS

Practice makes perfect! Once you are happy with this task, keep practising! Make up your own sets of NEWS2 or PEWS observations and continue building your confidence in calculating these. You can also look at the guidelines for accurate recordkeeping and documentation!

The NEWS2 and PEWS guidelines provide suggestions about how to respond to different NEWS2 or PEWS scores, depending on their severity. In the case of the patient described with a NEWS2 score of 1, the registered nurse in charge of their care should be informed of this score, and they are expected to assess the patient and identify whether increased monitoring or escalation of this patient's care is required (Royal College of Physicians, 2017). If you are concerned about a patient's condition, then you may, with your practice assessor or supervisor, be asked to complete an assessment called an A to E (meaning airway, breathing, circulation, disability, and exposure). The UK Resuscitation Council (2024) outlines in their guidelines what assessments each of these sections should contain. It is a structured and systematic method of assessing patients used by many multidisciplinary team members, including doctors and nurses. It enables clinicians to identify conditions and concerns that are most life-threatening so that these can be effectively treated or escalated to relevant professionals.

In some clinical areas, including accident and emergency, intensive care and high-dependency units, an A-E assessment is routinely completed on patients. However, in all care environments, regardless of their acuity, this assessment is essential to assist in prioritising patient care if you have concerns that they may be deteriorating. It is important as you progress through your course that you become confident in the fundamental principles of how to complete a detailed A-E assessment.

Important considerations

Technology and human factors. While you are in university, you will likely undertake theory and skills sessions to assist in learning to complete these observations and important aspects to consider, such as correct technique and how to identify the correct size of equipment needed for individual patients. Correctly and accurately completing assessments is essential to your role. Failure to perform techniques or use technology correctly could lead to issues such as patients being misdiagnosed, incorrectly treated or not escalated correctly, and may lead to further deterioration. For instance, you may need to size up the appropriate blood pressure cuff for your patients, or in children, you may need to identify which size pulse oximeter to use according to the child's weight to accurately measure oxygen saturations.

Here is some information detailing specific observations and the importance of accurate recording.

Respiratory rate. Practitioners calculate this by counting the number of breath cycles (one inspiration and one expiration) that a patient completes during a 1-minute period. It is important that you count for the entire minute (do not just count for 15 seconds and multiply by 4 or for 30 seconds and multiply by 2) because patients may have an irregular pattern of breathing. The respiratory rate has been recognised as one of the earliest indicators of deterioration and can assist practitioners in recognising when a patient is becoming unwell long before other vital signs might start to become deranged, such as heart rate and blood pressure (Hill and Annesley, 2020).

Oxygen saturations. You will generally use a pulse oximeter that is placed on patients' fingers to measure oxygen saturations. There can be occasions when a pulse oximeter may not accurately measure this, including if the probe is dirty, the patient's skin is cool, they have circulatory issues or they are wearing nail polish or have acrylic nails (Chan et al., 2013).

Heart rate. Depending upon the clinical environment you are in, you will see different ways of measuring the heart rate, or pulse. Sometimes devices are used to provide a digital reading, and in higher-dependency environments, you may also see patients connected to leads placed upon their chest which measure the heart rate. An important method for you to learn as a student nurse is how to manually check the pulse. This involves counting the radial pulse in the patient's wrist for 1 minute to identify the number of times the heart beats during this time. With the correct technique used, it will provide an accurate measurement of the pulse, and it will also provide important information that digital devices may not, such as whether the patient's heart is beating in a normal or irregular rhythm or if their pulse is weak or strong.

Blood pressure monitoring. Blood pressure can be measured either manually or electronically. On the ward, it is frequently recorded electronically, but there is still a human factor to consider when completing blood pressure monitoring in this manner, namely, that the cuff used is the correct size for your patient and positioned correctly. Failure to correctly size and position the cuff could lead to inaccurate results and therefore incorrect escalation of concerns.

ACVPU score. As students, you may be involved in measuring patients' conscious levels, called an ACVPU assessment. This stands for alert (A), confused (C), responsive to voice (V), responsive to pain (P) and unresponsive (U). It is important that you learn the appropriate methods for assessing what your patient's state of alertness is as well as what is 'normal' for them. This is because identification of any changes to a patient's neurological state away from their normal baseline could indicate a significant and acute deterioration, which needs to be identified and treated quickly.

Temperature. This is normally measured through a probe, which can be placed in a variety of different places in the body. Examples of locations include the ear, under the arm, in the mouth or rectally. It is essential that you are trained to use the different forms of probes, as incorrect placement may lead to inaccurate measurement.

Escalating concerns

Once we have gathered all this information through whichever assessment we have chosen, we need to think about what we are going to do with this information and may need to consider some of the following questions when deciding how we go about escalating any issues or concerns:

- Who do we need to share this information with?
- What was the purpose of the assessment we have just made?
- How urgently do we need to escalate our concerns?
- How do we get help?

Hospitals have different ways of summoning help. While some have a bleep system where pagers are used and the person you are paging calls the number you have paged them from, others have direct-dial numbers, and clinicians carry mobile telephones. If you are assessing a patient and identify that they are 'triggering' on the track-and-trigger score, many trusts will expect that care is escalated in line with the NEWS2 and PEWS recommendations.

With the expansion of IT and computerised systems, some hospitals have automated systems where people are notified when a patient's observations have changed and they are hitting a NEWS2 trigger point. When you start placement, it is worth spending some time finding out how you can get ahold of people and the escalation policy for the clinical area you are in. However, it is important to note that automated systems should not be relied upon if you have serious concerns about a patient and need an urgent review.

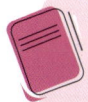

CASE STUDY

Calvin is a first-year nursing student who has been responsible for the care of Jordon over the past few days. Jordan is a 23-year-old male who was admitted for an abdominal surgery to repair a hernia. Jordan has autism and lives with a learning disability which impacts his oral communication.

He is well supported by his family and lives with his parents at home.

Today, Calvin notes that Jordan does not appear himself; he has seemed more tired than usual, and it is noted that he has been quite restless. His catheter was removed yesterday, and since then, he has been frequently incontinent of urine, and Calvin has noticed him

Continued

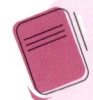

CASE STUDY—cont'd

rubbing his right side. His observations from the previous 4 hours are listed as follows:

	10:00	14:00
Respiratory rate	14 breaths per minute	19 breaths per minute
Oxygen saturations	97%	96%
Heart rate	68 bpm	85 bpm
Blood pressure	124/80	120/78
ACVPU	Alert	Alert
Temperature	37.0	37.6

When Calvin completes the NEWS2 chart, he identifies that Jordan is not 'triggering' an early warning score on any of the observations.

However, can Calvin note any subtle changes?

Jordan's respiratory rate, heart rate, and temperature are all trending upwards, and while he is not yet scoring on the NEWS2, combined with the signs listed in the earlier case study, he could be an example of a patient who is developing a urinary tract infection.

If left untreated, this could become a severe infection, and even sepsis, and early recognition is essential in successful treatment.

Who might Calvin ask to come and see Jordan if he has concerns about him?

_____

_____

_____

_____

_____

_____

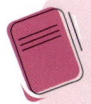

CASE STUDY

There are lots of healthcare professionals who Calvin might wish to refer to here. His practice assessor and supervisor will be able to assist, as well as the nurse in charge of the ward or unit where he is working. He might be advised to contact the medical team looking after Jordan to come and review him. They may ask Calvin and his assessor to complete a urine dip to identify whether there is a potential infection present, and he may also be asked to send this sample to the lab for further analysis. The doctors may ultimately prescribe some antibiotics to treat the infection, send some bloods off to check for infection markers and ask Calvin to complete Jordan's observations more frequently.

This case study highlights that while early warning scores are very helpful in increasing our confidence in clinical assessments, it is also important that alongside these tools, you use your clinical judgement, which will develop as you progress through your course. Do remember, if we can recognise slight differences in our patients' conditions which cause us to be concerned, then we should be escalating these concerns accordingly!

How to escalate effectively

What about if someone is really unwell or there is a cardiac arrest in the department you are in? Getting help in the ward area itself can be done by shouting for help—a loud, clear 'CAN I GET SOME HELP HERE' is usually effective in letting colleagues know you need help urgently. In acute hospitals, there is usually an emergency buzzer (Fig. 5.11) above the bed that you can push/pull to summon help from colleagues in the department; however, in situations like this, expert help is often also needed. In hospital, there is an emergency number to call; this is how you can contact the emergency team, sometimes known as the crash team or the medical emergency team. You will usually be asked by the operator what the emergency is and where it is; they will then arrange for help to be sent. For environments outside of the hospital or in places

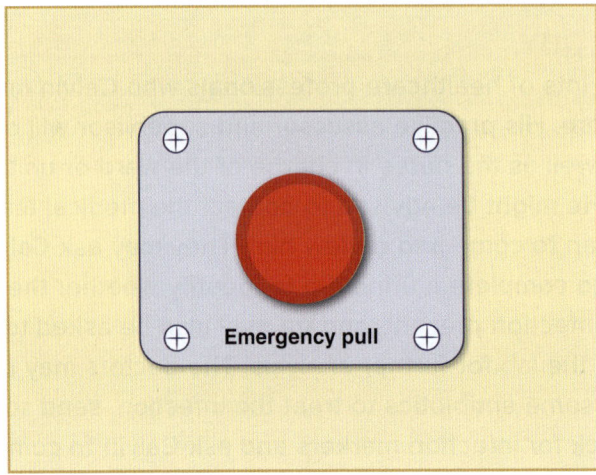

Fig. 5.11   Emergency buzzer found in clinical areas.

where there is no emergency team, there will be a policy to support how you summon help should it be required.

Handovers

CASE STUDY

Sarah is on placement on a surgical ward when her practice supervisor, Marie, is called into a bay by one of the healthcare support workers, as they are worried about one of the patients. Sarah is asked to complete a set of observations while Marie completes an A-E assessment of the patient. The patient has a temperature, is shivering and looks unwell. Once Marie has finished making her assessment of the patient, she tells Sarah to come along to listen to her call the on-call doctor.

'Hello, my name is Marie, I'm one of the staff nurses on the surgical ward/I am calling you about Mr Smith, one of the general surgical patients. He has a NEWS2 score of 6, is having episodes of rigors (shivering) and looks unwell.

He was admitted to the ward 2 days ago following an open appendectomy. He is a type 2 diabetic which is managed by diet

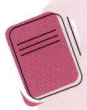

CASE STUDY—cont'd

only and has hypertension. Postop he has been stable, though pain management has been troublesome.

*'He looks unwell and is currently having rigors. **A:** self-maintained, **B:** saturations of 97% on air with a respiratory rate of 24 breaths per minute, **C:** BP is 140/75; he has a radial pulse with a rate of 125 beats per minute, **D:** he is alert and has a blood sugar of 9.7 mmol, **E:** he has a temperature of 39.2°C. There is redness around his dressing and increased tenderness around his wound; I am going to take the dressing down and swab the wound if needed.*

I am concerned he has an infection, and I would like you to come and review him urgently within the next 30 minutes'.

The doctor agrees to come and see the patient and asks Marie to complete a sepsis screen prior to their arrival.

Can you see how the information is broken down into clear chunks, sharing relevant points about the patient in a clear manner? This is useful in a number of ways: it allows Marie to share key clinical details with the on-call doctor, and it allows the doctor to consider this information and triage their workload, prioritising who they need to see more urgently or whether they need to ask for help and escalate their concerns to a more senior clinician.

This is an example of an SBAR handover, which stands for situation, background, assessment, recommendation. Some trusts use slightly different formats of this, such as SBAR/D, which includes a section called 'decisions'. It can be used effectively in many different patient scenarios, not just when a patient is acutely deteriorating and immediate help and support are required. SBAR/D was developed to encourage health professionals to be concise and objective when raising concerns about patient deterioration, and Fig. 5.12 provides further recommendations about what your handover should contain in each of these sections. Developing your handover skills is a priority as a nursing student working toward registration as detailed by the NMC (2018):

Order of priority	Application
S: Situation	Briefly identify yourself, the working area, the patient, current situation/concern and reason for the message.
B: Background	Provide context, e.g., patient's health status, reason for admission, current signs/symptoms and changes. Where necessary, consider any relevant previous medications, interventions, treatment, PMH and test results.
A: Assessment	Detail what current treatment and assessments you have completed for the patient; include the observations/MEWS/PEWS, etc., and any baseline observations to show a difference (repeat the observations as required). Where necessary, consider any relevant changes/updates to medications, interventions, treatment, PMH and test results.
R: Recommendation (also **R**equest, **R**epeat back, and **R**ecord)	You may be able to suggest a diagnosis based on your knowledge, skills and experience. Identify what is needed right now for the patient, what you want the health professional to do (as required) and what you will continue to do (as necessary). You can ask the other health professional to repeat the priority details back and identify when they will arrive. Document all the relevant details.
D: Decision (also **D**ocument)	What actions/inactions have been agreed by who and by when. 'Do' what you have to do, and wait for others to 'do' what they have advised. Document all the relevant details.

Fig. 5.12   SBAR/D handover. *NEWS,* National Early Warning Score; *PEWS,* Paediatric Early Warning Score; *PMH,* past medical history.

NMC

THE NMC SAYS

3.5 Demonstrate the ability to accurately process all information gathered during the assessment process to identify needs for individualised nursing care and develop person-centred evidence-base.

Have a look at the next case study:

CASE STUDY

Rajinder is a third-year student on her final placement with a community nursing team. She has gone to visit a patient with her practice assessor, who is letting her take the lead on this visit. They are visiting Ida, who has recently been discharged after a month-long stay in hospital for pneumonia. Ida is known to the community team, and the visit is to reassess her following her hospital stay. While speaking

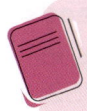

CASE STUDY—cont'd

with her, Rajinder notices that Ida appears to have lost weight. Ida explains that she hasn't had much of an appetite and is struggling to eat most of her meals. As part of this assessment, Rajinder uses a malnutrition universal screening tool (MUST) to risk assess for malnutrition in Ida. This assessment indicates that Ida is at high risk of malnutrition; because of this, one of the actions Rajinder needs to take is to refer Ida to a dietician for their input into the patient's care.

She phones the community dietician while her practice assessor listens in to refer the patient to them.

'Hi, my name is Rajinder. I am a third-year student nurse with the community nursing team and would like to refer someone to you for some support, please.

I have concerns about the patient's nutritional input; she appears to have lost a lot of weight, and she is struggling to eat more than half of most meals.

She was recently discharged from hospital following a month-long stay where she received treatment for a community-acquired pneumonia. She is known to the community team, as we have been helping manage her leg ulcers. She has carers visit at mealtimes to support her with her eating, and they have said she seems to be eating less. She has a history of previous stroke, ischaemic heart disease, peripheral vascular disease and type 2 diabetes, and she is being investigated for vascular dementia.

She is struggling to eat most of her meals, and I have commenced a food chart to keep track of this. Her MUST score today is 2, putting her risk of malnutrition as high. I've suggested to the patient and family that she has snacks frequently, asked for details on what foods she prefers and told her I would be referring her to you for some support.

I would like you to come and review her to see if what support you can provide to them, thanks'.

The dietician thanks Rajinder for her comprehensive assessment and the actions she has already carried out, agrees to add the patient to their list and will make a review when they are back on the ward the following day.

However, handing over this information is not the end of what we need to do. With a deteriorating patient, there may have been changes in their condition that need to be responded to. Thinking about NEWS2, an elevated score may mean that we need to escalate the frequency of their observations; it might be appropriate to move the patient to a more visible area of the ward, and the nurse in charge should be made aware that a patient in their department is deteriorating. Care plans will need commencing or updating. In the example in the first case study, Marie may need to commence care plans related to a wound infection and the patient having a temperature. When referring to other allied healthcare professionals, there may be further assessments they would like us to complete or monitoring they want us to commence, for instance, starting a food intake chart in the patient being referred to the dietician. If we look at the second case study, Rajinder will also need to document that she has made a referral to the dietician and ensure that the fact she has made this referral is shared with the rest of the community team and the patient's GP. This sharing of information helps the wider team know what's being done and avoids the duplication of work.

CONCLUSION

This chapter aimed to explore how to make the most of your time within clinical placements while providing you with top tips on how to learn clinical skills and assess a patient/service user. Learning within the clinical placement environments is a wonderful opportunity, and you will develop rapidly while on placements. Remember, you must practice within your limitations and never be afraid to ask your practice supervisors/assessors to explain procedures if you are unsure. We wish you all the best for your journey ahead.

💭 **Space for reader's own reflection:**

_____

_____

_____

_____

_____

_____

_____

_____

_____

_____

_____

_____

_____

_____

_____

_____

_____

_____

_____

_____

_____

_____

REFERENCES

Anderson, J.R., 1982. Acquisition of cognitive skill. Psychological Review, 89(4), 369–406. https://doi.org/10.1037/0033-295X.89.4.369

Chan, E.D., Chan, M.M., Chan, M.M., 2013. Pulse oximetry: understanding its basic principles facilitates appreciation of its limitations. Respir. Med. 107 (6), 789–799.

DeKeyser, R. 2007. Skill Acquisition Theory. In B. VanPatten & J. Williams (Eds.), Theories in second language acquisition: An introduction (pp. 97–113). Lawrence Erlbaum Associates Publishers.

Hello My Name Is. 2024. A campaign for more compassionate care. https://www.hellomynameis.org.uk/

Hill, B., Annesley, S.H., 2020. Monitoring respiratory rate in adults. Pract. Nurs. 31 (5), 206–211.

Mehrabian, A. 1972. Nonverbal Communication (1st ed.). Routledge. https://doi.org/10.4324/9781351308724

National Health Service England. 2023. National paediatric early warning system (PEWS) observation and escalation charts. https://www.england.nhs.uk/publication/national-pews-observation-and-escalation-charts/

National Patient Safety Agency. 2007. Recognising and responding appropriately to early signs of deterioration in hospitalised patients. https://www.england.nhs.uk/wp-content/uploads/2019/12/Patient_Safety_Alert_-_adoption_of_NEWS2.pdf

NICE. 2007. Guidance CG50: the acutely ill adults in hospital: recognising and responding to deterioration. https://www.nice.org.uk/guidance/cg50

Nursing and Midwifery Council. 2018. Future nurse: standards of proficiency for registered nurses. NMC, London.

Royal College of Nursing. 2018. Every nurse an e-nurse. RCN, London.

The National Confidential Enquiry into Patient Outcome and Death (NCEPOD). 2005. An acute problem? https://www.ncepod.org.uk/2005aap.html

The Resuscitation Council. 2024. The ABCDE approach. https://www.resus.org.uk/library/abcde-approach

The Royal College of Physicians. 2017. National Early Warning Score (NEWS) 2. https://www.rcplondon.ac.uk/projects/outputs/national-early-warning-score-news-2

World Health Organization. 2009. World Hand Hygiene Day. Save lives: clean your hands. https://www.who.int/campaigns/world-hand-hygiene-day

World Health Organization. n.d. Sepsis. https://www.who.int/health-topics/sepsis#tab=tab_1

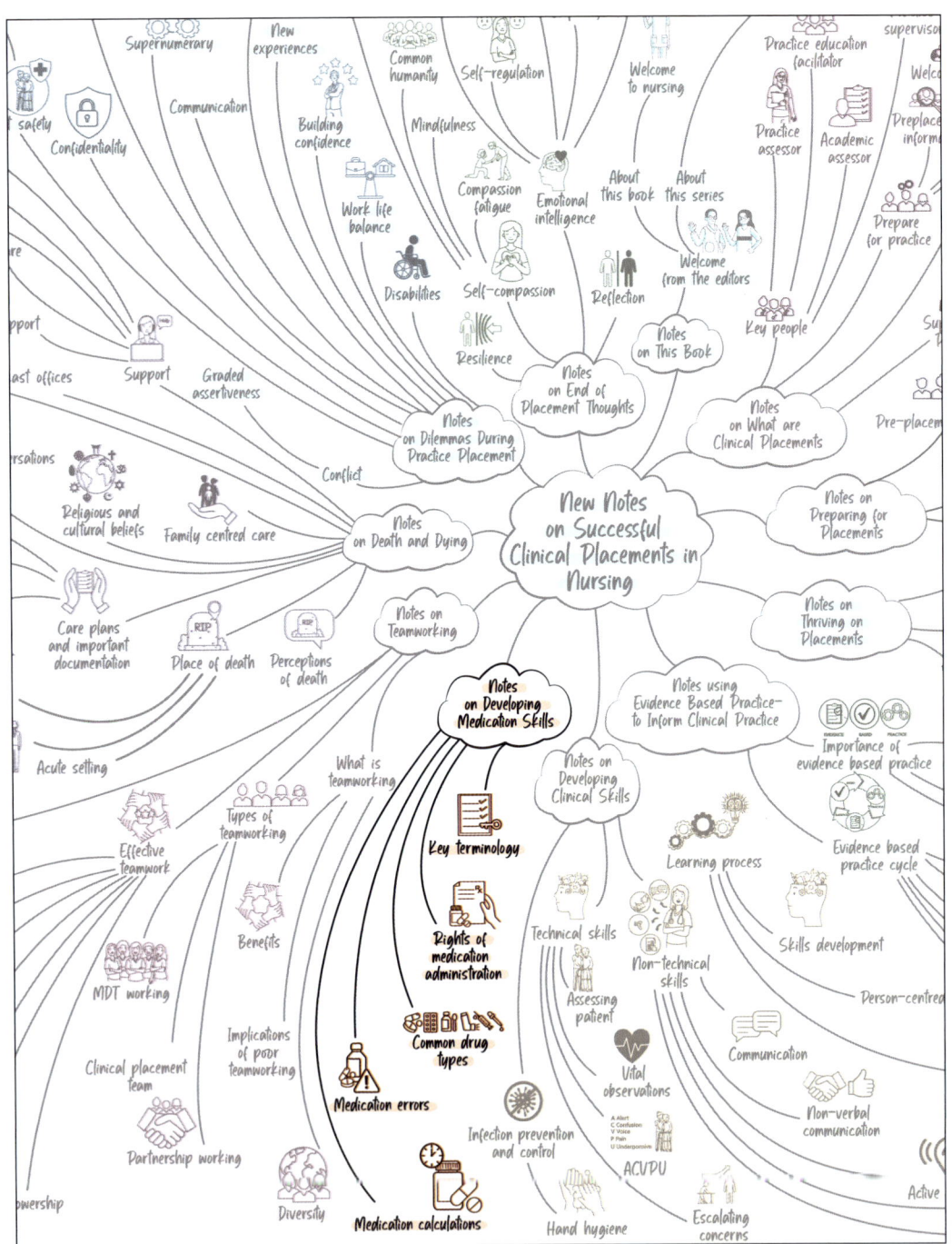

New Notes on Successful Clinical Placements in Nursing

Supernumerary
New experiences
Common humanity
Self-regulation
Welcome to nursing
Practice education facilitator
supervisor
Welc

safety
Confidentiality
Communication
Building confidence
Mindfulness
Compassion fatigue
Emotional intelligence
About this book
About this series
Practice assessor
Academic assessor
Preplace inform

re
Work life balance
Disabilities
Self-compassion
Reflection
Welcome from the editors
Prepare for practice

support
Support
Graded assertiveness
Resilience
Notes on This Book
Key people
Su

ast offices
Notes on End of Placement Thoughts
Notes on What are Clinical Placements
Pre-placem

rsations
Religious and cultural beliefs
Family centred care
Conflict
Notes on Dilemmas During Practice Placement
Notes on Death and Dying
Notes on Preparing for Placements

Care plans and important documentation
Place of death
Perceptions of death
Notes on Teamworking
Notes on Thriving on Placements

Acute setting
What is teamworking
Notes on Developing Medication Skills
Notes using Evidence Based Practice to Inform Clinical Practice
Importance of evidence based practice

Types of teamworking
Key terminology
Notes on Developing Clinical Skills
Learning process
Evidence based practice cycle

Effective teamwork
Benefits
Rights of medication administration
Technical skills
Non-technical skills
Skills development

MDT working
Common drug types
Assessing patient
Person-centred

Implications of poor teamworking
Medication errors
Vital observations
Communication

Clinical placement team
Infection prevention and control
Non-verbal communication

Partnership working
Diversity
Medication calculations
Hand hygiene
ACVPU
A Alert
C Confusion
V Voice
P Pain
U Underpromove
Escalating concerns
Active

owership

NOTES ON DEVELOPING MEDICATION SKILLS

Christie Roberts (she/her)

INTRODUCTION

Giving medications is often one of the most highly anticipated parts of clinical placements. However, it can also be anxiety provoking, and you may feel like there's far too much to cover during your time at university. Luckily, you don't need to have every detail from the British National Formulary (BNF) memorised!

Medication is a vital and safety-critical component of the nursing role. Nursing students and trainee nursing associates can give medications under supervision and will have related competencies required to undertake this. As a registered clinician, there may be further competencies to complete to allow you to administer medication independently. Registered nursing associates can administer medication similarly to registered nurses once they have undertaken relevant competencies that relate to understanding the principles of safe and effective administration (RCN, 2020). Any clinician, both registered and preregistration, should follow the principles laid out in the Nursing and Midwifery Council (NMC) code (NMC, 2018) to ensure that they are practising safely, effectively and professionally. In particular, section 18 of the NMC code applies to medication administration and covers actions including prescribing, dispensing and administering. You should read and become familiar with this section of the code before reading this chapter.

THE NMC SAYS

18 Advise on, prescribe, supply, dispense or administer medicines within the limits of your training and competence, the law, our guidance and other relevant policies, guidance and regulations.

This chapter will take you through some aspects of medication skills, including theory about the mechanism of action of medications, fundamental principles of medication administration, drug calculations and tips to help you learn medications and gain confidence to safely apply these skills in practice.

To start, there's some key terminology to familiarise yourself with. This will help you to understand how and why medications work and interact with the body.

Agonists and antagonists

Medications work following a 'lock and key' model, similar to enzymes. The medication will bind to cell receptor sites, as seen in Fig. 6.1, to either activate or block a response. These are known as agonists and antagonists (Neal, 2020). An agonist is a chemical substance that binds to a cell receptor to activate it and elicit a response (Fig. 6.2). An example is morphine binding to an opioid receptor as an agonist to provide an analgesic effect (Murphy et al., 2023).

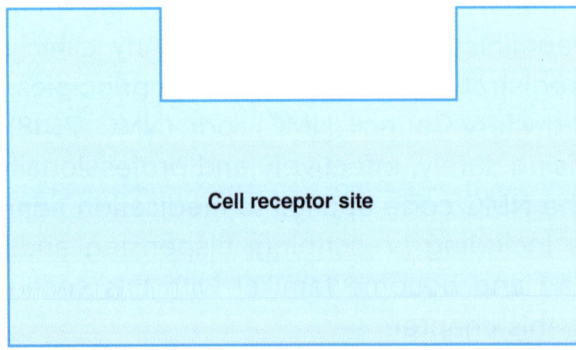

Cell receptor site

Fig. 6.1   Cell receptor site with no medication present.

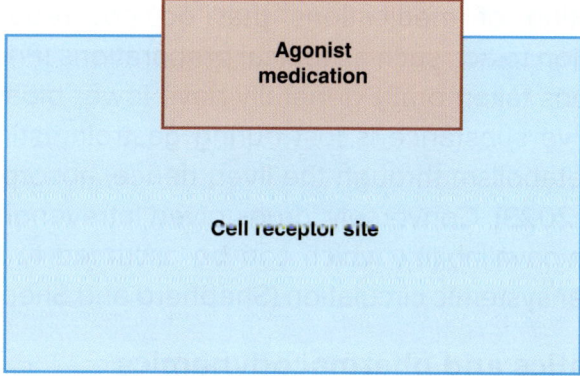

Fig. 6.2   Cell receptor site with agonist medication occupying it.

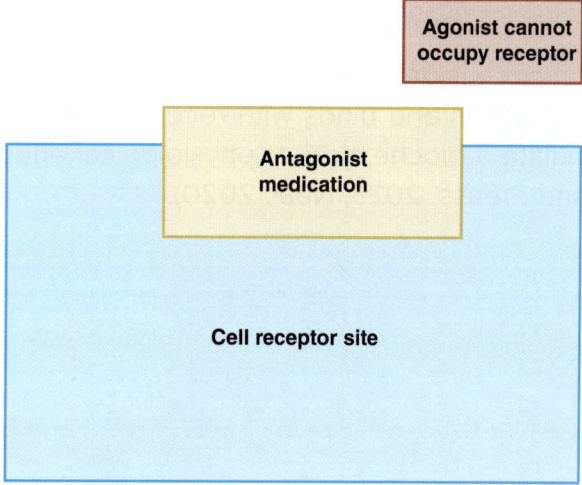

Fig. 6.3   Cell receptor site with antagonist medication occupying it.

An antagonist is a chemical substance that binds to a cell receptor without eliciting a response to prevent other substances binding to the site, therefore blocking a response (Fig. 6.3). An example is naloxone binding to an opioid receptor as an antagonist to block the effects of opioids such as morphine and reverse opioid overdoses (Theriot et al., 2023).

Bioavailability

Bioavailability is defined as the proportion of a medication that reaches the intended site of action in the body after administration (Martin and Law, 2021). It is typically the active amount that enters systemic circulation, with the exception of medications that do not require entry to systemic circulation to act, such as topical preparations (Price and Patel, 2023). Medications taken orally generally have lower bioavailability, as much of the active substance is lost during gastrointestinal digestion and first-pass metabolism through the liver; hence, absorption is lower (Price and Patel, 2023). Conversely, drugs given intravenously (IV) have a much higher bioavailability, which can be assumed to be 100%, as they directly enter systemic circulation (Shepherd and Shepherd, 2020).

Pharmacokinetics and pharmacodynamics

These are essential concepts to understand the effects of medication on the body. Pharmacodynamics relates to how the medication affects the body, while pharmacokinetics relates to how the body affects the medication.

Pharmacodynamics considers what happens when a medication reaches its primary site of action and binds with receptors, as seen in green in Fig. 6.4, to stimulate a biochemical or physiological effect on a cellular level (Grogan and Preuss, 2023; Neal, 2020).

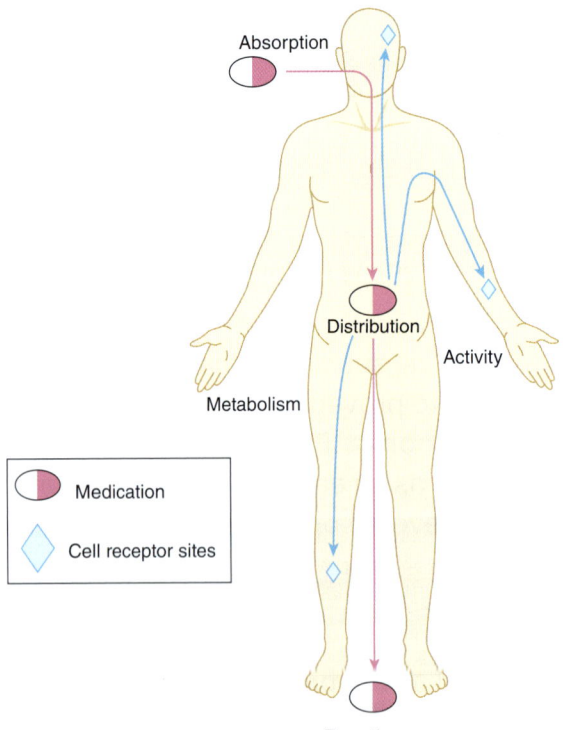

Fig. 6.4   **Pharmacodynamics and pharmacokinetics.**

Pharmacokinetics includes the absorption, distribution, metabolism and excretion of the drug (Grogan and Preuss, 2023; Martin and Law, 2021). These concepts are shown in blue in Fig. 6.4 and explained in the following table.

Absorption	After administration, the medication enters systemic circulation. This process can be impacted by the route of administration and formulation of the drug. Absorption also relates to bioavailability and can be affected by factors such as movement through the gastrointestinal tract and blood flow to an area of the body (Rang et al., 2016).
Distribution	The movement of the medication through body tissues and fluids to reach the intended site of action and cell receptor sites. This is also impacted by human physiology such as blood flow, as well as the biochemical properties of the medication, such as the ability to bind to proteins (Grogan and Preuss, 2023).
Metabolism	This occurs mainly through the liver but can also take place in the digestive tract and lungs. The metabolism can convert medication into a water-soluble form that can be excreted by the kidneys, or it can convert medications into an active form that can be used by the body. This is also known as biotransformation (Grogan and Preuss, 2023; Kebamo et al., 2015).
Excretion	The main routes for excretion of medication are via the kidneys, lungs and liver (Rang et al., 2016). Damage to the kidneys or liver can impact clearance of the medication from the body and can therefore impact the concentrations of medication in the body (Garza et al., 2023).

THE RIGHTS OF MEDICATION ADMINISTRATION

There are several guiding principles relating to medication administration, known as the '10 Rs' (Edwards and Axe, 2015).

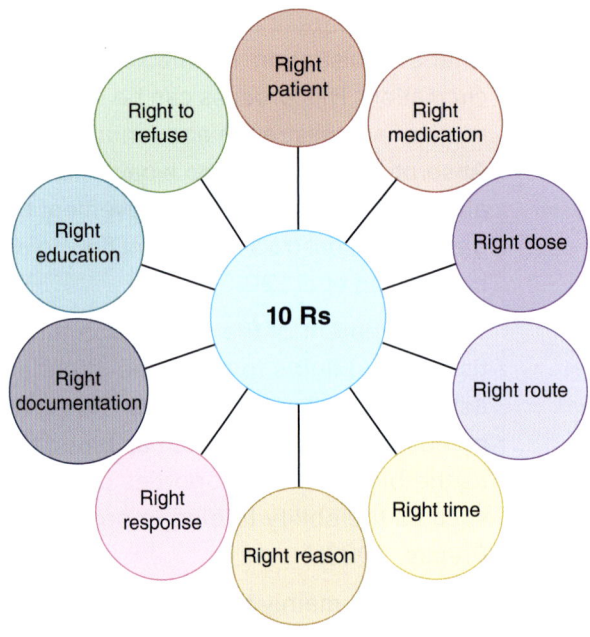

The 10 Rs.

TIPS

If you have any questions or concerns about a medication or a prescription, you should always check with another clinician, the prescriber or a pharmacist.

It is the responsibility of the registered clinician to check all of these factors prior to administering drugs to reduce the likelihood of any medication errors. Some medications, such as controlled drugs (CDs), will require a second check by another registered healthcare professional (RCN, 2020). In paediatrics, more medications could require a second check, but this will vary between clinical areas.

The second checker should check the drug, dose, time and route and confirm it against the prescription. The second check should be independent—the nurse should check all details and drug calculations as if they were preparing the medication themself, without sharing of information by the initial nurse (Westbrook et al., 2021). Although this process can be time consuming, it is essential to reduce medication errors.

'Double checking very much depends on where you work! In ICU, everything is double checked down to feeds and saline flushes. Depends on which ward and how strict they are, but generally it would be CDs and IVs for definite. There's a bit of a grey area on other meds'.

Sorcha Canterbury, registered paediatric nurse

Right patient

Positive patient identification is defined by the Healthcare Safety Investigation Branch (2022a) as 'the correct identification of a patient to ensure that the right patient receives the care meant for them'. Misidentification of your patient can lead to medication errors.

Multiple methods can be used to ensure that you have the right patient, including obtaining verbal confirmation of patient details where possible. Ideally, two identifiers should be used, such as name, date of birth or NHS number (NHS Digital, 2018). Room or bed number should never be used as an identifier (WHO, 2007).

These identifiers should be checked against the patient's wristband if they are in an acute setting and double checked against the medication administration record (MAR) or electronic patient record. In community settings, nursing homes or psychiatric wards, patients are unlikely to be wearing a wristband, so details should be confirmed verbally and checked against MARs. Medication records or prescription charts are often kept in patients' homes if medication is being administered in the community, for example, by district nurses, and this should have patient identifiers indicated against which to confirm details.

Some areas may have photographs of service users attached to records or care plans as an additional method to confirm identity, although this should not be used as the sole method for ensuring you are giving medication to the right patient.

'Our care plans will have a photograph of the resident and a section on medications which will explain how the resident likes to take their medications. Also includes any allergies and if there's any pathways in place for covert administration'.

Sylvie Angela, registered care home nurse

Positive patient identification is especially important in clinical areas with high turnovers of patients or where patients may be moving to different bed spaces within the clinical area, as the risk of having the wrong patient is higher.

It is always best to ask for the information from the patient instead of asking for confirmation: asking 'What is your date of birth?' is better than asking 'Is your date of birth the 3rd of March 1983?' The latter has the possibility of your patient just agreeing with what you have said, even if it is incorrect. Particular attention should be given to patients with the same or similar names and matching dates of birth (WHO, 2007).

'On one placement, we had two patients admitted in adjacent bed spaces. They had the same name, and their birthdates were exactly 1 month apart. We ended up moving one patient to a different bay to reduce the risk of making an error and made sure to double check that any team member knew exactly which patient they were referring to'.

Christie Roberts, registered nurse

Some patients, such as young children or people with dementia, may not be able to provide verbal confirmation. In these cases, you could check with a family member or caregiver who could confirm the patient's identity on their behalf.

When confirming the patient's identity, you should also ask if the patient has any allergies they are aware of. You may see 'NKDA' written on patient records. This means 'no known drug allergies'.

Right medication

The BNF is an easy, quick and reliable way to check medications. It is available in book format, online or via an app. Print versions of the BNF and the BNF for children are being phased out and will no longer be available after 2023, but the BNF can still be accessed online. The online versions, available on the internet or via the app, are updated monthly, so they contain the most up-to-date information.

TIPS

If you want your own print copy of the BNF, ask your local pharmacy if they have any old copies that they don't need. It probably won't be the most up-to-date version, but it should still be relatively recent and can be useful for familiarising yourself with the format.

The BNF provides all the information you might need about a medication, including indications, contraindications and cautions, dose guidance, interactions, side effects, pregnancy and breastfeeding information, and directions for administration. An indication is what the medication can be used for, and a contraindication is a reason that a medication could not be used. For example, aspirin is indicated for cardiovascular disease as secondary prevention for adults but is contraindicated for children under 16 due to the risk of Reye syndrome (BNF, 2023a).

You won't be expected to know every medication off the top of your head, but there are ways to learn groups of medications so that you can recognise them more easily. For example, beta blockers end in the suffix -lol (such as propranolol, labetalol, bisoprolol and atenolol), so when you see a medication ending in -lol, you can quickly recognise it as a beta blocker.

Some common prefixes and suffixes are listed as follows. Try and think of more examples of medications that fit into these groups.

Prefix/suffix	Drug group	Example medication
Pred-, -onide or -sone	Corticosteroid	Prednisolone, budesonide, dexamethasone
Cef- or ceph-	Cephalosporin antibiotic	Ceftriaxone
-cillin	Penicillin antibiotic	Amoxicillin
-pril	ACE inhibitor	Ramipril
-ridone	Atypical antipsychotic	Rispiridone
-lol	Beta blocker	Propranolol
-dipine	Calcium channel blocker	Amlodipine
-pam	Benzodiazepine	Lorazepam
-sartan	Angiotensin receptor blocker	Losartan
-mab	Monoclonal antibodies	Rituximab
-tidine	H2 agonist	Ranitidine
-prazole	Proton pump inhibitor	Lansoprazole
-pram or -ine	SSRI	Citalopram, sertraline
-arin	Anticoagulant	Warfarin
-cycline	Tetracycline antibiotic	Doxycycline
-fenac or -profen	Nonsteroidal antiinflammatory drug	Diclofenac, ibuprofen
-floxacin	Quinolone antibiotic	Ciprofloxacin
-mycin	Macrolide antibiotic	Clarithromycin
-azole	Antifungal	Fluconazole
-semide	Loop diuretic	Furosemide
-tyline	Tricyclic antidepressant	Amitriptyline
-vir	Antiviral	Tenofovir

ACE, Angiotensin-converting enzyme; SSRI, selective serotonin reuptake inhibitor.

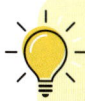

TIPS

Some medication names can give you hints about how they work. For example, direct oral anticoagulants help to prevent blood clots by inhibiting factor Xa in the clotting cascade. Therefore the medication names all have 'xa' in them: apixaban, edoxaban, rivaroxaban.

When preparing a medication for administration, you should check the drug name, dose, formulation and expiry date, and double check these against the prescription. Some medications, such as controlled drugs (CDs), may require a second check by another registered healthcare professional. Following these steps to check that you have the right medication will help to reduce the incidence of drug errors.

The term 'CDs' refers to a group of medications subject to tighter control and regulation due to them being high-risk medications with greater susceptibility to cause harm, be misused or become addicted to (NICE, 2016). Some examples include morphine, oxycodone, ketamine, midazolam and pregabalin (Home Office, 2022). In hospital and care home settings, these drugs will be locked away in a separate cupboard or trolley from other medications, have a separate book (known as a CD register, or CDR) that is used to sign for the medication, require a countersignature from a second healthcare professional for administration and will require counting on regular occasions to ensure that none are missing. Any CDs that are dispensed but then not used and so are wasted must be destroyed in a specific way and witnessed by a second member of staff (NICE, 2016). These medications are considered high risk, so particular care should be taken when prescribing, preparing or administering them.

Right dose

Medication will usually be prescribed in doses ranging from micrograms to milligrams or grams. The conversion between these units is important to ensure the correct dose is being given.

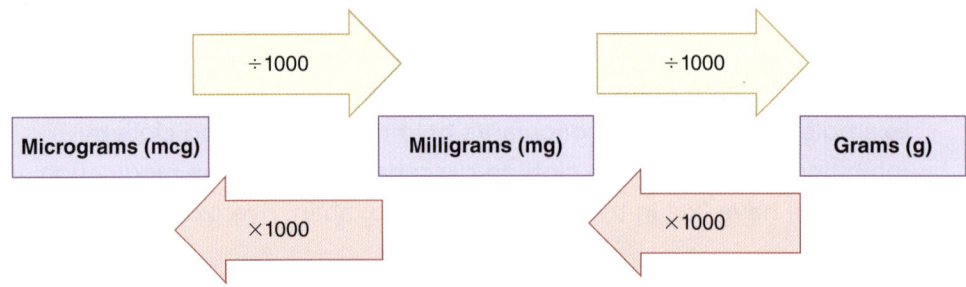

The formulation of the medication should be specified: tablets, capsules, oral solutions or suspensions, solutions for injection and so on (NICE, 2023a). Tablets can be split in half along the score line using a pill cutter. Dosages in capsules cannot be divided. Tablets and the contents of capsules can sometimes be dissolved in water to enable a patient to take them—medications are not usually licensed for this, so be sure to check before dissolving medications.

Extended- or modified-release medications should not be crushed or dissolved, as this can lead to a change in the manner of absorption and the dose being absorbed too quickly or not at all (Shepherd and Shepherd, 2020). Delaying absorption by using an extended-release formulation can help prolong the systemic effects of the medication (Rang et al., 2016). Pharmacists can always help if there is any confusion about the formulation of a medication or how it should be given.

Some dosages are weight dependent, particularly for paediatric medicines. For children, most medications require personalised prescriptions based on weight (Healthcare Safety Investigation Branch, 2022b). It is important to have an up-to-date weight for all patients to reduce the incidence of dose errors.

You may see the maximum dose per day written in the BNF or in a prescription. This can be written as just the dose or as the dose per weight.

Using paracetamol as an example, the BNF (2023b) states that up to 4000 mg, or 4 g, of IV paracetamol can be given per day for a patient weighing over 51 kg and above. However, in a patient up to 51 kg, the maximum IV dose is 60 mg/kg. Therefore if your patient weighed 50 kg, this would be 3000 mg, or 3 g, per day.

Right route

There are many different routes of administration, which all have different abbreviations that you should familiarise yourself with. The most common routes are summarised in the following sections. The 'P' before many of them stands for 'per', which just means 'by'. Routes of administration can be classed as enteral, where the drug enters via the digestive tract; parenteral, where the drug bypasses the skin, mucous membranes and digestive tract; or topical (Kim and De Jesus, 2023).

Enteral

- Oral: PO (per oral). Medication is delivered through the mouth or via an enteral feeding tube, such as a nasogastric tube or percutaneous endoscopic gastrostomy tube (CQC, 2023a).
- Rectal: PR (per rectum). Medication is delivered through the rectum via a suppository or enema following digital rectal examination (RCN, 2019).
- Buccal: Medication is placed between the gum and cheek in the mouth.
- Sublingual: Medication is placed under the tongue as a tablet or liquid/spray.

Parenteral

- Intramuscular: IM. Medication is delivered via injection into a muscle. The most common IM sites are the deltoid, ventrogluteal, vastus lateralis and rectus femoris (Shepherd, 2018a).
- IV. Medication is delivered into a vein through a peripheral cannula or central line.
- Subcutaneous: SC or sub-Q. Medication is delivered via injection into subcutaneous fat, usually in the abdomen, upper arm or thigh (Shepherd, 2018b).
- Intraosseous: IO. Medication is delivered into a bone through an IO cannula. This is most commonly used in emergencies when IV access is not available (Dornhofer and Kellar, 2022).

Topical

- Vaginal: PV (per vaginal). Medication is delivered through the vaginal cavity via creams, gels or pessaries.
- Transdermal: Medications are delivered into a localised area or systemic circulation via a cream, ointment or patch (Shepherd and Shepherd, 2020).
- Inhaled: Medications are nebulised from a liquid and delivered as a fine mist or via an inhaler (Asthma and Lung UK, 2023).
- Nasal: Medication is delivered via a cream or ointment applied to the inside of the nose.
- Ophthalmic: Medication is delivered directly into the eyes via eye drops or ointments.

Routes of administration such as rectal, vaginal, nasal and buccal allow medications to be absorbed by mucous membranes, which typically have a thin epithelial layer and are highly vascularised, enabling medications to act locally or be absorbed into systemic circulation (Le, 2022). Enteral medications are absorbed within the gastrointestinal system, and parenteral medications enter straight into the bloodstream or tissues, bypassing the digestive tract (Shepherd and Shepherd, 2020).

Many medications can be given in multiple forms. For example, paracetamol is available as a tablet, capsule, effervescent tablet, orodispersible tablet, oral suspension, oral solution, solution for infusion and rectal suppository.

The route of administration and formulation can impact on the bioavailability of the medication. As previously discussed, this is the proportion of medication that reaches the correct site of action in the body. Oral medications typically have a lower bioavailability, as some active substance is lost during digestion and metabolism, so less is available to be used. IV medication typically has 100% bioavailability, as the medication goes straight into systemic circulation, so all of the medication that is given can be used by the body.

Therefore different dosages may be required when switching between drug formulations, such as converting from IV to oral routes of administration; for example, typical doses of propranolol, a beta blocker, are 1 mg when given IV but 40 mg and above when given orally (BNF, 2023c; Cyriac and James, 2014; Shepherd and Shepherd, 2020).

Right time

There are even more abbreviations for the timings of medication doses! These come from Latin and are summarised here.

OD: once daily
BD: twice daily
TDS: three times daily
QDS: four times daily
Mane: in the morning, am
Nocte: in the evening, pm
Stat: immediately
PRN: *pro re nata*, or as required

Doses that are taken more than once daily will often have periods of time required between doses. For example, a BD dose, which is required twice daily, will usually have a 12-hour window between doses, so it could be scheduled for 8 a.m. and 8 p.m. Any PRN medications should have the minimum interval between doses specified (NICE, 2023a).

TIPS

You may see documentation that says 'q2h' or similar; this means every 2 hours.

Certain medications are considered time specific and must be given at the same time every day to promote safety and effectiveness. One example is medications for Parkinson disease. These medications should be given within a 30-minute administration window each day to avoid development of complications such as acute akinesia (NICE, 2018). Delays in medication administration can lead to decrease quality of life and increased symptom burden for patients (Saleem et al., 2023). Other time-specific medications include bisphosphonates and medications containing paracetamol (CQC, 2023b).

Some medications should be taken with food, such as NSAIDs that can cause gastric irritation if taken on an empty stomach (Moore et al., 2015) or fast-acting insulins that could cause low blood sugar (NHS, 2021a). This should be taken into consideration when the medication is prescribed, and dose timings may need to be altered to ensure that food is available around the same time as the medication. It is also necessary to consider medication that should be given on an empty stomach, as this can limit absorption, and any foods that can interact with medications (NHS, 2021b). A common example is grapefruit and selective serotonin reuptake inhibitors due to an inhibitory effect on a vital enzyme required for metabolism of selective serotonin reuptake inhibitors (DeCou et al., 2015).

Right reason

Why is this medication prescribed for this patient? Ideally, the indication for the medication should be listed in the prescription, for example, 'nitrofurantoin: for urinary tract infection', and this allows you to know exactly why this medication has been prescribed for this patient, as it may not always be immediately clear from the medication itself.

Specific parameters should also be given so that you are able to ascertain when the medication should be given. An example could be amlodipine for hypertension, with a specified target systolic blood pressure of 120 mmHg, or oxygen therapy to aim for oxygen saturations >94%. This also gives you an idea of when it would be suitable to hold the medication, such as if oxygen saturations are already above 94% on room air, additional oxygen would not be required.

Administering or holding medication can rely on clinical judgement, and rationale for giving or not giving a prescribed medication should be clearly documented.

Right response

Some medications may require monitoring pre- and postdose. For example, if rapid-acting insulin is prescribed to bring blood glucose levels down, you should check the blood sugar before and after giving the medication to ensure that it is working. Checking vital signs prior to giving the medication will also ensure that the medication is being given appropriately; if the blood sugar level is on the low side, you may decide that it's appropriate to hold the medication, as administration could lead to hypoglycaemia.

After giving medication, it's important to watch out for any adverse effects or allergic reactions. This is particularly important for new medications that the patient has not received before and high-risk medications such as opioids and antibiotics (Gilkey et al., 2022). For example, opioid medications such as morphine can cause respiratory depression, so the patient's respiratory rate should be monitored accordingly.

TIPS

If you are keeping a list of medications you've seen used in practice, add in any common side effects or reactions to look out for. This can then be used to inform your patients of what they may need to look out for.

A drug allergy is distinct from a known side effect, a toxicity reaction from drug overdose and drug sensitivity or intolerance (Allergy UK,

2023). An allergic reaction will usually occur within a few hours of taking the medication, and symptoms can include rashes, itching, nausea and vomiting, blurred vision and headaches. In rare cases, anaphylaxis can occur, which can be life-threatening due to multiorgan dysfunction. Signs include airway swelling, with difficulty breathing, hypotension and loss of consciousness (Allergy UK, 2023). Anaphylaxis is usually treated with a combination of adrenaline, antihistamines and steroids (NHS, 2023).

Sometimes, patients may consider a negative symptom experienced after taking a medication to be indicative of a drug allergy. However, these are usually known side effects (Hanson and Haddad, 2022). An example is antibiotics causing an upset stomach or diarrhoea. This may be uncomfortable or distressing to a patient but is not considered a drug reaction or a reason to not give the medication if it is clinically required.

The effects of some medications can be altered—increased or decreased—in patients with poor kidney or liver function, known as renal or hepatic impairments. This can mean that medication is filtered from the blood less effectively and with reduced excretion, leading to a buildup in the body and potential drug toxicity, or it might mean that medications are less effective due to impaired metabolism (NICE, 2023b; NICE, 2023c).

Right documentation

This can relate to both the prescription being documented correctly and to your documentation after administering the medication.

All medications, including oxygen therapy, enteral or parenteral feeds, and IV flushes, should be prescribed. Medication should not be administered without a written prescription unless in an emergency. This prescription should include, as a minimum, the medication name (either the generic drug name or a specific brand), dose, frequency of administration and route of administration (NICE, 2023a).

TIPS

Some medications must be prescribed by specific brand name. Tacrolimus, an immunosuppressant drug, is an example. Brands include Adoport, Prograf, Modigraf, Advagraf, Dalliport and Envarsus (BNF, 2023c). Patients should not switch between brands of tacrolimus, as this can affect the clinical effectiveness.

Some medications are given under patient group directions (PGD) and do not require a prescription for each specific patient. This includes medications such as immunisations and naloxone (Mitchell, 2021; NHS England, 2023a). These medications can be delivered once a PGD is signed by a doctor or dentist and a pharmacist. It is the responsibility of the clinician to ensure that the PGD is up to date and valid (NHS England, 2023a). Nursing associates are not currently able to administer medications under a PGD; a signed prescription is required (Health Education England, 2018; RCN, 2020).

After administering medication, this should be documented in a MAR or electronic patient record. Documentation should include the date, time, drug and dose being given, your name and the name of the clinician providing second checking if applicable. After administering medications, they should be signed for immediately to reduce the risk of the dose being repeated (Black Country Partnership NHS Foundation Trust, 2019). Records should not be signed prior to the patient taking the medication.

If a medication is being given late, the reason for this should be documented, for example, if the previous dose was given late, your dose had to be delayed to ensure an appropriate gap. If the patient has declined the medication, this should also be documented with the reason for doing so.

Nurses have overall legal liability for medications given to their patients, and it's important to remember that if it isn't documented, it didn't happen (RCN, 2020)!

Patients should always be observed taking medication to ensure that it is being taken and being taken appropriately and therefore documented correctly. In some cases, patients may have responsibility for their own medications. If this is the case, you should ask the patient to inform you if and when they are taking the medication so that this can be documented.

NMC

THE NMC SAYS

10.1 Complete all records at the time or as soon as possible after an event, recording if the notes are written some time after the event.

Right education

Empowering and educating patients about their medications are an essential part of nursing practice. Does the patient know what medications they are taking and why? Do they know about potential side effects to look out for?

Medication counselling should occur during any consultation with healthcare professionals where medication is being initiated, titrated or discontinued. Commonly, patient education will occur when a patient is being discharged from hospital; the registered nurse should go through the discharge letter with the patient, double check any medications that are being given and ensure that the patient knows what to take and when. This is particularly important for new medications that the patient has not taken at home before. The information leaflet that comes with the medication can be an important source of information, and further information may be available on the NHS website.

Many NHS trusts will have a medication helpline available that patients can call if required for more information about their medications, and this should be highlighted to patients before they are discharged if available (Williams et al., 2020).

Providing adequate information on medicines for patients can be vital for promoting adherence to treatment plans. A combination of patient counselling and written information has been shown to improve medication adherence and improve compliance with taking prescribed medications

(Taibanguay et al., 2019). Patients may have different requirements for education depending on their personal learning and communication styles, so a range of options should be presented and discussed with the patient and any caregivers, from written information to verbal directions and use of any existing resources such as patient information leaflets (PILs). Translation services should be used if required to ensure that language is not a barrier to the patient receiving adequate education. Services such as language line can be utilised to ensure that patient understanding of medication education is optimised (Bowen et al., 2017).

NMC

THE NMC SAYS

3.3 Act in partnership with those receiving care, helping them to access relevant health and social care, information and support when they need it.

Right to refuse

Patients should provide informed consent prior to you administering medications. This requires them to have all required information about a medication, understand this information and use it to make an informed decision (NHS, 2022). In a typical situation, patients retain the right to refuse medication once they are provided with all relevant information, such as what the medication is indicated for, the potential risks and benefits of the medication and possible outcomes if the medication is given or not given. If a medication is declined by a patient, this should be clearly documented. This forms part of the NMC code: to support and respect patients declining care or treatment and make sure this is documented.

NMC

THE NMC SAYS

2.5 Respect, support and document a person's right to accept or refuse care and treatment.

4.2 Make sure that you get properly informed consent and document it before carrying out any action.

There are some situations in which it may not be possible to obtain consent prior to administration of medication, including emergencies and situations in which the patient does not have the capacity to accept or decline the specific medication in the absence of a lasting power of attorney. In such cases, medication and treatment may be given in the patient's best interests at the discretion of the healthcare professional following a capacity assessment (NHS, 2022; NICE, 2019).

Consent for medications should be sought from children where appropriate. If possible, consent should be sought directly from the patient after assessing if the young person is deemed 'Gillick competent', but parents or guardians may be required to provide consent from children up to the age of 16 (British Medical Association, 2023).

Covert administration refers to medication being given to a person without their knowledge or consent, which could include medication being disguised in food or drink or given via a feeding tube without telling the patient (CQC, 2022). For covert administration to be used, the person must be deemed to not have the capacity to make a decision around taking the medication, and the medication should be deemed essential to the health and wellbeing of the patient (CQC, 2022). Covert administration should always be a last resort, the least restrictive option and in the best interests of the patient. Covert administration should also be a multidisciplinary team decision, involving family members or significant others where appropriate. A deprivation of liberties safeguard may be required (Cardiff and Vale UHB, 2017).

Prior to using covert administration, you should speak with the patient and undertake a mental capacity assessment to understand why they may be refusing the medication and try to problem solve; for example, would changing the formulation from a tablet to a liquid enable the patient to take the medication? Do they understand why the medication is required? Are there side effects that the patient finds unmanageable that could be addressed?

It's also important to consider whether altering the medication to be able to give it covertly would alter the mechanism of action of the medication. For example, crushing a tablet to conceal it within food could impact the rate of absorption (CQC, 2022). It is advisable to consult a pharmacist before altering or concealing any medications, as pharmacists can provide information on the safest way to do this.

TIPS

If disguising medication within food or drink, you must consider whether the patient is receiving a full dose of the medication. What happens if the patient does not finish the food or drink that the medication is concealed in?

Tips and tricks for learning medications

One way to familiarise yourself with medications is by taking the PIL from the box of medications to read and learn more about it. Just make sure that the box is empty before taking the PIL, as others may need to refer to it. Some people keep these and file them away and use them for learning throughout their course.

'I started collecting medicine information leaflets in my first year of my nursing degree after seeing them just get thrown away after the medicine box is empty...I made up a folder at home where I've been collecting leaflets, and it's become a portfolio of medication knowledge that I enjoy sharing with other students on placement. It'll also help as I move into my first newly qualified nursing (NQN) post this year'.

Amy Bishop, student nurse

Pronouncing medication names can be tricky, especially if you've not heard them said aloud before or don't use the medication commonly. YouTube videos that give pronunciations of the drug name or Google Translate can be useful to familiarise yourself with the pronunciation. Some medications have names that not everyone agrees on the pronunciation; clopidogrel is one, where some will say clo-PID-o-grel, and others will say clopi-DOG-rel. In this case, the pronunciation doesn't matter too much, as either is accepted.

'My first placement as a student nurse was in neuro rehab. Nearly every patient was on levetiracetam, and I had no idea how to pronounce it because everyone used to refer to it by the brand name, Keppra.
I listened to YouTube video on repeat just saying it over and over, and by the next shift, I could actually pronounce it'.

Christie Roberts, registered nurse

You should get the opportunity to practise giving medications via oral, SC, IM and IV routes in simulation sessions at university, and this will give you a good foundation for providing medication in practice.

Once on placement, get involved with drug rounds when you can. You might start initially by simply observing, and this can give you an overview of how a medication round works and any common medications that are given frequently in a clinical area. After this, you should get involved where possible and within your scope of practice (for example, not giving IV medications prior to undertaking relevant competencies). Involvement with medication administration is likely to form part of your placement competencies or national curriculum, and getting experience with medication rounds will help to improve your confidence and clinical skills.

'I choose a couple of medications I would see on the ward and then read up on them and start dispensing them with my supervisor'.

Ellie Cowl, student nurse

The following is a table of medication groups with some examples. You may wish to add to this list as you encounter different medications and add any other details such as common side effects, formulation options, indications, and contraindications or cautions.

Medication group	Medication subgroup	Examples
Analgesics	Opioids	Fentanyl
	Nonopioids	Paracetamol
	NSAIDs	Ibuprofen
	Adjuvants	Amitriptyline
Antacids	Histamine H2 receptor antagonists	Ranitidine
	Proton pump inhibitors	Omeprazole
Antiarrhythmics	Sodium channel blockers	Amiodarone
	Beta blockers	Carvedilol
	Potassium channel blockers	Dofetilide
	Calcium channel blockers	Amlodipine
	Cardiac glycosides	Digoxin
Antibiotics	Penicillins	Amoxicillin
	Cephalosporins	Ceftazidime
	Aminoglycosides	Gentamicin
	Tetracyclines	Doxycycline
	Macrolides	Erythromycin
	Fluoroquinolones	Levofloxacin
Anticholinergics	Antimuscarinics	Tolterodine
	Antinicotinics	Atracurium
Anticoagulants	DOACs	Apixaban
	Vitamin K antagonists	Warfarin
	Antiplatelets	Clopidogrel
	LMWH	Tinzaparin
Anticonvulsants	GABA enhancers	Phenobarbital
	Glutamate blockers	Levetiracetam
	Carbonic anhydrase inhibitors	Diclofenamide

Continued

Medication group	Medication subgroup	Examples
Antidepressants	SSRIs	Citalopram
	SNRIs	Venlafaxine
	NaSSAs	Mirtazapine
	TCAs	Lofepramine
	MAOIs	Isocarboxazid
Antiemetics	Dopamine agonists	Droperidol
	Antihistamines	Promethazine
	Serotonin/5-HT3 receptor antagonists	Ondansetron
Antifungals		Fluconazole
Antihistamines	First generation (sedating)	Chlorphenamine
	Second generation (nonsedating)	Fexofenadine
Antihyperglycaemics	Biguanides	Metformin
	Thiazolidinediones	Pigolitazone
	Sulfonylureas	Gliclazide
	Meglitinides	Liraglutide
	Insulins	Insulin degludec
Antihypertensives	ACEIs	Lisinopril
	Calcium channel blockers	Amlodipine
	ARBs	Losartan
	Beta blockers	Atenolol
	Alpha blockers	Doxazosin
Antipsychotics	First generation (typical)	Haloperidol
	Second generation (atypical)	Clozapine
Beta-1 agonists		Dobutamine
Bronchodilators	Beta-2 agonists	Albuterol
	Anticholinergics/antimuscarinics	Ipratropium bromide
	Leukotriene receptor antagonists	Montelukast

Medication group	Medication subgroup	Examples
DMARDs	Conventional synthetic	Methotrexate
	Biologic	Adalimumab
	Targeted synthetic	Tofacitinib
Diuretics	Loop	Furosemide
	Potassium sparing	Spironolactone
	Thiazides	Hydrochlorothiazide
Laxatives	Bulk forming	Ispaghula husk
	Osmotic	Lactulose
	Stimulant	Bisacodyl
	Stool softening	Docusate
Sedatives	Benzodiazepines	Lorazepam
	Barbiturates	Pentobarbital
	Hypnotics	Zolpidem
	Opioids	Morphine
Statins		Atorvastatin

ACEIs, Angiotensin-converting enzyme inhibitors; ARBs, angiotensin receptor blockers; DMARDs, disease-modifying antirheumatic drugs; DOACs, direct oral anticoagulants; LMWH, low-molecular-weight heparins; MAOIs, monoamine oxidase inhibitors; NaSSAs, noradrenergic and specific serotonergic antidepressants; SNRIs, serotonin and norepinephrine reuptake inhibitors; SSRIs, selective serotonin reuptake inhibitors; TCAs, tricyclic antidepressants.

Medication errors

Medication errors can arise from individual mistakes or systemic failures, including prescription errors, human factors or fatigue. Many nurses will make a medication error at some point in their careers. Fortunately, the majority of medication errors will lead to little or no harm. However, some can lead to very poor outcomes and even fatality. Serious consequences from medication errors are more likely in children, owing to them having less physiological reserve to manage a medication error, and in patients with known drug allergies (Edwards and Axe, 2015; Marufu et al., 2022).

If you do make a medication error, the most important thing to do is to report it and be open and honest about it, remembering that patient safety is the priority. The NMC outlines a duty of candour which outlines explaining the mistake to the patient and their family, carers or advocate, apologising for the mistake and acting to ensure that harms or potential harms are addressed and mitigated (NMC, 2018). A 'just culture' in the clinical environment should allow people to feel comfortable to speak up when mistakes happen rather than fearing blame or retribution (NHS England, 2023b). This kind of open and honest culture should allow mistakes and errors to be documented and escalated to reduce the risk of further similar mistakes and to ensure that learning can take place from the incident to improve patient safety and staff competence. One of the key responses is that you personally learn from it and reflect on it to consider why it happened and what you could do differently next time to prevent it from happening again.

NMC

THE NMC SAYS

14.2 Explain fully and promptly what has happened, including the likely effects, and apologise to the person affected and, where appropriate, their advocate, family or carers.

Human factors can contribute to medication errors. These include things such as similar-looking medication packaging, as shown, medications with similar-sounding names and medications being put back into the wrong place, such as a drug in the wrong box or a box in the wrong place in a medicine cabinet or trolley. This highlights the importance of fully focusing when dealing with medications. Medication rounds are considered as protected times in many settings, and some nurses may wear tabards with 'medication round in progress' or similar written on them so that they are not disturbed when preparing and dispensing medications.

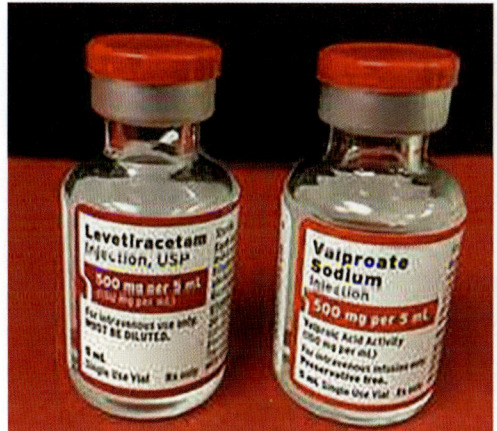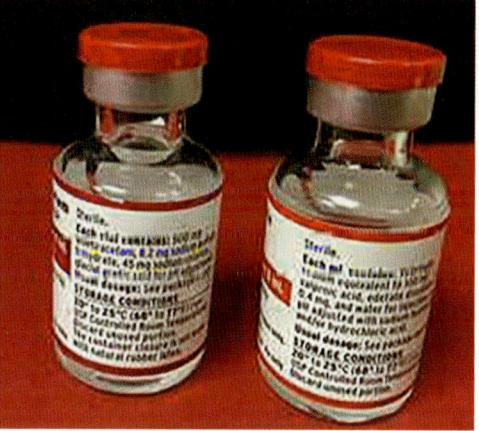

Levetiracetam and sodium valproate vials (Institute of Safe Medical Practices, 2016).

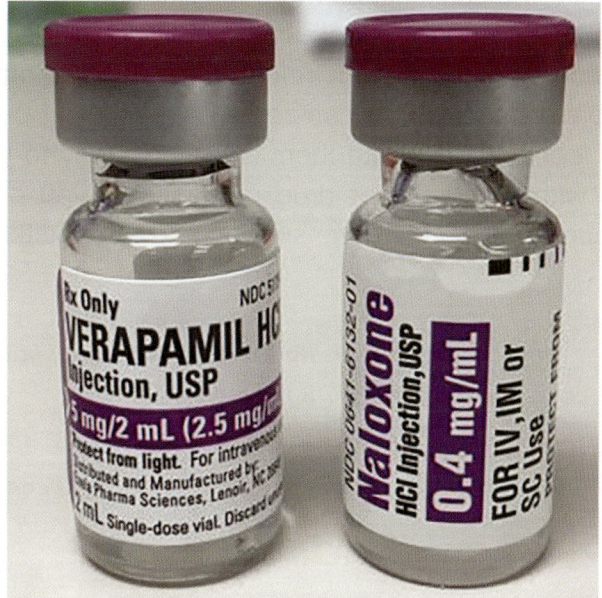

Verapamil and Naloxone vials (Institute of Safe Medical Practices, 2018).

The Medicines and Healthcare products Regulatory Authority (MHRA) has warned of cases where patients have suffered serious negative outcomes due to medications with names that sound similar. They list sulfadiazine, an antibiotic, and sulfasalazine, a disease-modifying antirheumatic drug, as one case where harm has been reported after mixing up the two drugs (MHRA, 2018). This highlights the importance of vigilance when reading prescriptions and preparing medications.

The Yellow Card reporting scheme is operated by the MHRA and acts as potential safety concerns relating to medications and medical devices. Any concerns about adverse drug reactions can be reported by healthcare professionals or the public. The reporting system can be accessed online by searching for 'MHRA Yellow Card'.

Medication calculations

The universal advice to ace your drug calculation exam, from students to registered nurses alike, is to practise. Doing as many sample questions as you can will make the calculations more familiar and increase your confidence. Student nurses and trainee nursing associates will be required to pass a medication calculation exam before qualifying, and often these tests will have a 100% pass rate. This can seem daunting, but practising questions until you feel confident with them is the best way to prepare. If you are struggling with numeracy or drug calculations, you could speak to someone at your university to ask for support and any additional resources.

 'I remember drug calculations using the NHS formula. I find this easier to remember, as most nurses work for the NHS.

What you NEED/what you HAVE × how it is SUPPLIED

Natalie Elliott, registered community nurse

The following are some sample questions with answers below them. You may wish to revise the theory behind medication calculations first, including conversion calculations and IV drop rates, before trying the questions. If you're stuck on any questions, you may want to brainstorm with a study group to understand how to get to the correct answer.

QUESTIONS

1. Convert 2 g into milligrams.

_____

_____

_____

_____

2. Convert 500 mcg into milligrams.

_____

_____

_____

_____

3. Convert 800 mg into grams.

_____

_____

_____

_____

4. Convert 1.2 mg into micrograms.

_____

_____

_____

_____

5. Convert 1.9 L into millilitres.

_____

_____

_____

_____

6. Your patient is prescribed 750 mg of naproxen. How many 375-mg tablets should they be given?

_____

_____

_____

_____

7. Your patient is given 2.5 tablets of clozapine to take orally. If one tablet is 100 mg, what is the total dose the patient is receiving?

_____

_____

_____

_____

8. Your paediatric patient is prescribed erythromycin at a dose of 40 mg/kg/day in four equal doses. The child weighs 15 kg. Calculate a single dose for the patient.

_____

_____

_____

_____

9. Your patient, who weighs 33 kg, has been prescribed levetiracetam. The initial dose is 10 mg/kg once daily. How much levetiracetam should be given?

_____

_____

_____

_____

10. Your patient is prescribed 150 mg of pregabalin daily, divided into three doses. You have 25-mg pregabalin capsules in stock. How many capsules should be given for a single dose?

11. Your patient is prescribed 10 mg of baclofen oral solution three times daily. The medication is available as 5 mg/5 mL. Calculate how many millilitres should be given for a single dose.

12. Your paediatric patient is prescribed amoxicillin oral solution. The prescription states the medication is prepared to 20 mg/kg, and the patient weighs 9 kg. How many milligrams of amoxicillin should be given?

13. The amoxicillin in the previous question is available as 30 mg/mL. Calculate how many millilitres of amoxicillin should be given.

_____

_____

_____

_____

14. Five hundred milligrams of acyclovir is reconstituted in 20 mL of sterile water. Your patient is prescribed 400 mg. How many millilitres of reconstituted acyclovir should be withdrawn from the vial for administration?

_____

_____

_____

_____

15. A loading dose of IV vancomycin is prescribed for your patient, who weighs 65 kg. The dose requires a concentration of 25 mg/kg. How many milligrams of vancomycin should be given to achieve this concentration?

_____

_____

_____

_____

16. Your patient, who weighs 90 kg, is prescribed IV voriconazole. The medication should be infused at 3 mg/kg/hour. What is the maximum amount of voriconazole that can be infused in 1 hour?

_____

_____

_____

_____

17. Your patient has an IV infusion of Hartmann solution. The total volume of the infusion is 1 L, and it is running at 250 mL/hour. How long will the infusion take to finish?

_____

_____

_____

_____

18. Calculate the flow rate in millilitres/hour for 250 mL of fluid to run over 2 hours.

_____

_____

_____

_____

19. Your patient has an infusion of 5% glucose running at 75 mL/hour. How much fluid will the patient receive over 6 hours?

_____

_____

_____

_____

20. A patient is prescribed 1 U of blood (250 mL) to be transfused over 2 hours. The IV-giving set runs at 20 drops/mL. Calculate the drip rate in drops per minute (hint: you can calculate this using a drop rate denominator or the extended equation).

_____

_____

_____

ANSWERS

1. 2000 mg
2. 0.5 mg
3. 0.8 g
4. 1200 mcg
5. 1900 mL
6. Two tablets (375 mg × 2 = 750 mg)
7. 250 mg (100 mg × 2.5 tablets = 250 mg)
8. 150 mg (40 mg/kg × 15 kg = 600 mg in four divided doses, so one dose = 150 mg)
9. 330 mg (10 mg/kg × 33 kg = 330 mg)
10. 2 capsules (150 mg in three divided doses, so one dose = 50 mg. 50 mg = 2 × 25 mg capsules)
11. 10 mL (5 mg is in 5 mL, so 10 mg is in 10 mL)
12. 180 mg (20 mg for 1 kg, so 20 mg × 9 kg = 180 mg)
13. 6 mL (30 mg in 1 mL, so 180 mg in 6 mL)
14. 16 mL (500 mg in 20 mL reconstituted, divide by 5 to find 100 mg in 4 mL, × 4 to get 400 mg in 16 mL)
15. 1625 mg (65 kg × 25 mg/kg = 1625 mg)
16. 270 mg (3 mg × 90 kg × 1 hour = 270 mg)
17. 4 hours (1000 mL divided by 250 mL/hour = 4 hours)
18. 125 mL/hour (250 mL divided by 2 hours = 125 mL/hour)
19. 450 mL (75 mL/hour × 6 hours = 450 mL)
20. 42 drops/minute (drop rate denominator: 125 mL/hour divided by 3 = 41.6, rounded up to 42 drops/minute. Extended equation: 250 mL × 20 drops/mL divided by 2 hours × 60 minutes = 5000 divided by 120 = 41.6, rounded up to 42 drops/minute)

CONCLUSION

Critical thinking and clinical judgement are required in medicine management, and experience with medication administration will enhance these factors related to decision making (Hanson and Haddad, 2022). As a student, you should always be supervised while administering medications, so this should be seen as a safe space to develop your skills and knowledge, and once registered, you may be required to undertake further competencies, particularly for medications such as cancer therapies and blood products.

Space for reader's own reflection:

_____

_____

_____

_____

_____

_____

_____

_____

_____

_____

_____

_____

_____

_____

_____

_____

_____

_____

_____

REFERENCES

Allergy UK. 2023. Drug allergy. https://www.allergyuk.org/types-of-allergies/drug-allergy/. [Accessed June 27, 2023]

Asthma and Lung UK. 2023. Nebulisers. https://www.asthmaandlung.org.uk/symptoms-tests-treatments/treatments/nebulisers#:~:text=it%20for%20you.-,What%20is%20a%20nebuliser%3F,through%20a%20facemask%20or%20mouthpiece. [Accessed June 28, 2023]

Black Country Partnership NHS Foundation Trust. 2019. Administration of medicines. https://www.bcpft.nhs.uk/documents/policies/m/975-medicines-administration/file. [Accessed July 6, 2023]

BNF. 2023a. Aspirin. https://bnf.nice.org.uk/drugs/aspirin. [Accessed July 10, 2023]

BNF. 2023b. Paracetamol. https://bnf.nice.org.uk/drugs/paracetamol/#hepatic-impairment. [Accessed June 27, 2023]

BNF. 2023c. Propranolol hydrochloride. https://bnf.nice.org.uk/drugs/propranolol-hydrochloride/. [Accessed September 10, 2023]

BNF. 2023c. Tacrolimus. https://bnf.nice.org.uk/drugs/tacrolimus/#:~:text=To%20ensure%20maintenance%20of%20therapeutic,dispensed%20by%20brand%20name%20only. [Accessed July 2, 2023]

Bowen, J., Rotz, M.E., Patterson, B.J., Sen, S., 2017. 'Nurses' attitudes and behaviors on patient medication education. Pharm. Pract. (Granada) 15 (2), 930.

British Medical Association. 2023. Children and young people toolkit: a toolkit for doctors. https://www.bma.org.uk/media/4666/bma-children-and-young-people-ethics-toolkit-oct-2021.pdf. [Accessed June 26, 2023]

Cardiff and Vale UHB. 2017. Covert medication guidance, decision tool and record. https://cavuhb.nhs.wales/files/policies-procedures-and-guidelines/patient-safety-and-quality/c-patient-safety/final-v-1-2-covert-medication-administration-guidance-and-decision-tool-covert-medication-administration-guidance-and-decision-tool-pdf/#:~:text=If%20the%20person%20is%20in,review%20can%20be%20carried%20out. [Accessed March 17, 2024]

CQC. 2022. Covert administration of medicines. https://www.cqc.org.uk/guidance-providers/adult-social-care/covert-administration-medicines#:~:text=Covert%20administration%20is%20when%20medicines,they%20are%20taking%20a%20medicine. [Accessed March 17, 2024]

CQC. 2023a. Enteral feeding and medicines administration. https://www.cqc.org.uk/guidance-providers/adult-social-care/enteral-feeding-medicines-administration#:~:text=Enteral%20feeding%20tubes%20provide%20access,person%20has%20difficulty%20in%20swallowing. [Accessed June 28, 2023]

CQC. 2023b. Time sensitive medicines. https://www.cqc.org.uk/guidance-providers/adult-social-care/time-sensitive-medicines. [Accessed March 16, 2024]

Cyriac, J., James, E., 2014. Switch over from intravenous to oral therapy: a concise overview. J. Pharmacol. Pharmacother. 5 (2), 83–87.

DeCou, J., Biergenheier, N., Dull, R., 2015. CYP3A4: the workhorse. In Marcucci, C., et al., (Eds.), A case approach to perioperative drug-drug interactions. Springer, New York, pp. 37–40.

Dornhofer, P., Kellar, J., 2022. Intraosseous vascular access. https://www.ncbi.nlm.nih.gov/books/NBK554373/#:~:text=Intraosseous%20(IO)%20vascular%20

access%20refers,not%20easily%20obtained%20in%20the. [Accessed June 29 2023]

Edwards, S., Axe, S., 2015. The 10 'R's' of safe multidisciplinary drug administration. Nurse Prescribing 13 (8), 352–360.

Garza, A., Park, S., Kocz, R., 2023. Drug elimination. https://www.ncbi.nlm.nih.gov/books/NBK547662/. [Accessed October 5, 2023]

Gilkey, T., Trinidad, J., Kovalchin, C., Minta, A., Rosenbach, M., Kaffenberger, B.H., 2022. Defining drugs that are high-risk associations for drug reactions within the hospital setting. J. Clin. Aesthet. Dermatol. 15 (6), 59–64.

Grogan, S., Preuss, C., 2023. Pharmacokinetics. https://www.ncbi.nlm.nih.gov/books/NBK557744/#:~:text=Pharmacokinetics%20(PK)%20is%20the%20study,on%20the%20body%20more%20closely. [Accessed September 15, 2023]

Hanson, A., Haddad, L., 2022. Nursing rights of medication administration. https://www.ncbi.nlm.nih.gov/books/NBK560654/. [Accessed July 2, 2023]

Healthcare Safety Investigation Branch. 2022a. Positive patient identification. https://www.hsib.org.uk/investigations-and-reports/positive-patient-identification/#:~:text=Positive%20patient%20identification%20is%20the,in%20routine%20or%20emergency%20situations. [Accessed June 26, 2023]

Healthcare Safety Investigation Branch. 2022b. Weight-based medication errors in children. https://www.hsib.org.uk/investigations-and-reports/weight-based-medication-errors-in-children/. [Accessed July 2, 2023]

Home Office. 2022. List of most commonly encountered drugs currently controlled under the misuse of drugs legislation. https://www.gov.uk/government/publications/controlled-drugs-list—2/list-of-most-commonly-encountered-drugs-currently-controlled-under-the-misuse-of-drugs-legislation. [Accessed July10, 2023]

Institute for Safe Medical Practices. 2016. Acute Care ISMP medication safety alert. https://www.ismp.org/sites/default/files/attachments/2018-03/20160421.pdf. [Accessed June 29, 2023]

Institute for Safe Medical Practices. 2018. Verapamil-Naloxone look-alike vials. https://www.ismp.org/alerts/verapamil-naloxone-look-alike-vials. [Accessed June 29, 2023]

Kebamo, S., Tesema, S., Geleta, B., 2015. The role of biotransformation in drug discovery and development. J. Drug Metab. Toxicol. 6 (5), 196. Doi: 10.4172/2157-7609.1000196.

Kim, J., De Jesus, O., 2023. Medication routes of administration. https://www.ncbi.nlm.nih.gov/books/NBK568677/. [Accessed June 26, 2023]

Le, J., 2022. Drug absorption. https://www.msdmanuals.com/en-gb/professional/clinical-pharmacology/pharmacokinetics/drug-absorption. [Accessed June 29, 2023]

Martin, E., Law, J., (Eds.). A dictionary of nursing, eighth ed. Oxford University Press, Oxford.

Marufu, T.C., Bower, R., R.N., Hendron, E., Manning, J.C., R.N., 2022. Nursing interventions to reduce medication errors in paediatrics and neonates: systematic review and meta-analysis. J. Pediatr. Nurs. 62, e139–e147.

MHRA. 2018. Drug-name confusion: reminder to be vigilant for potential errors. https://www.gov.uk/drug-safety-update/drug-name-confusion-reminder-to-be-vigilant-for-potential-errors. [Accessed July 4, 2023]

Mitchell, G., 2021. Proposal to give more nurses right to hand out overdose reversal medication. https://www.nursingtimes.net/news/public-health/proposal-to-give-more-nurses-right-to-hand-out-overdose-reversal-medicine-04-08-2021/. [Accessed July 2, 2023]

Moore, R.A., Derry, S., Wiffen, P.J., Straube, S., 2015. Effects of food of pharmacokinetics of immediate release oral formulations of aspirin, dipyrone, paracetamol and NSAIDs- a systematic review. Br. J. Clin. Pharmacol. 80 (3), 381–388.

Murphy, P., Bechmann, S., Barrett, M., 2023. Morphine. https://www.ncbi.nlm.nih.gov/books/NBK526115/. [Accessed September 3, 2023]

Neal, M., 2020. Medical pharmacology at a glance, ninth ed. Wiley-Blackwell, New Jersey.

NHS. 2021a. About insulin. https://www.nhs.uk/conditions/type-1-diabetes/managing-insulin/about-insulin/. [Accessed June 27, 2023]

NHS. 2021b. Why must some medicines be taken on an empty stomach? https://www.nhs.uk/common-health-questions/medicines/why-must-some-medicines-be-taken-on-an-empty-stomach/. [Accessed July 2, 2023]

NHS. 2022. Consent to treatment. https://www.nhs.uk/conditions/consent-to-treatment/#:~:text=capacity%20%E2%80%93%20the%20person%20must%20be,to%20make%20an%20informed%20decision. [Accessed June 26, 2023]

NHS. 2023. Anaphylaxis. https://www.nhs.uk/conditions/anaphylaxis/. [Accessed June 27, 2023]

NHS Digital. 2018. ISB 0099: Patient identifiers for identity bands. https://digital.nhs.uk/binaries/content/assets/website-assets/data-and-information/information-standards/standards-and-collections/isb-0099-patient-identifiers-for-identity-bands/042009v2.pdf. [Accessed June 26, 2023]

NHS England. 2023a. Patient Group Directions (PGD). https://www.england.nhs.uk/east-of-england/publication/patient-group-directions-pgd/. [Accessed July 2, 2023]

NHS England. 2023b. A just culture guide. https://www.england.nhs.uk/patient-safety/a-just-culture-guide/. [Accessed July 10, 2023]

NICE. 2016. Controlled drugs: safe use and management. https://www.nice.org.uk/guidance/ng46/evidence/full-guideline-pdf-2427186353. [Accessed July 10, 2023]

NICE. 2018. Parkinson's disease. https://www.nice.org.uk/guidance/qs164/chapter/Quality-statement-4-Levodopa-in-hospital-or-a-care-home. [Accessed March 16, 2024]

NICE. 2019. Giving medicines covertly. https://www.nice.org.uk/about/nice-communities/social-care/quick-guides/giving-medicines-covertly#download-this-guide. [Accessed June 26, 2023]

NICE. 2023a. Prescription writing. https://bnf.nice.org.uk/medicines-guidance/prescription-writing/. [Accessed July 2, 2023]

NICE. 2023b. Prescribing in renal impairment. https://bnf.nice.org.uk/medicines-guidance/prescribing-in-renal-impairment/. [Accessed June 27, 2023]

NICE. 2023c. Prescribing in hepatic impairment. https://bnf.nice.org.uk/medicines-guidance/prescribing-in-hepatic-impairment/. [Accessed June 27, 2023]

NMC. 2018. The Code. https://www.nmc.org.uk/globalassets/sitedocuments/nmc-publications/nmc-code.pdf. [Accessed July 4, 2023]

Price, G., Patel, D., 2023. Drug bioavailability. https://www.ncbi.nlm.nih.gov/books/NBK557852/. [Accessed September 3, 2023]

Rang, H., Ritter, J., Flower, R., Henderson, G., 2016. Rang & Dale's pharmacology, eighth ed. Elsevier, Amsterdam.

RCN. 2019. Bowel care. https://www.rcn.org.uk/-/media/Royal-College-Of-Nursing/Documents/Publications/2019/September/007 522.pdf. [Accessed June 28, 2023]

RCN. 2020. Medicines management. https://www.rcn.org.uk/-/media/royal-college-of-nursing/documents/publications/2020/january/009-018.pdf. [Accessed June 29, 2023]

Saleem, A., Ungcharoen, N., Bell, F., Storton, J., Bibi, H., 2023. Improving Parkinson's medicine administration in hospitals: the impact of an out of hours drug box. Cureus 15 (11), e48447. Doi: 10.7759/cureus.48447. PMID: 38050523; PMCID: PMC10693925.

Shepherd, E., 2018a. Injection technique 1: administering drugs via the Intramuscular route. Nursing Times. 114 (8). https://www.nursingtimes.net/assessment-skills/injection-technique-1-administering-drugs-via-the-intramuscular-route-23-07-2018/

Shepherd, E., 2018b. Injection technique 2: administering drugs via the subcutaneous route. Nursing Times 114 (9). https://www.nursingtimes.net/assessment-skills/injection-technique-2-administering-drugs-via-the-subcutaneous-route-28-08-2018/

Shepherd, M., Shepherd, E., 2020. Medicines administration 1: understanding routes of administration. Nursing Times 116 (6), 42–44.

Taibanguay, N., Chaiamnuay, S., Asavatanabodee, P., Narongroeknawin, P., 2019. Effect of patient education on medication adherence of patients with rheumatoid arthritis: a randomized controlled trial. Patient Prefer. Adherence 13, 119–129.

Theriot, J., Sabir, S., Azadfard, M., 2023. Opioid antagonists. https://www.ncbi.nlm.nih.gov/books/NBK537079/. [Accessed September 3, 2023]

WHO. 2007. Patient identification. https://cdn.who.int/media/docs/default-source/patient-safety/patient-safety-solutions/ps-solution2-patient-identification.pdf?sfvrsn=ff81d7f9_6. [Accessed June 26, 2023]

Williams, M., Jordan, A., Scott, J., Jones, M., 2020. A systematic review examining the characteristics of users of NHS patient medicines helpline services, and the types of enquiries they make. Eur. J. Hosp. Pharm. 27 (6), 323–329.

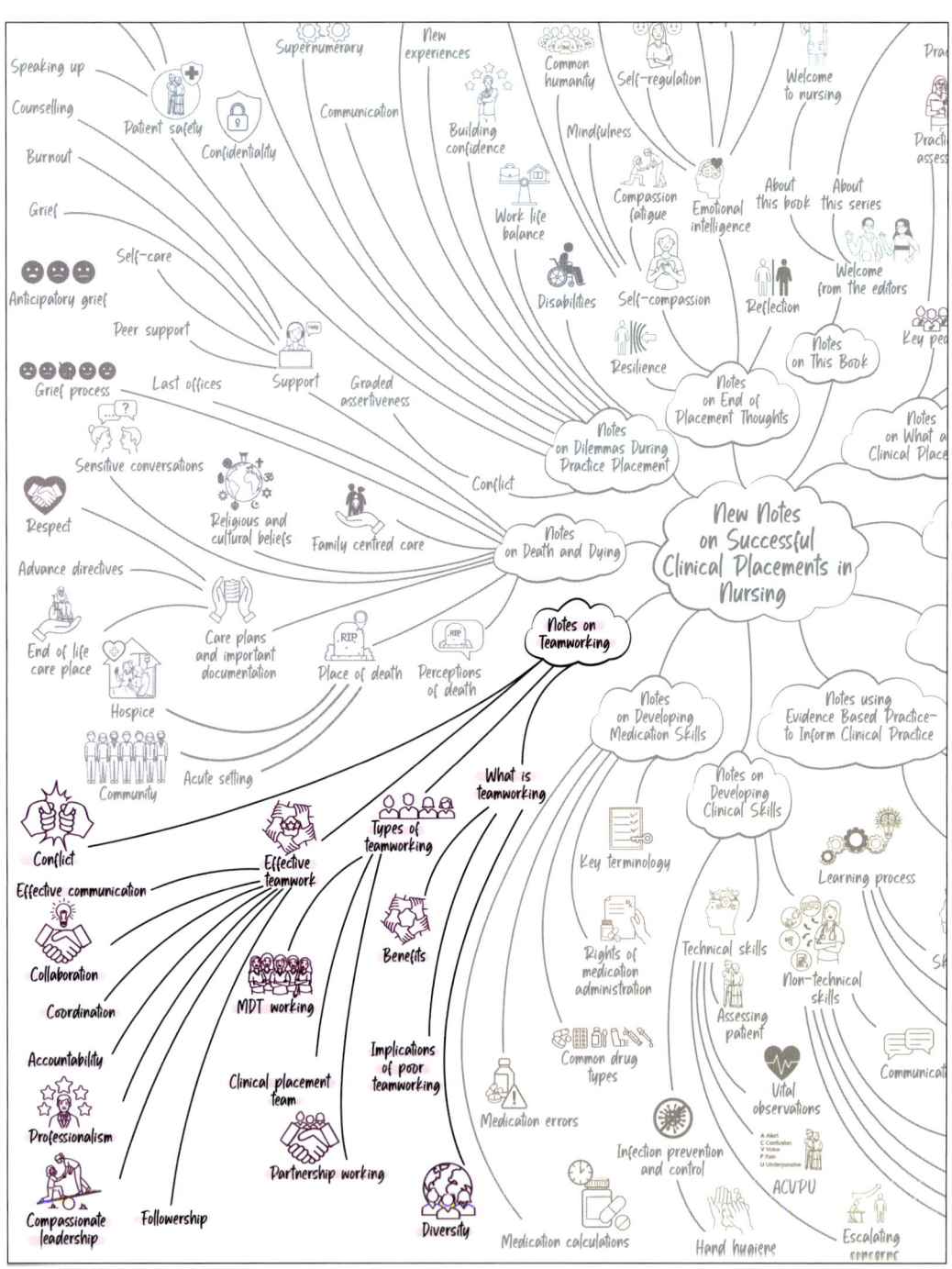

NOTES ON TEAMWORKING

Paul Jebb (he/him)

INTRODUCTION

Professionalism in nursing and midwifery is realised through purposeful relationships and underpinned by environments that facilitate professional practice. Professional nurses and midwives demonstrate and embrace accountability for their actions (NMC, 2018). However, healthcare professionals do not work alone; they all form part of a wider team to deliver person-centred care to those they have responsibility for. Understanding teamwork is essential for all registered nurses, registered nursing associates, registered midwives and their students so they can ensure care is delivered to people, the best outcomes are met and a quality experience of care is delivered. Teamwork across healthcare is essential in order to meet the needs of those in our care and be certain that healthcare professionals are working together collaboratively with the patient at the heart of decision making, care delivery and patient outcomes.

NMC

THE NMC SAYS

8 Work cooperatively.

To achieve this, you must:

8.1 Respect the skills, expertise and contributions of your colleagues, referring matters to them when appropriate.

8.2 Maintain effective communication with colleagues.

8.3 Keep colleagues informed when you are sharing the care of individuals with other health and care professionals and staff.

Continued

NMC

> **8.4** Work with colleagues to evaluate the quality of your work and that of the team.
>
> **8.5** Work with colleagues to preserve the safety of those receiving care.
>
> **8.6** Share information to identify and reduce risk.
>
> **8.7** Be supportive of colleagues who are encountering health or performance problems. However, this support must never compromise or be at the expense of patient or public safety.

Teamwork is fundamental to healthcare delivery, and at the centre of those teams are people who are receiving care and their loved ones/carers. The benefits of teamwork include improving patient safety, ensuring an effective experience of care, enhancing communication across the team and supporting the individual professional's personal and professional development.

WHAT IS TEAM WORKING?

The use of team is commonplace across our communities; we are a team in most aspects of our daily lives where we all need to reach a common goal or outcome. This is no different in healthcare where all professionals will work as a team to deliver the care to individuals to optimise their health or to ensure they have a pain-free, dignified end of life.

Katzenbach and Smith (cited in Climer, 2016) talk about a team as being: 'a small number of people with complementary skills who are committed to a common purpose, performance goals, and approach for which they hold themselves mutually accountable'.

As a nursing student, understanding other team members' roles is fundamental to care being coordinated and professionals understanding their responsibilities in minimising the delineation of responsibilities.

Teamwork in healthcare is essential so that the healthcare professional team members can deliver safe, effective and high-quality care to individuals. Understanding teamwork is key when working in highly skilled, diverse teams, which can be very varied across organisations and across the United Kingdom. Delivering safe, quality care should be at the centre of every healthcare team's goals, focusing on the person themselves and their individual goals. And when there are conflicts in care delivery, team members need to be able to discuss these openly with the primary focus being the outcomes for the patient.

Perry (2022) highlights one key to a successful team is when individuals realise that working together on a project is more effective than working alone. Great teamwork is about working together and collaborating to come up with better approaches in healthcare. This can be a constantly moving goal as people change, and as emotional beings who at times struggle to reach our goals due to the pressures of everyday life, doing things as part of a team and not just separate tasks at one time can bring those tasks together to not only reach the expected outcome but be beneficial to us as individuals in overcoming any physical or psychological challenges.

The NMC (2018) highlights the professional standards of practice and behaviour for nurses, midwives and nursing associates, and it identifies as a key area that all those on the NMC register must listen to people and respond to their preferences and concerns, including working in partnership with people to make sure they deliver care effectively. To practise effectively, the Code (NMC, 2018) goes on to describe how registrants need to assess and deliver or advise on treatment on the basis of the best evidence available and best practice while communicating effectively, keeping clear and accurate records and sharing skills, knowledge and experience where appropriate; this will support the communication across the whole team and ensure each team member is aware of what actions have been delivered and discussed and what the outcomes of these were.

A whole section within the NMC Code (section 8) highlights the need to work cooperatively, including:

- Respect the skills, expertise and contributions of your colleagues, referring matters to them when appropriate.

- Maintain effective communication with colleagues.
- Keep colleagues informed when you are sharing the care of individuals with other health and care professionals and staff.
- Work with colleagues to evaluate the quality of your work and that of the team.
- Work with colleagues to preserve the safety of those receiving care.
- Share information to identify and reduce risk.
- Be supportive of colleagues who are encountering health or performance problems. However, this support must never compromise or be at the expense of patient or public safety.

The NMC (2018) also highlights a key aspect of team working is learning from each other as well as learning from each other to benefit those who are in receipt of the care being delivered; this should be done by:

- Providing honest, accurate and constructive feedback to colleagues.
- Gathering and reflecting on feedback from a variety of sources, using it to improve your practice and performance.
- Dealing with differences of professional opinion with colleagues by discussion and informed debate, respecting their views and opinions and behaving in a professional way at all times.
- Supporting students' and colleagues' learning to help them develop their professional competence and confidence.

'Working within the community is challenging for many reasons; one of which is lone working. Despite lone working, oddly, teamworking and teamwork are of great importance in community and district nursing. I am a trainee district nurse and community charge nurse in a community and district nursing team in Scotland. Within the team I lead, there are five registered nurses, including myself, and two healthcare support workers and a caseload of just over 100 patients.

Something that makes community nursing a challenge can be geography. The team that I am in, due to the area, rural Scotland, we can spend more time traveling to a visit/patient than we actually do with the patient in the visit. Each morning because of this, alongside lone working policies and procedures, all staff check in with me to say they are safe, on duty and have arrived at their first visit. This might not seem significant, but it is. It allows me to know who is safe and if people have made it to where they need to be. Without this knowledge, I would not know where all the team members were.

Each day, one of the team allocates the following day's work. This is not always me, and often we do this collectively as a team because it's key we recognise each others' skill sets, experience, exposure and, what some people might find odd, preferences. Preferences are important. Now skill, experience and exposure sometimes will and should supersede preference, so, for example, not allowing yourself to deskill, but as a confident and complementary team, we recognise each other has preferences such as wounds, catheter care or end-of-life care, for example, so why would we not want to send the best person to the job? To us as a team, it makes sense. Collectively and proactively allocating the following day's work allows us to come together as a team and make decisions, give feedback and updates, and share vital information for the day ahead.

Another key element of our teamworking is the fact we come together each afternoon to have a debrief and 'handover'. I say 'handover', as we don't actually hand over the care, but we give a rundown of all the visits we have attended that far on that day so that we are all on the same page regarding the patients on the caseloads, care plans, progress, needs, wants and such. This allows the members of the team to visit patients having a solid grounding of what the recent plan and actions have been. We also as suggested have a debrief of what has gone well and what hasn't, both professionally and personally, so that we can all offer one another support and suggestions if needed/wanted.

Sometimes we don't manage to deliver the care or treatment as planned or desired for a wealth of reasons. This is why our daily debrief handover is key, as we are able to see if others in the team can support

Continued

or suggest: perhaps a joint visit or a new visit with a new set of eyes, so to speak, but this is also something that links back to the staff all checking in each morning because then we all are aware who is on shift, and if struggling, we can actually seek support from the best person on any given day. This goes back to that collective delegation and allocation, as, if I know someone on duty is the best at wounds, and someone is struggling, I know I could send them together, for example. We all complement one another by bouncing off each others' own individual but important skill sets.

Every 2 months, our team meets to have a more formal meeting. Patients tend not to be discussed at this meeting, and it's an opportunity for me to share any key updates, changes and the like, but most importantly, the staff members are able to share worries, concerns, complications and the like. The meeting, is very informal and allows all to have a space to share thoughts, ideas, suggestions and such. The staff really value this time and opportunity, and it allows me as the team leader to give people a sense of voice and ownership and set them goals, challenges and opportunities.

An example of teamwork in action is as below:

1. *Patient assessment and care planning:*
   - *A district/community nurse visits an elderly patient at home.*
   - *The nurse collaborates with other team members, such as health-care assistants and social workers.*
   - *They discuss the patient's needs, preferences and goals.*
   - *Together, they create a comprehensive care plan that addresses physical, emotional and social aspects.*
2. *Coordination and communication:*
   - *The district/community nurse communicates with the patient's family, general GP and community pharmacist.*
   - *They share relevant information about medications, wound care and mobility.*
   - *Effective communication ensures seamless transitions between healthcare settings.*

3. *Holistic approach:*
- *The district/community nurse coordinates with occupational therapists and physiotherapists.*
- *They assess the patient's home environment, safety and mobility aids.*
- *By working together, they enhance the patient's overall wellbeing.*

4. *Supportive care:*
- *The district/community nurse collaborates with palliative care teams.*
- *They provide pain management, emotional support and end-of-life care.*
- *The interdisciplinary team ensures the patient's comfort and dignity.*

In summary, district and community nursing relies on teamwork to address diverse patient needs, promote continuity of care and enhance patient outcomes'.

Brian Webster, trainee district nurse

Benefits of team working

The key to ensuring the benefits of teamwork are recognised is to have effective team working, and then the benefits that this can bring to all team members as well as to the person recovering the care and their family/carers can be recognised. Perry (2022) highlighted four benefits of teamwork, including:

- A source of motivation and inspiration: The team members will see success and be able to motivate others to drive forward to reach greater outcomes.
- More productive conflict management: Working as a team brings with it the advantages of open communication, being more respectful, appreciating others' roles and views as well as great productivity. Diverse viewpoints are good to discuss openly.
- More meaningful team development: Knowing each other's skills and how they can complement each other's areas of expertise,

enabling professional relationships to flourish and open up opportunities for students to learn more and gain more mentoring and coaching to enhance personal development

- Bigger goals: Great teams achieve great things; they will not want to stay still for long and will want to challenge themselves more to achieve greater outcomes for individuals.

Implications of poor team working

At times, team working can break down. This is for many reasons; one relates to culture, not just organisation culture, but also the team culture and potentially subcultures within that team.

The impact of a team that does not perform well cannot be underestimated, not only on the team or the organisation but also on individuals within that team. The behaviours that people are often coerced into adopting in order to manage around the vagaries of dysfunctional teams or to militate against the lack of effective team working are highly destructive, suck energy from all around and have a hugely detrimental impact on morale and performance (Lynus, 2013). As defined in Climer (2016), team members having mutual accountability will determine the culture within a team; if this mutual accountability is lost, then the team may become dysfunctional and underperforming.

Patrick Lencioni (cited in the NHS Leadership Academy document 'Introduction to Team Development') describes five dysfunctions of a team, including:

- Focusing on personal success, status and ego before team success
- Ducking the responsibility to call peers on counterproductive behaviour, which sets low standards
- Feigning buy-in for group decisions creates ambiguity throughout the organisation
- Seeking artificial harmony over constructive passionate debate
- Unwilling to be vulnerable within the group

Across the NHS and healthcare in general, you may see some, if not all, of these behaviours; as a nursing student, you will need to reflect on the actions of these team members and also think about what impact this has had on you, other team members and patient care.

The report of the mid staff NHS foundation trust public enquiry (Francis, 2013) highlighted teamwork as a theme. The report recommended a need for effective teamwork between all the different disciplines and services that together provide the collective care often required by an elderly patient; the report highlighted that the contribution of cleaners, maintenance staff and catering staff all needed to be recognised and valued.

Teamwork within healthcare is wider than nursing and medical teams. All services across healthcare, whether patient facing or support services, need to identify their role within patient care and be able to articulate the impact they have on the delivery of high-quality care to patients; this is teamwork. As nursing teams, we also need to recognise, value and celebrate the wider role teams have in care delivery.

Diversity in teams

Diversity within healthcare is paramount, and our workforce needs to reflect the communities we serve; this includes within teams. Diversity will ensure people are treated as equals as well as ensuring that their individual care needs are met with dignity and respect. When a diverse healthcare team cares for patients, the patients are more likely to be open and honest with their care when they see professionals who understand their beliefs and cultural identity; this will lead to quality care, compassionate care and better outcomes for the individual patient (Murphy, 2023).

Murphy (2023) went on to describe three examples of qualities and behaviours of culturally competent health professionals.

Not only do we need to ensure diversity across the people delivering care; we also need to think of the diversity of teams and what will really matter to the patient and support them in meeting their outcomes and nursing needs.

They understand their patients	• Barriers such as a difference in language are treated not as added difficulty to the job or fault of a patient but rather just as an issue that needs to be resolved.

Staff members know how to respect different backgrounds	• Past experiences of their patients don't affect the quality of their services at all. They recognise any unconscious biases they have so that they can prevent them from affecting their work.

They have cultural knowledge that leads them to a more empathic approach when giving care.	• They are also willing to learn more about different cultures to widen their ideas about the diverse people they meet.

TYPES OF TEAM WORKING

Healthcare has many teams that ensure quality care is delivered to patients. These teams will deliver direct clinical care, support the delivery of clinical care or support those who are delivering the care to enable them to develop and continuously improve the care that is delivered to their patient group. At the centre of this must always be the patient and, if appropriate, their carer/family members, as they are fundamental in the decision making.

Clinical placement team

Many healthcare providers working with education establishments will have developed clinical placement teams; these are made of healthcare professionals from different backgrounds, mainly nursing, to act as clinical facilitators and placement support coordinators. These teams support students while they are on a clinical placement within their organisations. Their role is to ensure that all learners have the opportunity to access learning and succeed on their placements, giving clinical and emotional support when needed. All students need to make sure that they are aware of their clinical placement team and access them for support and for the team members to share their knowledge of the placement area as well as support the student to identify learning opportunities and support materials.

Multidisciplinary team working

Multidisciplinary teams (MDTs) are teams consisting of individuals drawn from different disciplines who come together to achieve a common goal, whether that be a project to introduce a new role, redesign of a patient pathway or provide care in a different way (Health Education England, 2021). Within clinical care, these could include the nurse, physiotherapist, dietician, speech and language therapist, medical teams and many others.

MDT working is not a new concept and has been seen across the wider NHS. MDT working offers an opportunity to improve quality by drawing on a broader range of skills and competencies, as the workforce shortage means that the whole team needs to work smarter together to maximise outcomes and job satisfaction.

> What sort of people do you think make up the MDT? Take time to reflect on the MDT working that you have been involved in and who made up that team. How did they communicate effectively?
>
> _____
>
> _____
>
> _____
>
> _____
>
> _____
>
> _____

Partnership working

Effective teamwork within healthcare can have a massive impact on patient safety and care outcomes. The need for effective and diverse teams is increasing due to the increasing complexities of care as well as increasing comorbidities. No one professional group can solely deliver quality care that satisfies the patients' needs and/or expectations.

Healthcare has advanced significantly, not just within care delivery but also with the use of technology and digital advancements; the global demand for quality means that we have to also be aware of our own professional development and have a great focus on a person-centred approach (Babiker et al., 2014).

As registered nurses, we need to be able to place the patient in the centre of care and deliver care that matters to them, with who matters to them—the patients and their care are fundamental members of the team delivering care to a person in whatever settings care is being delivered.

EFFECTIVE TEAMWORK

Effective team working has three principles to ensure they are effective (West, 2019):

- Clear shared objectives: This is so everyone is rowing in the same direction. If this isn't the case, the team can become disjointed and be moving in all directions other than forward.
- Working interdependently: A team needs to be independent and be able to work by clear guidelines to achieve its aims without being watched or micromanaged by others.
- Meet regularly: This communication is vital to ensure the shared objectives are clear and continue to develop.

If these three areas meet the research undertaken by West, the outcomes go on to suggest that teams will be more effective and innovate more, as well as enhance the health and wellbeing of team members, including by lower levels of stress, absenteeism and turnover.

These outcomes depend on the quality of team working and particularly whether there is a team climate of psychological safety.

Faubion (2023) highlighted that effective teamwork in nursing is centred around the client and involves shared goals focused on measurable outcomes. The following are examples of key elements that help promote good teamwork among nurses specifically.

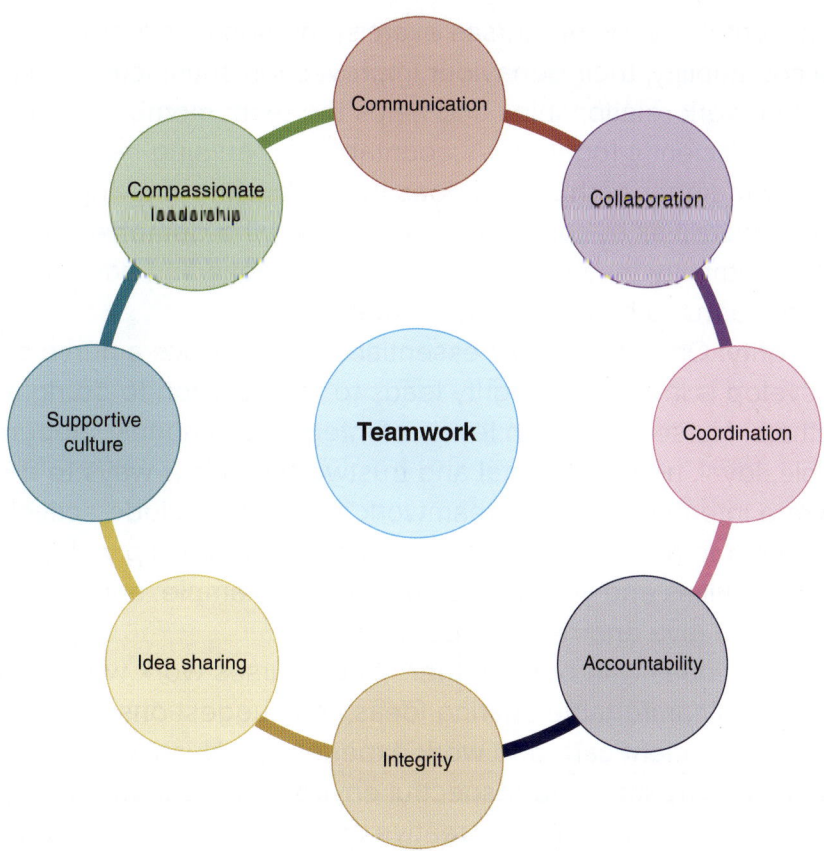

- Communication: One of the most essential elements of good teamwork is communication. The way nurses communicate with one another can positively or negatively impact not only the quality of patient care but also the relationships within the healthcare team.
- Collaboration: Teamwork in nursing requires collaborative care coordination. When nurses work together, each team member's skills and strengths can be utilised to achieve high-quality patient care and improved patient and workplace satisfaction.
- Coordination: Care coordination is essential to improving how healthcare systems work for patients, promoting improved safety and efficiency. When implemented correctly, care coordination will positively impact outcomes for patients, nurses and other members of the interdisciplinary healthcare team.

- Accountability: When nurses exercise personal and professional accountability, their behaviour improves job satisfaction, fosters better work relationships and helps the team members work more efficiently together. Accountability in nursing helps ensure every member of the team does their job without giving their responsibilities to someone else. Nurses who demonstrate accountability take ownership for their actions and accept instructions to help improve, as needed.

- Integrity: One of the most essential characteristics a nurse can develop is integrity. Integrity leads to the decision to do right by others. Nurses with high levels of integrity are honest, dependable, loyal, nonjudgmental and trustworthy. A few ways to demonstrate integrity and build teamwork in nursing include actively working to build and maintain a trusting relationship with patients, their families and your peers; leading by example; and being willing to give and receive feedback.

- Sharing ideas with one another: When nurses work well together, they feel comfortable sharing ideas and suggestions to help improve patient care and work experiences. Nurses who share ideas in a trusting and respectful environment encourage colleagues to become more creative and promote more productive planning sessions, which positively impacts every aspect of patient care and employee experiences.

- Being supportive of others: Nursing is a rewarding career, but it can also be stressful. Having a strong team environment where support for peers is practised can help build bonds of reliance and dependability. Showing support for coworkers is an excellent way to build strong teams in nursing.

- Compassionate leadership: Compassionate leaders will support the team to develop themselves, and therefore they become increasingly productive and deliver great outcomes for their patients, service users and clients. This in turn enhances workplace morale along with ensuring an open culture for clients and relatives/carers to ask questions, seek clarification and support the delivery of safe, effective quality care.

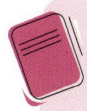

CASE STUDY

Jamie was starting his first clinical placement on a busy surgical ward, and he was both excited and intimidated. He quickly realised how crucial teamwork was in this fast-paced environment.

In his first week, he was paired with Nurse Amy, his practice assessor. She was great at explaining the ward's routines and patient care procedures, stressing the importance of communication and collaboration. She encouraged him to ask questions and get involved.

In his second week, a patient named Mr Smith, who had just had major surgery, suddenly showed signs of sepsis. It was a tense situation that required immediate action.

Nurse Amy quickly assessed the situation and activated the emergency protocol.

She assigned tasks to the team: one nurse called the rapid response team, another gathered emergency supplies and Jamie monitored Mr Smith's vitals and tried to keep him calm.

The charge nurse coordinated with the doctors and kept everyone updated on the situation.

The rapid response team arrived, and it was amazing to see how smoothly the doctors and nurses worked together to stabilise Mr. Smith, each playing their part perfectly.

Afterwards, Nurse Amy and the charge nurse held a debriefing session to discuss what went well and what could be improved. This was an eye opener for Jamie. Key lessons included:

- Clear roles: Knowing everyone's role helped manage the emergency efficiently.
- Communication: Effective, concise communication was crucial.
- Support: The debriefing session was a great way to reflect and learn as a team.

Effective communication

Effective communication is essential not only with patients, carers and family members but also with other team members and members of the MDT while also maintaining confidentiality and respecting the privacy of others. This is highlighted in the code (NMC, 2018).

NMC

THE NMC SAYS

5 Respect people's right to privacy and confidentiality.

When communicating with people, we also need to think about health literacy, which is whether people have the knowledge, skills, understanding and confidence they need to be able to use health and care information and services. This needs to be constantly considered, as people's understanding can fluctuate depending on their own capacity to understand.

Good communication across healthcare teams is essential and means approaching every interaction differently to enable team members to understand other team members' and people's concerns, experiences and opinions to ensure they can make informed decisions and choices relating to their care and treatment. This includes using verbal and non-verbal communication skills along with active listening and patient teach-back techniques.

Ten effective communication skills for nurses, as identified by the University of St Augustine for Health Sciences (2020), are summarised in the following diagram:

Improvement and innovation in the NHS requires a foundation of trust, psychological safety, open communication, strategic clarity and processes.

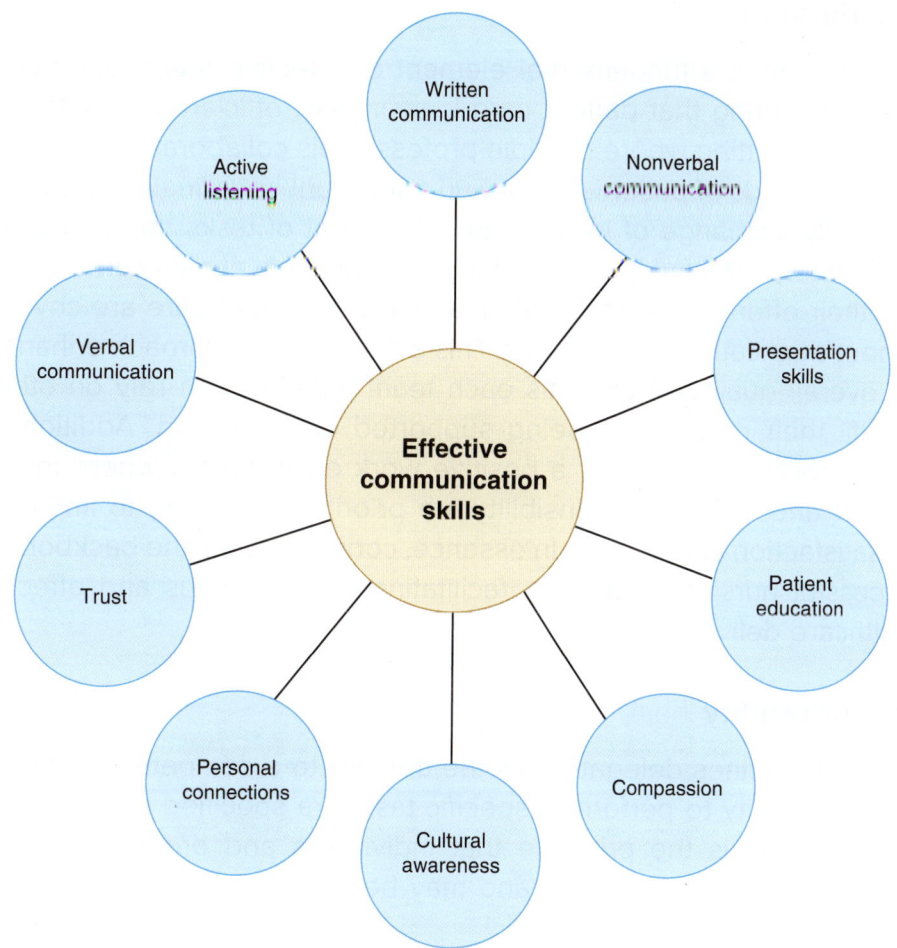

Collaboration

Collaboration is a partnership, and by working in collaboration, we, as nurses and healthcare professionals, can enhance the outcomes for our patients, as a team supporting the delivery of care to meet their needs. A collaborative approach can improve communication, save time, reduce duplication of effort, improve working relationships and provide a better experience for people who use health and social care services. Each professional expert will bring specific knowledge, skills and insight that will impact the patient and their healthcare outcomes. No one professional group has the monopoly on care delivery, but as a registered nurse, you will be expected to coordinate care across many disciplines, ensuring that care is delivered in a timely, professional way to meet the individual's needs.

Coordination

Coordination is a fundamental element of effective teamwork among nurses, ensuring that patient care is seamless, efficient and safe. In a healthcare setting where multiple professionals collaborate to meet the complex needs of patients, clear and consistent coordination allows for the timely exchange of information, alignment of tasks and avoidance of errors. By effectively coordinating their actions, nurses can synchronise their efforts, ensuring that all aspects of patient care are covered without duplication or oversight. This collaborative approach enhances the overall quality of care, as each team member can rely on others to fulfil their roles while being supported on their own. Additionally, good coordination fosters a positive work environment where mutual respect and shared responsibility are prioritised, leading to improved job satisfaction and morale. In essence, coordination is the backbone of successful nursing teamwork, facilitating a harmonious and effective healthcare delivery system.

Accountability

The NMC defines delegation as the transfer to a competent individual of the authority to perform a specific task in a specified situation, and accountability is the principle that individuals and organisations are responsible for their actions and may be required to explain them to others.

The person in overall charge of the nursing care is the registered nurse, but they cannot perform every intervention or activity, and therefore they will need to delegate aspects of care to colleagues (Royal College of Nursing, 2023).

Working as part of the MDT, you may find that some tasks will be delegated to you. The NMC goes on to highlight that:

Delegation of an activity may be from:

- One registered professional to another.
- A registered professional to an unregulated member of staff.
- A registered or unregistered person to a carer or family member.

The NMC code (NMC, 2018) highlights delegation as an area that nurses, midwives and nursing associates need to consider carefully, and if individuals are delegating a task, they take the responsibility to make sure that:

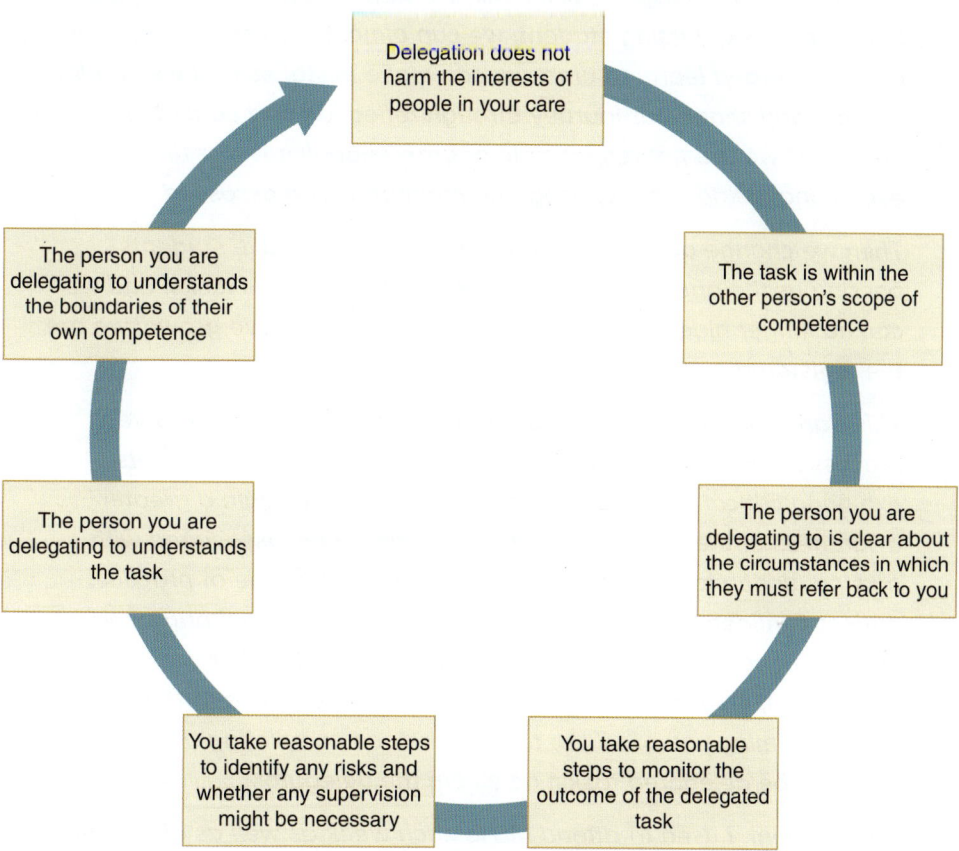

These seven points need to also be considered by the person who is having a task delegated to them, and if the delegation is appropriate and in the client's best interest in relation to nursing students and other students, permission must be given for the delegation or educational event to take place.

The NMC (2018) sets out the responsibilities of people on the professional register when they accept a delegated task. It states that nurses, midwives and nursing associates must act, as appropriate

'As a nursing student, I have many memories of answering the phone or seeing various professionals on the wards, and most of them asked the same thing of me. "Can I speak to the nurse in charge, please?"

I would duly hand them over or redirect them to said person and continue my supervised tasks. Little did I know how protected I was back then. As a nursing student, we can almost hide behind our mentor; we are afforded learning time, we can make mistakes and we continue to grow and shape our journey through reflection and education. That is not to say we are not responsible or professional; it is just that everything we do is supervised and monitored and assessed.

Then we change our tunic from white to blue and have students passing us the phone and professionals delegating us tasks, and we can no longer hide behind our student badge. We have grown; we are the registered nurse.

This transition from nursing student to registered nurse is a 3-year process involving skills labs, placements, university assignments, exploring critical theories and nursing practice. We gain a greater awareness of the legal and ethical responsibilities associated with nursing: understanding and adhering to the NMC code of practice, patient confidentiality, informed consent, capacity, monitoring and implementing care. Yet nothing prepares you for the first time you sit in a handover, wearing blue, a shift sheet in front of you and the leaving team informing you of all the tasks that need completing that shift. I used to be delegated tasks; now I am the delegator.

As a student, I used to attend MDTs each week as well as discharge meetings, medication reviews, best interest, initial care programme approach (CPAs). I would sit on the chairs on the outskirts of the meeting, as the table was full of professionals, doctors, consultants , physios, nurses and social workers. I would listen intently, take notes, listing some unknown terminology or new medication so I could research it later. The registered nurse would be documenting actions and outcomes and was an integral part of the MDT.

The first time I sat at the table was the moment I realised I was a registered nurse. Ignore the fact I had been qualified for 4 weeks and *that I was regularly doing medications and updating care plans and risk assessments in my role. I was in this meeting as a registered nurse and was responsible for discussing and coordinating the nursing care of all of the patients on the ward.*

Fear, trepidation, feelings of anxiousness—totally unfounded, yet at the time, I was in a room with all these highly educated professionals, and what if I messed up?

Looking back now, this was ridiculous, yet it is a fear felt by many newly registered nurses, and it is only when we speak in these meetings, when we somehow use our voice and all these nursing terminologies escape that we really do actually know what we are doing. That the 3 years of education and placements have ingrained the knowledge in our subconscious and that we will add to it, we will gain experience and our confidence and competence grow.

A consultant asked me to write a tribunal report for my patient, a report documenting my reasons as to why or if the patient should continue to be detained under the mental health act. This report would be read by myself at a mental health tribunal alongside reports of others involved in the patient's care. A difficult task, notably as the patient would be present at the tribunal, and I had built up a good rapport with them, I was their advocate and I had to write why they should stay in hospital; even though it was for the patient's own benefit, I felt I would be breaking their trust in me.

Nursing requires a balance of empathy and professional detachment. Cultivating compassion while managing emotional boundaries ensures we provide empathetic care without becoming overwhelmed, a fact that was not lost on me and enabled me to write the report. The patient remained in hospital, recovered and was discharged back home, and I felt responsible in part.

The transition from student to registered nurse is a transformative journey that involves adapting to new responsibilities and continuing to embrace learning and personal and professional development. There are significant challenges faced along the way, yet it is through these challenges that we grow, we adapt, we overcome, we continuously reflect on self'.

Steven Jowell, newly registered nurse

Think of when you have been on placement or worked in a clinical setting:

- What different teams were you aware of, and what professionals made up these teams?
- Who coordinated the care for the patient?
- What was their specific role, and how was this carried out? What leadership skills did you identify?
- How were different members of the team contacted?
- Were there nurses in the team? What was their role? How did they collaborate with others to deliver quality care?

What are your thoughts on the questions given here?

_____

_____

_____

_____

_____

_____

Professionalism

Professionalism in nursing means something different to everyone, but there are some common factors involved in this, including providing quality care, respect for others, advocacy and responsibility.

Showing the skills of professionalism in what we do, what we wear and how we deliver ourselves has many benefits; it not only helps us build confidence with our clients but it also helps safeguard their health and wellbeing by empowering them to make better life choices with information that they can trust.

Nursing is a profession that requires a lot of trust from people as they completely surrender to the care of nurses and the wider MDT. With excellent nursing care comes more positive outcomes, as the nurses' professionalism helps make nursing a worthy and noble profession in the eye of the public.

A great nurse is someone who knows their own values and also how to make sure these values shine through their everyday practice and how to define empathy and professionalism, and they consistently demonstrate their commitment to delivering safe, quality, effective care.

As a nursing student on a placement, you, too, need to be aware of professionalism, values-based care and, importantly, the values you hold and the standards you expect to be delivered. You need to look at those who are on the MDT and reflect on their values and the impact that has on the care being delivered as well as on the outcomes to the client and the team dynamics. This relates to the NMC code regarding practising effectively.

Kay (2023) highlighted that there are many ways to achieve more as a registered nurse, a team player and an individual. For example, demonstrating professionalism in nursing through:

Advocate for patients: In general, not being afraid to support patients in public and always look out for their welfare within the multidisciplinary team. Thinking of patients as they would think of themselves is a rare and precious quality.	Teamwork: This requires nurses to work with other healthcare professionals, with the motto of always thinking of their patients first, which demonstrates their commitment and professionalism to nursing.
	Person receiving care	
Effective communication: For excellent teamwork, it is necessary to know how to communicate ideas in the best possible way so that any receiver can understand, comprehend and apply what needs to be done.	Deliver the best possible care: By providing impeccable care, nurses can demonstrate that they are genuinely committed to their patients and the institution they represent.

Kay also went on to highlight the need for teams to be able to:

- Have a positive attitude. Nothing reflects professionalism more than maintaining a positive attitude. Nurses can do this by being confident in the care they provide and the team they have.

- Maintain integrity and principles. No matter how many complex cases they handle, nurses must stand by their principles and do their best to demonstrate their commitment to their profession.

These attributes can be a challenge with increasing workforce challenges that we see across the United Kingdom. As registered nurses, we need to be aware of our accountability and that we need to make sure we highlight any concerns or incidents that will put the safety of clients at risk; this includes staffing levels to meet the needs of the people who are receiving care.

Part of being a professional is also the need to constantly update and improve our skills; using the code and reflecting on our practice can support this as you move forward to being a registered nurse. Revalidation is an essential part of that professionalism. This includes reflection, professional conversations, professional development, gaining feedback on your practice and delivering a set number of hours in your area of practice; in turn, this will support each registered nurse to maintain their knowledge, skills and professionalism to enable the public to receive safe, effective care.

Compassionate leadership

The role of compassionate leadership in creating the right conditions for MDT working is fundamental (West, 2021). Compassionate leadership in practice involves attending to, understanding, empathising with and helping those we lead.

Attending means being present with, and attending to, those we lead—'listening with fascination'—so we can understand others' challenges and look at how we can support them to drive compassion forward and be role models of leadership behaviours. Nursing students need to recognise these for when they become registered nurse, they, too, can be compassionate leaders in the field of their work with the intent to help others and deliver high-quality, compassionate care.

Nursing and, indeed, healthcare in general, is highly emotive; we are dealing with people whose emotions could be at their highest level, and also as emotional beings, we need to think and learn how to manage these emotional responses. When working as part of a team, it's important to look after others and ensure they are supported. This experience can build a sense of belonging and, importantly, safety in the workplace. Compassionate leaders who model such behaviours have a powerful influence in shaping the team's climate (West, 2021).

To be a team member and deliver compassionate leadership, we also need to be aware of the diverse roles of team members and what unique skills and experiences each member brings to that team, identifying the opportunities and challenges multicultural teams can bring, but this may also bring along enhanced decision-making capabilities—all improving the quality of care that will be delivered to people and enhancing the value of the team members and the roles they play as a fundamental member of an MDT. Building relationships also enables you to build trust within and across teams, resulting in good team working.

Reflect on the leaders you have interacted with across nursing and other professional groups, how have they displayed compassion and how has their leadership impacted the patient, their carer or family members, or other staff members.

_____

_____

_____

_____

_____

'As a nurse manager, I have learned that compassionate leadership is the heartbeat of our healthcare system. It's not just about making decisions or guiding a team; it's about identifying the human element in every action we take. Compassionate leadership means actively listening, not just to what is said but to what is left unspoken—the fears,

Continued

the struggles and the hopes of those we care for and those we work with. It's offering empathy, not as a solution but as a presence, letting others know they are seen and valued.

In my role, I've witnessed the impact of small acts of kindness, whether it's taking an extra moment to comfort a resident or ensuring a colleague feels supported in a time of personal crisis. Compassionate leadership is rooted in these everyday gestures, building trust and resilience within a team. It encourages open communication, where mistakes are met with learning, not judgement or blame, and where everyone feels empowered to contribute. Ultimately, compassionate leadership fosters a culture where both residents and staff thrive because it prioritises the wellbeing of the whole person—body, mind and spirit—in every interaction'.

Krishnaprasad Mullekattu, registered nurse, home manager

The role of followers

Being a follower does not imply a passive role; where there are leaders, there must be followers. The notion of followership is aligning ourselves and our values with another person who can also support us in our own development (Jebb, 2021). We have seen over the COVID-19 pandemic why followership matters, and we, as leaders in our feelings, must take this seriously. Everyone has been tested to the limit. But where the notion of followership was strong, leaders not only inspired and influenced, but they in turn were also inspired and influenced by those in their teams; leaders and followers go hand in hand and complement each other. The leader/follower relationship is essential within healthcare, which in turn will support us to reflect and develop ourselves and can challenge us.

CONFLICT

Conflict is an unavoidable aspect of any collaborative environment, and the healthcare profession is no exception. Due to the high-pressure nature of healthcare, diverse teams and the critical importance of patient care, conflicts can frequently arise among nursing staff, between nurses and other healthcare professionals, or with patients and their families. Understanding and effectively managing conflict is crucial for nursing students, as it not only impacts personal wellbeing but also the quality of care provided to patients. By developing strong conflict reso lution skills, nursing students can enhance their professional relation ships, foster a positive work environment and ultimately contribute to better patient outcomes.

What does conflict look like?

Conflict in a nursing environment can manifest in various forms and degrees of intensity, ranging from minor disagreements to severe disputes. These conflicts often include verbal disagreements such as open arguments or debates between colleagues or between nurses and patients/families. Nonverbal tension may be evident through body language such as crossed arms, avoidance of eye contact and tense facial expressions. Passive-aggressive behaviour such as sarcastic remarks, deliberate procrastination and withholding information can also contribute to conflict. Additionally, conflicts may arise from professional discrepancies, such as differences in opinion regarding patient care plans, ethical issues or procedural methods. Emotional reactions, including increased stress, frustration, anger or feelings of being undervalued or misunderstood, further indicate underlying conflicts. Lastly, breakdowns in communication, such as misunderstandings, lack of clear instructions or complete communication failures, are common signs of conflict within nursing teams.

'During a clinical placement, my team, we were receiving a handover from the nightshift, and the charge nurse was asking really difficult questions to the nurse handing over. You could tell this was causing the staff nurse to be nervous, and she became flustered. This caused the charge nurse to continually roll her eyes and huff anytime her questions weren't answered. It made me feel really awkward'.

Natalie Elliott, RN

Why does it happen?

Conflict arises in nursing for a variety of reasons, often stemming from the high-stakes, high-stress nature of healthcare. Common causes include diverse perspectives among nurses due to their different backgrounds and training, which can lead to varying opinions on patient care. The demanding nature of nursing also contributes, as high stress levels can result in burnout. This is evident by irritability and interpersonal conflict. Communication breakdowns, whether due to miscommunication or lack of communication altogether, frequently lead to misunderstandings and disagreements among team members. Additionally, competition for limited resources such as time, equipment and staff can create tension among colleagues. Hierarchical structures within healthcare settings may exacerbate conflicts related to authority and decision-making processes. Furthermore, personal differences, including individual personality traits and personal issues, can contribute to interpersonal tensions within nursing teams. Lastly, ethical dilemmas in patient care often present complex challenges that can lead to disagreements and conflicts among healthcare professionals.

'One placement, a staff nurse stormed onto our ward shouting and balling because we had borrowed the bladder scanner and hadn't returned it promptly'.

Anonymous nursing student

Tips to deal with conflict

Addressing conflict effectively is a crucial skill for nursing students to develop. But how can we do it effectively?

TIPS

Develop strong communication skills: Practise active listening by paying full attention, acknowledging the speaker's perspective and avoiding interruptions. Ensure that messages are clear and understood, using simple and direct language. Be mindful of body language, facial expressions and tone of voice, aiming to convey openness and respect.

NMC

THE NMC SAYS

7.3 Use a range of verbal and non-verbal communication methods, and consider cultural sensitivities, to better understand and respond to people's personal and health needs.

TIPS

Cultivate emotional intelligence: Recognise your own emotional triggers and responses to conflict. Practice techniques to manage emotions such as deep breathing or taking a brief pause before responding. Try to understand the feelings and perspectives of others involved in the conflict.

Engage in conflict resolution techniques: Tackle conflicts early before they escalate into bigger problems. Focus on areas of agreement and work collaboratively towards a mutually acceptable solution. Use 'I' statements: Express your feelings and concerns without blaming others. For example, 'I feel frustrated when...' instead of 'You always...'.

NMC

THE NMC SAYS

9.3 Deal with differences of professional opinion with colleagues by discussion and informed debate, respecting their views and opinions and behaving in a professional way at all times.

TIPS

Leverage teamwork and collaboration: Encourage open dialogue and team-based problem solving. Value the contributions and perspectives of all team members, recognising that diversity can enhance patient care.

NMC

THE NMC SAYS

2.1 Work in partnership with people to make sure you deliver care effectively.

Conflict is an inevitable part of nursing, but this is no excuse for incivility given the complexities and pressures of the environment we work in. However, by understanding what conflict looks like, recognising the potential causes and employing effective strategies to address it, nursing students can turn potential challenges into opportunities for growth and improved team dynamics. Developing these skills not only enhances personal resilience and professional effectiveness but also contributes to a more supportive and collaborative healthcare environment, ultimately leading to better patient outcomes.

CONCLUSION

Teamwork is fundamental in healthcare; as stated, no professional group can deliver care to meet the patient's holistic needs without each other. Care needs to be assessed, prescribed and coordinated by the registered nurse in collaboration with other professional disciplines. These disciplines will assess the patients' needs and deliver the care needed specific to their speciality, with the registered nurse advocating for the patients' needs so they receive the care they need.

Space for reader's own reflection:

_____

_____

_____

_____

_____

_____

_____

_____

_____

_____

_____

_____

_____

_____

_____

_____

_____

_____

_____

_____

_____

_____

_____

_____

REFERENCES

Babiker, A., Husseini, M., Nemri, A., Al Fryah, A., 2014. Health care professional development: Working as a team to improve patient care. Sudan. J. Paediatr. 14 (2), 9–16. https://www.ncbi.nlm.nih.gov/pmc/articles/PMC4949805/pdf/sjp-14-9.pdf

Climer, A., 2016. The deliberate creative episode 33: the difference between teams and working groups. https://climerconsulting.com/episode-33-the-difference-between-teams-and-working-groups/#:~:text=Katzenbach%20and%20Smith%20give%20this,to%20actually%20be%20a%20team

Faubion, D., 2023. What is teamwork in nursing? Nursing Press.Org https://www.nursing-process.org/teamwork-in-nursing.html

Francis, R., 2013. Report of the Mid Staffordshire NHS foundation trust public enquiry, executive summary. UK Stationary Office, London.

Health Education England. 2021. Working differently together: progressing a one workforce approach https://www.hee.nhs.uk/sites/default/files/documents/HEE_MDT_Toolkit_V1.1.pdf

Jebb, P., 2021. Wherever there are followers there must be leaders RCN Bulletin. RCN London.

Kay, M., 2023. Professionalism in Nursing: what it is and why it matters. NURSA. https://nursa.com/blog/professionalism-in-nursing-what-it-is-and-why-it-matters

Lynus, K. Introduction to team development. 2013. NHS Leadership Academy https://www.leadershipacademy.nhs.uk/wp-content/uploads/2013/04/7428f23d7207f39da1eda97adbd7bf34.pdf

Murphy, K., 2023. United in healthcare: why diversity is a key component of compassionate care. Nursing Career, Healthcare Employers. PRS Global.

Nursing & Midwifery Council. Delegation and accountability. https://www.nmc.org.uk/globalassets/sitedocuments/nmc-publications/delegation-and-accountability-supplementary-information-to-the-nmc-code.pdf

Nursing & Midwifery Council. 2018a. Enabling professionalism. https://www.nmc.org.uk/globalassets/sitedocuments/other-publications/enabling-professionalism.pdf

Nursing & Midwifery Council. 2018b. The code. https://www.nmc.org.uk/standards/code/read-the-code-online/

Perry, E., 2022. What will make or break your next role? Find out why teamwork matters. Blog https://www.betterup.com/blog/what-is-teamwork

Professor Michael West. 2021. Teamworking, psychological safety and compassionate leadership. NHS Employers. https://www.nhsemployers.org/articles/teamworking-psychological-safety-and-compassionate-leadership

Professor Michael West: what is the difference between a real team and a pseudo team [video file]. September 2019. https://www.youtube.com/watch?v=bqipJlb1oMM

Royal College of Nursing (RCN). 2023. Accountability and Delegation Pocket Guide. UK. https://www.rcn.org.uk/Professional-Development/Accountability-and-delegation/Guide

University of St Augustine For Health Sciences. February 2020. The importance of effective communication in nursing. USA. https://www.usa.edu/blog/communication-in-nursing/

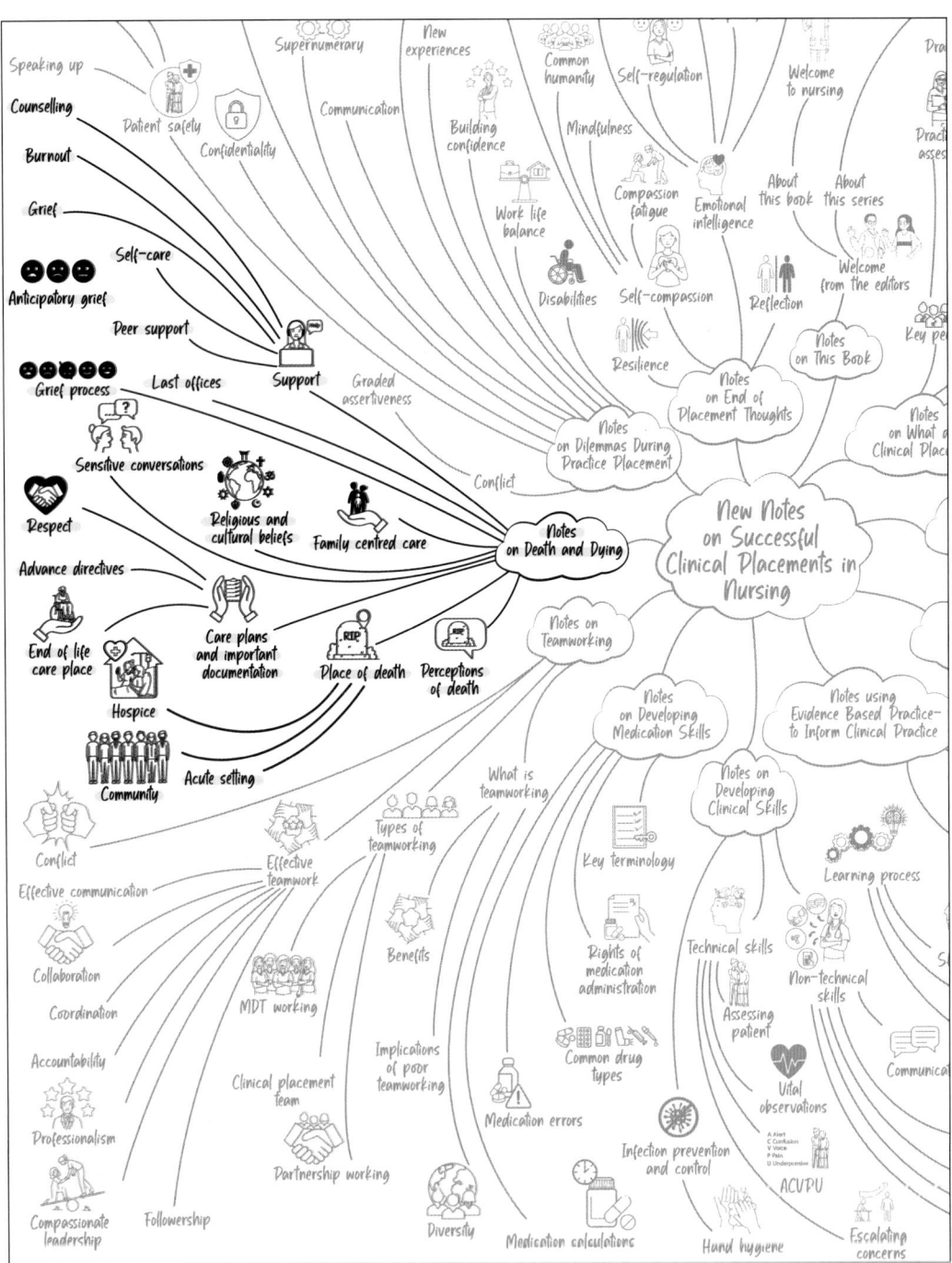

NOTES ON DEATH AND DYING

Elisha Woolf (she/her)

INTRODUCTION

This chapter covers one of the most sensitive subjects in nursing; however, we cannot stress enough the value of reading it. One of the only guarantees in life is death; however, it is a subject that is often avoided. In nursing, we are faced with it often throughout our careers, and it is something you will likely be exposed to on placement. This chapter will cover how death is a natural process and will talk about what you can expect to see patients go through, from both psychological and physiological points of view. How death and dying can be in different settings will be explored. It will also look into how family can be affected and how they can be supported. It will look at what sort of documentation you may come across, who completes this and how it can help with patient care. It will also cover sensitive conversations; these can be distressing and hard to process, so we cover what you might expect to help you to prepare for these. We also look at a nursing student's experience on placement as an insight into their personal experience. Finally, we explore how you can best support yourself while on placement and where to go in terms of support, with some useful information that you can access in your own time. There is space for reflection at the end.

DYING: A NATURAL PROCESS

Dying is a subject often skirted around, seen as a taboo subject that's been historically difficult to talk about because of the emotions it triggers within us and others. Dying is a natural process and one that we see often in healthcare. It is likely that as a nursing student, you will have the privilege of caring for someone in their last days or hours and even be involved in sensitive conversations with patients and their families.

If we strip back the complexities of the feelings surrounding dying, humans have contemplated their mortality for thousands of years. Death was celebrated in ancient Egypt. They had such elaborate funeral practices; they believed that when they died, their spiritual body would continue to exist in the afterlife, and there was an entire ritual to aid the dead to negotiate the underworld journey to eternal life and immortality after death. Death was prepared for in ritual and seen as a part of life, as normal as birth. However, now the words 'death', 'dead' or 'dying' are replaced with 'passed away', 'gone' or 'lost', almost as though the words themselves are frightening or we are afraid to say what has happened. It's as though, socially, we have forgotten about the practicalities of death and what happens to people when they die.

Death in contemporary times is perceived differently:

> 'The death rate remains 100 per cent, and the pattern of the final days, and the way we actually die, are unchanged. What is different is that we have lost the familiarity we once had with that process, and we have lost the vocabulary and etiquette that served us so well in past times, when death was acknowledged to be inevitable. Instead of dying in a dear and familiar room with people we love around us, we now die in ambulances and emergency rooms and intensive care units, our loved ones separated from us by the machinery of life preservation'.

> **(Mannix, 2018)**

In medicine, doctors train for years to essentially stop people from dying. People come to hospital to get well again; they are given treatment, antibiotics and medicines. They have scans, X-rays and a multitude of blood tests, surgeries and investigations, and then when people die, it is sometimes seen as a medical disaster. How could this have happened with modern medicine and the technology we have now? Yes, people do get better, and they leave hospital or are discharged for care in the community. However, there are times when people don't get better and die in hospital, the community, their own homes or hospices, and people can die suddenly, leaving many unanswered questions.

Many people will go their entire lives without seeing another person die. So what happens when someone is dying? There is a pattern of events that are similar. We often see people becoming more and more tired. They will start to find it harder to find energy to do things. People will recharge by sleeping more and eating and drinking less, and as time goes by, they will be more asleep than they are awake. They will stop eating and drinking. There may be times for medications or visitors that we can wake people for and other times there are periods when we can't wake people. This is because they are not asleep; they are unconscious. Sometimes people wake from unconsciousness and tell the people around them they have had a wonderful sleep. They didn't know they were unconscious, but they knew they were peaceful. So when someone is at the very end of their life, they don't recognise they are unconscious. If they are in a deep unconscious state, the brain is only driving the breathing. Sometimes this breathing is quick or slow, sometimes with pauses. Sometimes there are 'sighs' and 'groans', but the person can't feel their throat because they are deeply unconscious. Sometimes the lungs rattle from fluid, but the patient is not drowning or choking. Then there will be a last breath in and a last breath out. There is no sudden panic or rush of pain. Only quiet and peace (NHS, 2023c).

In summary, 'ordinary dying' may include some of the following aspects:

- Becoming very tired and sleeping a lot.
- Finding it difficult to swallow or take medicines orally.
- Not interested in or stopping eating.
- Not wanting to drink as much or stopping drinking.
- Feeling hot or cold to touch.
- Become confused; they may not know where they are.
- They may feel emotional.
- They may not want to see or talk to people.
- They may lose interest in what is going on around them.
- They may not be strong enough to leave their bed.
- They may not be able to physically go to the toilet themselves and may want to wear pads instead.
- They may be upset or become restless.

- They will become unconscious—they look like they are asleep but are not easy to wake up.
- Their breathing pattern will change; there may be noise or more shallow breaths. Sometimes there are gaps in the breathing until it stops.

(ICU Steps, 2023)

This is broken down simply, but these elements of dying are present in all deaths in some way. Some last longer than others; every situation is different, depending on the circumstances surrounding each person. Death is individual to each patient, depending on a nonexhaustive number of factors. These factors are assessed on an individual basis when considering end-of-life or palliative care for a patient, and this assessment is often carried out by a wider multidisciplinary group of allied health professionals, including nurses, so that the patient's decisions or best interests come first. Depending on the trust or area you have a placement at, will depend on how the care plan is formulated. However, end-of-life/palliative care has the patient and their family at the heart of it. This allows all their needs to be met, not only from a from a medical point of view but also any psychological and spiritual needs.

End-of-life care or palliative care doesn't just mean when death is imminent. It can be for people who are in the last months or years of their lives. Its main aim is to help patients live as well as possible until they die and for them to die with dignity. Their wishes and preferences should be taken into consideration when their care is planned. They should also aim to support family, carers and other people who are important to them. Patients have a right to express their wishes about where they want to receive their care, whether this is at home, hospital or hospice.

DEATH IN AN ACUTE HOSPITAL SETTING

Dying at hospital can look different depending on what area you may have your placement in. This section aims to talk about some different areas you may be exposed to, what death might look like in those areas and the feelings/emotions that can come with those experiences. In this section, we will look at the emergency department, a medical ward and intensive care.

The emergency department

The emergency department is quite a hectic place. Emotions are high; often people have been brought in via ambulance after suddenly deteriorating at home. Family members are distressed, and there's a lot of activity from medical staff, ambulance staff and nurses around a patient. It can be difficult to get an idea of what exactly is going on at times. Resus (short for resuscitation; usually an area of the emergency department where patients are the sickest and need immediate care with close monitoring) can be a very stressful environment with a lot of activity and sudden deterioration.

This can be a place where there are a lot of emotions; staff is very busy trying to make people well or stable enough to be moved to a different area of the hospital for their treatment to continue. Resus in the emergency department is particularly busy, and death in this department can come suddenly; this is often shocking and distressing. The staff members are specifically trained to deal with emergency situations and patients' families in these instances, and debriefs are usually able to be arranged after something particularly traumatic. Communication in these situations is key; if you ever feel like you need a debrief or would like to talk about a situation, it is important to talk to a member of staff or practice assessor to talk it through to gain better understanding. Debriefs are not uncommon and should be actively encouraged for reflection.

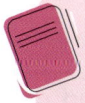

CASE STUDY

Greta is a registered nurse who has been qualified for 2 years. Greta was asked to help in resus for a couple of hours on a night shift, and a nursing student, Sarah, on shift with her wanted to come along to get some experience.

The phone rang for a prealert from the ambulance service to say they were bringing in a gentleman who had been found in his car unconscious; he'd suffered a cardiac arrest. They were still delivering chest compressions and were bringing him through. They said 5 minutes. A team was assembled, and everyone was given a role. Greta took the role of scribe with Sarah, as Sarah had never

Continued

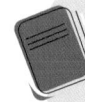

CASE STUDY—cont'd

witnessed a cardiac arrest and didn't know what to expect. Greta very quickly explained there was going to be a lot going on and she would do her best to answer questions and explain as things were happening. The doors opened, and the ambulance crew brought in the gentleman on the stretcher. He was quickly transferred onto a resus trolley, and advanced life support continued. As Greta closely documented the times of all defibrillator shocks and adrenaline administrations, the phone rang; it was the gentleman's family, his wife and daughter. A doctor spoke: 'Pop them in the family room for now, and I'll come through and speak to them right away'. He hastened away to speak to them while all attempts were made to bring their husband and father back. His family wanted to come and see him while we were resuscitating him. Greta thought this was quite unusual, as witnessing a cardiac arrest is quite traumatic, but she explained to Sarah it was their wish. His wife came and sat beside him, held his hand and spoke quietly in his ear. All the while, chest compressions continued; it was as though no one else was in the room. She was asked to let go and stood back as another shock was delivered. A doctor knelt beside her and touched her hand gently. He spoke with kindness and compassion and explained that, unfortunately, despite all their attempts, his heart wasn't making any effort to try and restart and that even if they were to continue, the likelihood of it starting again now would be very low, so they were going to make the decision to stop, if that was okay with them. His wife, even though she was clearly very upset, accepted this. She said they have had a wonderful life together, and he wouldn't have wanted to suffer at all. She said her goodbyes and left with her daughter with a doctor to explain what would happen next. Resuscitation was stopped. Greta and Sarah were offered a debrief with the consultant in charge, and they went through the entire series of events and were offered further support. Greta and Sarah were called to go back to their original place of work. The walk back gave Greta time to reflect, and she chatted to Sarah about how they both felt. Greta encouraged an open dialogue if they needed to talk about it again in the future.

Debriefing is very important and shouldn't be underrated; it allows you time to ask questions such as:

- What did you do well?
- What do you think could have been improved?
- How do you think you communicated?
- How do you feel after being involved in the scenario?

It encourages reflection and insight after challenging situations (Parry et al., 2022).

There are also support services for healthcare providers; they differ slightly depending on what trust or area you are in. Usually there are health and wellbeing teams, counselling, confidential phone lines and information accessible via the trust or area that can be accessed for further help if needed.

The ward

On a ward, the atmosphere can be quite different; sometimes patients are transferred from other parts of the hospital to a ward so they can have some space in a side room away from the hustle and bustle. They can have their family come to visit, and it is a way to create a more peaceful environment. Moving to a ward may have to happen for several reasons:

- Death is imminent, and there is not enough time to get the patient home, as they might die en route.
- A palliative care ambulance is booked and not available for part of the day, depending on the service.
- The patient doesn't want to go home and away from the hospital because they are worried about a delay in treatment should they need it, for example, a delay in anticipatory or just-in-case medications. When patients are placed on an end-of-life or palliative care pathway, medications to help with breathlessness, pain or anxiety, to name a few, are prescribed as anticipatory or just-in-case medications. These medications are quickly accessible in hospital by a bedside nurse, and therefore patients worry that if

they are in pain or struggling, they won't get them as quickly at home, as they may not be able to administer them to themselves, their family could be away or a district nurse might have to be called out to administer the medication.

Care of people who are dying on the ward does have some advantages if it isn't possible for patients to go home. Patients can have open visits, so their family, friends and loved ones can stay with them; sometimes they can even have their pets come and visit. Anticipatory medications are readily available. Care plans can be made immediately and implemented by all members of the team. Nurses are always available for care, repositioning, mouth care, medications and any other needs.

Hospitals have specialist palliative care teams that work alongside to help all hospital staff care for people nearing the end of their lives. These teams are specialists working on individualised care plans for pain and symptom control. They work together with bedside nurses to make sure these care plans are implemented, so the care given to patients is the best they can offer. If there are any changes that need to be made to care plans, this is usually a more streamlined service with immediate effect and minimal disruption to the patients' care, giving the best possible patient-centred care.

It is important to note, however, that wards are still very busy places, and despite the hospital and staff doing the best that they can, sometimes not all allowances can be made. Nursing staff will always want to do things within the best of their ability, but many factors may be outside their control. For example, they may not be able to get a side room for a patient due to bed pressures, only a couple of family members may be able to visit at any one time due to space and some wards may have rooms for family to rest at night, but these may need to be used during the day by staff and other patients' family members. There are often limited washing facilities and parking. So, while the staff may do their best to accommodate all of the patients' and families' needs, it may not always be possible. This can lead to feelings of letting people down and not feeling like the very best is being done despite factors being beyond their control.

Intensive care

An intensive care unit is quite a different environment to experience death. When someone comes to intensive care, it is not always clear if they are going to get better or not. It usually depends on how well someone is responding to treatment. It is often a very stressful, fast-paced environment and can be quite traumatic at times when emotions are high. Intensive care often means that people require life-sustaining treatment that often needs multiple-organ support. So when a patient's family is told the news that their family or friend is dying, it doesn't look like ordinary dying as mentioned earlier because machines and medication are keeping them alive. This can be confusing and can often lead to questions such as, 'How do you know that they are at the end of their life if they don't look like it?'

If someone is becoming more ill in intensive care, they may need more oxygen or medication; they may be placed on a ventilator or dialysis because their lungs and kidneys are failing. Blood tests may indicate how much help they need with their breathing and blood pressure. Patients are monitored closely, so when there are subtle changes in their blood or breathing or their response to treatment starts to decline, then the intensive care team will start to think about the patient's best interest (if they are sedated or unconscious). Treatment in intensive care can be very stressful for patients and can cause long-term harm to their bodies from which the person may not recover. Confusion, restlessness and becoming upset are very common, and patients may not understand where they are or what is happening to them. The treatments can also be very uncomfortable. Sometimes it is not in the patient's best interest to continue with treatment if they are dying. However, what is important to remember is that they will still be cared for, and identifying that they are at the end of their life means they will get the right care to help them.

Conversations between the intensive care team and the family can be sensitive. When it has been identified that the patient is not getting better and is going to die, a conversation is held with the family; this often involves a run through of events that are likely to happen next.

For example, if a person is on a ventilator and on medication supporting their heart and blood pressure and medication keeping them asleep, then it will be explained that the medication keeping them asleep will be kept on, but any medication sustaining their heart or blood pressure will be switched off. With regards to the ventilator, this will be either switched off or the settings changed so the patient is breathing on their own with minimal support. The monitors are switched either off or on night mode so they won't sound anymore, and the family can sit with their loved one for as long as they like. Unfortunately, when life support is switched off, it is difficult to tell how long a person will take to die; however, it is important to note that throughout that time, they will remain comfortable, pain free and always cared for with respect.

One of the questions that may be asked in intensive care, depending on the circumstances of the patient, is the subject of organ donation. This is usually broached by the medical team; they would then refer to a specialist nurse team that deals with organ donations. This is after every effort has been made to save the patient's life, and then conversations begin with the patient's family. There are strict criteria in place in the United Kingdom to help those caring for the dying, and organs are never removed from a patient until their death has been confirmed in line with those criteria. As they are so strict, most people do not die in circumstances that make it possible for them to donate their organs. Only around 1 in 100 people who die in the United Kingdom are able to be donors. Typically, donors will have to have died in an intensive care unit or emergency department (NHS Blood and Transplant, 2023).

Within the hospital, there are also bereavement teams that are accessible for every family member or friend of the dying person. These teams put together information which is usually handed to the bereaved once their relative or friend has died. These are special packs that are put together with any information they may require to access, such as chaplaincy, counselling, when they will receive a death certificate and guidance for funeral planning as well as contact numbers.

Death of a person in an acute setting can be traumatic, sudden and heartbreaking. Emotions are often high. While this is the case and you may experience it in some of the placements you are allocated, it is important to remember that despite what circumstance or scenario you might find yourself in, the staff around you is there to support you. They were new once too; there is a lot to take in, not only the care you are delivering but the care and compassion needed for the patient's family. Be kind to yourself, and always ask for a debrief, even if you feel like it's not needed. It's important to talk things through. We discuss this more later in the chapter on how to deal with death as a nursing student and helpful resources, should you need them.

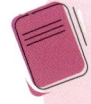

CASE STUDY

Sony is a registered nurse who has been qualified and working in intensive care for 5 years. Sony reflects on the death of someone she was caring for:

'The first time I withdrew (stopped) treatment on a patient, I was brand new to intensive care, and sadly, the patient I was caring for one night was dying. All treatment options had been exhausted, and they were completely reliant on the oxygen we were giving them. They had fallen into a coma, unrousable, not showing any signs of pain. Their family was there, and they said that their loved one wouldn't want to suffer anymore and were confident, despite everything we had done, that enough was enough, and it was time to say goodbye. I had to explain that when I took the oxygen off, it was likely they would die quite soon after and to be prepared for that. I assured them that if there were any signs of pain or discomfort, I would be in straightaway to give appropriate medication. The family agreed and asked me to stop the oxygen coming through the ventilator and take off the patient's mask. I silenced the monitors, took off the patient's mask and switched off the ventilator. The patient took three slow breaths and slipped away

Continued

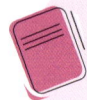

CASE STUDY—cont'd

before I'd left the room. I could see on the monitoring that the patient's heart had stopped. The patient's family looked at me. "We didn't think it would be that quick!" "I'm so sorry to say that they have died; I'm incredibly sorry for your loss", I responded. The family, despite their surprise, seemed relieved that it was all over so quick. "She couldn't have suffered anymore", they said. They stayed for a short time to say their final goodbyes, thanked me for my time and care, and they left. I reflected in sadness and relief but also how strange and quick it had all been. Sometimes you think scenarios are going to go one way, and they are the complete opposite. One I will never forget'.

What are your thoughts on Sony's experience?

_____

_____

_____

_____

_____

_____

Death in a community setting

You might have a placement in the community. This could be with a team of community nurses, in a nursing/care home or residential homes, or a hospice. Generally, when asked, if people had a choice, they would prefer to die at home (Office for National Statistics, 2013). Many people would choose to spend most time at home but to die in a hospice, an appropriate choice for many—yet many of our hospice services would struggle currently to meet this preference, especially for patients without cancer (Thomas, 2023). Nurses in the community are able to build a therapeutic relationship with their patients. You might have a chance to get to know patients and their families better. You might be working with a nurse who has known the family for years, and this can have more of an impact when a patient dies. This continuity of a relationship can have a profound effect on you, and many community teams have bereavement support for carers, nurses and nursing students.

Within the community, there are specialist teams, specialist Macmillan nurses for cancer care, specialist palliative nurses, specialist respiratory nurses and community matrons. These all specialise in specific areas but can add to the holistic care approach that is so important in end-of-life care (The Queen's Nursing Institute, 2015).

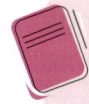

CASE STUDY

Tanya is a second-year nursing student. While on placement with a community district nurse team, Tanya had the opportunity to work with a Macmillan nurse, Chrissie, for a day. The opportunity provided great insight into the important care Macmillan nurses do. Some of the patients on Chrissie's caseload, she had known for years, and she explained to Tanya that she had built such a strong therapeutic relationship with them that she found it quite hard at times to process it all when they died. Despite years of experience and knowledge in the area, Chrissie was affected by every one of them. It really made Tanya think about the emotional toll of Chrissie's job. However, it was clear that the love of the job and impact Chrissie must have on patients was so important that it took precedence over her own feelings. Tanya asked Chrissie what help she accessed to support her. She said that her team had a counsellor who was available on certain days of the week. She said she'd accessed the service before, and it was great knowing that if she ever needed it, it was there for her.

> What support could you use to help with the emotional toll of caring for people who are dying?
>
> _____
>
> _____
>
> _____
>
> _____
>
> _____
>
> _____

Hospice

If you are allocated a placement in a hospice, you might have feelings of apprehension; you might feel like it's something you don't think you'll be able to do. There is a lot more to hospice care than dying and end-of-life care.

Hospice care can either be in a hospice setting, or it can be accessed in a patient's home with a 'hospice-at-home' team; hospice-at-home services aim to enable patients with advanced illnesses to be cared for at their own homes and die at home if that is their preference (National Association for Hospice at Home, 2024). Hospice care has an entire team dedicated to holistic patient care, such as doctors, nurses, physiotherapist, occupational therapists, complementary therapists, community teams and volunteers.

Patients do not just come to a hospice to spend their last weeks or days of life; they also come for respite and pain and symptom management. Hospice care can provide respite for families who are caring for their loved ones at home. Patients can go to a hospice for a couple of weeks to be cared for while their family has a short break. Pain management is often a need for many patients reaching the end of their life, depending on their diagnosis. Hospice care nurses are very experienced in pain and symptom management. Hospice care focuses on quality of life, giving care to patients that is holistic, comfortable and, importantly, as symptom free as possible.

Going into a hospice placement, you might feel unprepared or lack confidence (Murnane et al., 2023). You might be asking questions such as 'How will I cope', 'how will I manage in conversations with bad news' or 'how will I feel when I see someone die or see a body for the first time?' Here are some tips to help you prepare for a placement in a hospice or community hospice team:

There are small bite-size courses that are available as continuing professional development with some unions for free if you are a member. This might be a good place to start.	Write down the things you are most anxious about, and talk to someone about how you are feeling before you start.
If there is anything you would like to overcome for this placement, put it as one of your objectives, and your practice assessor or supervisor could help you with it.	Take time to identify the signs of self-anxiety and stress, so if these do happen, you can nip it in the bud before you start to spiral.
Start practicing some mindfulness techniques before you go to placement so that if you do find yourself in a situation where you are struggling to cope, you have something to help you, for example, grounding techniques and square breathing (choosing a square or rectangular object and taking a moment to follow the edges with your eyes, breathing in along one edge and breathing out along the next. Repeat for as long as necessary).	Identify early healthy coping mechanisms that will help you when you are feeling stressed, such as getting plenty of sleep, going for a walk or even just sitting outside to get some fresh air, can give you clarity.

Whether you have the opportunity to be placed in an acute hospital or a community setting, it is important to remember that the main goal of any end-of-life or palliative care for patients is to give the best possible care to facilitate a good quality of life that is as symptom free as possible. This is only possible by collaborating with the wider healthcare team to give comprehensive care to both the patient and their family, giving both patient- and family-centred care.

FAMILY-CENTRED CARE

It is important to involve and support families through the dying process as well as the patient. The way this is done will look similar across the areas you will have placement in. They may look like:

- Informal chats by the bedside.
- Telephone calls to check in and see how they are doing and how things are progressing.
- Time away from the patient in a family room to have more in-depth sensitive conversations.
- Families staying overnight with patients by the beside or on the ward/unit.
- Making cups of tea and coffee for family members.
- Answering questions.
- Repeating what doctors have discussed because the family was upset and couldn't listen anymore.
- Sometimes the family might just want to give you a hug.

Having a family-centred approach to care is embedded in practice, particularly at the end of life. From formal meetings to care planning and decision making, consideration for the family to be involved as much as possible is a must (Bloomer et al., 2022). We must remember that the family that is left behind will remember how they were treated and the care their loved one received. The nursing staff and wider healthcare team should address the needs of the family early on, and it should be continually monitored; this can even be continued after the death of the patient. Both hospital and community teams often have protocols in place to contact the family after the death of a loved one; this can include a phone call from bereavement teams, medical examiners or the district nursing team that cared for the patient to check on the family after a death.

CARE PLANS AND IMPORTANT DOCUMENTATION _

Nursing documentation is one of the most important parts of nursing as is stated by the Nursing and Midwifery Council (NMC) code of conduct:

THE NMC SAYS

10 Keep clear and accurate records relevant to your practice.

Care planning for individualised care is at the heart of what we do to ensure that patients are cared for in the best possible way, ensuring their wishes are respected or, if the patient is not able to communicate their wants and needs, that the care and interventions provided are done in the person's best interests. This section looks at the types of documents and care plans you may come across in your placements.

End-of-life care plans

As mentioned previously, end-of-life care refers to the support patients receive in their last days, months or years of their lives. The NHS considers people to be at the end of their life if they have 12 or fewer months left to live (NHS, 2022). However, this prediction is not always possible (Taylor, 2022). An end-of-life care plan may include some of the following points:

- Once it's been recognised that a person may die within the coming hours, days or longer, early communication and decisions about care are made with the person's needs and wishes at the heart of the care plan. This is reviewed and revised regularly. It might include questions such as where they would like to die and if they have any religious needs that need to be fulfilled.
- Any communication that has taken place between staff and the patient, plus the people important to them, is clearly documented.

- The dying person should be involved as much as possible; it should be identified as soon as possible who and what are important to them. They should be listened to and their needs respected.
- The care plan should be tailored to the dying person specifically and should be delivered with compassion.
- Some care plans come with a bundle for morning, afternoon and night reviews. They may also have pages for syringe driver pre-scriptions and anticipatory medications. Online care plans are also available in some areas so that many members of the wider multidisciplinary team can have access and make changes remotely, enabling reduced delays in patient care.

Advance care plans and advance directives

Some people may want to express their wishes about what happens to them if they ever become unable to speak for themselves. They can make an advance statement; this is a statement written by the person that sets their preferences, wishes, beliefs and values regarding their future care (NHS, 2023b). An advance statement is not the same as an advance decision or directive. An advance decision/directive is known as a living will or advance decision to refuse treatment. These are legal in the United Kingdom (except Scotland) if they meet a certain criteria (NHS, 2023a; NHS Lothian, 2024).

A person's decision about their care can then be incorporated into a care plan, and these are sometimes called advance care plans. Some people will have thought about what they would like the end of their life to look like, and they may have this documented. These can sometimes include information such as:

- Preference for their care and treatment and what needs to be prioritised.
- Decisions about resuscitation.
- Where they would like to be looked after in their last days and if they want to be taken to hospital or a hospice.
- The people they want to have with them when they die.
- Their spiritual or religious needs or beliefs and how these should be considered.
- Who they want to make decisions for them if they become unable to make decisions or communicate for themselves.

If the advance decision is binding legally (not in Scotland), it takes precedence over decisions made in the patient's best interest by other people. However, it must be valid. Its validity depends on the following points:

- The patient must be over 18 years old and have the capacity to make, understand and communicate their decision when they made it
- The patient specifies clearly which treatments they wish to refuse.
- The patient explains the circumstances in which they wish to refuse them.
- It is signed by the patient, and this must be signed by a witness if the patient wants to refuse life-sustaining treatment.
- The patient has made the advance decision of their own accord, without any harassment by anyone else.
- The patient has not said or done anything that would contradict the advance decision since they made it (for example, saying that they have changed their mind).

Some patients may also have instructed to have a lasting power of attorney. This is legally binding, and it allows for someone other than a medical professional to make decisions about a patient's care and welfare should they become unable to make decisions for themselves in the future (NHS, 2023b).

ReSPECT documentation

Patients receiving end-of-life or palliative care may have a Recommended Summary Plan for Emergency Care and Treatment (ReSPECT) form included with their care plan.

A ReSPECT form (Fig. 8.1) is a document that creates personalised recommendations for a person's clinical care and treatment in a future emergency where the person is unable to make or express choices. Usually these are put in place through recommendations of the medical team or healthcare professional. It can document levels and ceilings of care—for example, if a patient is for ward-based care, full escalation to intensive care or resuscitation, including cardiopulmonary resuscitation, or not. It takes their wishes into consideration, or medical professionals implement them in the patients' best interests if they are unable to make decisions for themselves, after conversations with their family or carers.

ReSPECT — Recommended Summary Plan for Emergency Care and Treatment

1. This plan belongs to:

Preferred name

Date completed

Full name

Date of birth

Address

NHS/CHI/Health and care number

The ReSPECT process starts with conversations between a person and a healthcare professional. The ReSPECT form is a clinical record of agreed recommendations. It is not a legally binding document.

2. Shared understanding of my health and current condition

Summary of relevant information for this plan including diagnoses and relevant personal circumstances:

Details of other relevant care planning documents and where to find them (e.g. Advance or Anticipatory Care Plan; Advance Decision to Refuse Treatment or Advance Directive; Emergency plan for the carer):

I have a legal welfare proxy in place (e.g. registered welfare attorney, person with parental responsibility) - if yes provide details in Section 8   ☐ Yes   ☐ No

3. What matters to me in decisions about my treatment and care in an emergency

Living as long as possible matters most to me   Quality of life and comfort matters most to me

What I most value:

What I most fear / wish to avoid:

4. Clinical recommendations for emergency care and treatment

Prioritise extending life	**or** Balance extending life with comfort and valued outcomes **or**	Prioritise comfort
clinician signature	clinician signature	clinician signature

Now provide clinical guidance on specific realistic interventions that may or may not be wanted or clinically appropriate (including being taken or admitted to hospital +/- receiving life support) and your reasoning for this guidance:

SPECIMEN COPY - NOT FOR USE

CPR attempts recommended Adult or child	For modified CPR **Child only, as detailed above**	CPR attempts **NOT** recommended Adult or child
clinician signature	clinician signature	clinician signature

www.respectprocess.org.uk

Version 3.0 © Resuscitation Council UK

Fig. 8.1 Example of a ReSPECT form, version 3 (Resuscitation Council UK, 2020). (Source: Resuscitation Council UK introduces version 3 of ReSPECT Plan. Available at https://www.resus.org.uk/about-us/news-and-events/resuscitation-council-uk-introduces-version-3-respect-plan).

5. Capacity for involvement in making this plan

Does the person have capacity to participate in making recommendations on this plan? Document the full capacity assessment in the clinical record.

☐ Yes
☐ No

→ If no, in what way does this person lack capacity?

If the person lacks capacity a ReSPECT conversation must take place with the family and/or legal welfare proxy

6. Involvement in making this plan

The clinician(s) signing this plan is/are confirming that (select A,B or C, OR complete section D below):

☐ **A** This person has the mental capacity to participate in making these recommendations. They have been fully involved in this plan.

☐ **B** This person does not have the mental capacity, even with support, to participate in making these recommendations. Their past and present views, where ascertainable, have been taken into account. The plan has been made, where applicable, in consultation with their legal proxy, or where no proxy, with relevant family members/friends.

☐ **C** This person is less than 18 years old (16 in Scotland) and (please select 1 or 2, and also 3 as applicable or explain in section D below):

☐ **1** They have sufficient maturity and understanding to participate in making this plan

☐ **2** They do not have sufficient maturity and understanding to participate in this plan. Their views, when known, have been taken into account.

☐ **3** Those holding parental responsibility have been fully involved in discussing and making this plan.

D If no other option has been selected, valid reasons must be stated here: (Document full explanation in the clinical record.)

7. Clinicians' signatures

Grade/speciality	Clinician name	GMC/NMC/HCPC no.	Signature	Date & time

Senior responsible clinician:

8. Emergency contacts and those involved in discussing this plan

Name (tick if involved in planning)		Role and relationship	Emergency contact no.	Signature
Primary emergency contact:	☐			optional
	☐			optional
	☐			optional
	☐			optional
	☐			optional

9. Plan reviewed (e.g. for change of care setting) and remains relevant

Review date	Grade/speciality	Clinician name	GMC/NMC/HCPC No.	Signature

SPECIMEN COPY - NOT FOR USE

If this page is on a separate sheet from the first page: Name: DoB: ID number:

www.respectprocess.org.uk

Fig. 8.1, cont'd

In emergencies, rapid decisions may need to be made, and the patient may not be well enough to discuss what is important to them at that moment. Many treatments that are life sustaining for some may cause harm, discomfort and loss of dignity, so it's important to have these discussions early if possible. If it's not possible, as it isn't always, depending on the circumstances, it should be done with people who would act in the best interest of the patient, so this is usually with their family, medical team and nurses looking after them (Resus Council, 2023).

This is me

'This is me' is a simple document that has been endorsed by the Royal College of Nursing since 2010 (Alzheimer's Society, 2023). It was initially introduced as part of dementia care or for anyone experiencing delirium, but it can be used as part of end-of-life or palliative care as well. It's a support tool that can be used to record details about a person who can't easily share information about themselves and can help people caring for the dying person understand who the person really is and how to care for them. It includes:

- What the person prefers to be called.
- What areas they have lived in.
- Carer's name or the person who knows them best.
- The people who are important to them.
- Hobbies and interests they have or had.
- Little things that matter every day (for example, TV programmes, reading, coffee in the morning; do they become upset if they don't have these things in place?)
- Routines that are important, for example, first thing in the morning and last thing at night.
- What are the things they must have with or around them? For example, photos of their loved ones near them.
- Anything else that they would like you to know about what matters to them, for example, their favourite music, culture.
- What may worry or upset them?
- What makes them feel anxious?
- How is best to help them with decisions about their care?
- What helps them sleep well?

- How do they usually move around?
- What matters to them about food and drink?
- Where have they lived?
- What jobs have they done?
- Special occasions that are meaningful to them.

These questions are formulated and laid out in a booklet or online, so they are easily accessible for anyone caring for them and add to the holistic approach for well-rounded care.

Patient diaries

In some intensive care departments, patients have a diary. This is written by staff, and patients' families are encouraged to contribute day to day too. The idea is that during their stay, there is a sequence to the events that may have happened to them. Patients often have days or sometimes weeks where they are put into a medically induced coma. They are sedated, but there is evidence that sometimes they hear sounds and remember voices while they are 'asleep'. Of course, sadly, sometimes people don't get better when they are brought to intensive care, and they die. It is at this point that the patient's diary can be offered to the family for them to keep. Sometimes it brings comfort to them knowing they were cared for with an extrapersonal touch.

Religious and cultural beliefs

A person's religion and culture are central to their very being; they can have a direct effect on their needs, behaviour and often their attitude to illness and treatment. They also affect how they wish to be cared for in death. Not all people wish for the same things, so it is important to try and discuss these with them and family if possible. People will often have something to say about their spirituality; everyone is unique. It is good practice to ask patients if possible and particularly their family. Recognising these early on and addressing any spiritual concerns they may have could have a big impact on how they feel mentally but also build a rapport with them. In hospitals, there is usually a hospital chaplain that can help too (National Health and Wellbeing Team, NHS England and NHS Improvement, 2020).

It is important to take into consideration that not everyone has the same beliefs and to be sensitive to this, particularly in the care during and after dying.

CASE STUDY

Toby is a newly qualified nurse who has been caring for a patient over several shifts in a row. The patient was in a coma and not able to speak for themselves. Toby got to know their family a little, and they explained that it was important for the patient to be surrounded by certain types of crystals; it was important to them and helped the family feel more at ease knowing they were there. They wanted a particular crystal placed on the chest of the patient when they died to help with, as the patient's family said, 'passing to the next realm', and so of course this was facilitated. It made Toby think that even though the meaning of these things weren't important to him, seeing how much it meant to the family really made him want to reassure them that their wishes were respected. Not only did it mean Toby was able to build a better professional rapport with them but it instilled trust from the family to know that Toby was respecting the patient's wishes and doing everything he could to help the patient and family spiritually, too, by the smallest of gestures.

Sensitive conversations and bereavement

Communicating sensitive news and information and being involved in these conversations can be very hard. As a nursing student, you may be privy to these conversations, depending on the patients you are looking after. It's difficult to know what to expect; they can be difficult to navigate, and there is usually a lot of emotion in these conversations. In this section, we have broken down what you might expect from these conversations, who is involved, how families or carers may be supported and how you can support yourself too.

The environment should be a comfortable private place.

| If it's in person, usually a family room, a separate room away from hustle and bustle. | If they are on the phone, ask if It is a good time to talk and if they are somewhere where they can sit and be as comfortable as possible. |

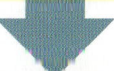

The conversation will usually be led by members of the team who have had significant involvement in the care of the patient.

| They will be fully informed of all circumstances surrounding their care. | They will be able to answer any questions the family or carers might have. |

The conversation should begin with engagement and empathy from the beginning.

| It should start by asking the family, carers and/or patient what they already know, expect and feel. | Then it should be established if they have someone to talk to after or if they are with someone who can support them. |

(MacMillan Cancer Support, 2023)

The persons leading the conversation will then bring the people in the room towards understanding of the situation.

| How things are, what has happened, the results of an investigation. | What is going to happen or what is likely to happen going forward. |

Clear terms should always be used.

| For example, death, dying, died or going to die. | Depending on the situation, gentler terms might be used, but it must be clear that they can't be misunderstood. |

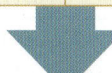

Reassurance should be offered at this point—an expression of sympathy and kindness.

| Silence at this time can seem uncomfortable; however, it gives people time to think of any questions and process what has been said. | Once questions have been answered, people should be informed about what happens next and then have time for any further questions. |

(MacMillan Cancer Support, 2023)

There are usually a lot of emotions, too, for all involved, such as:

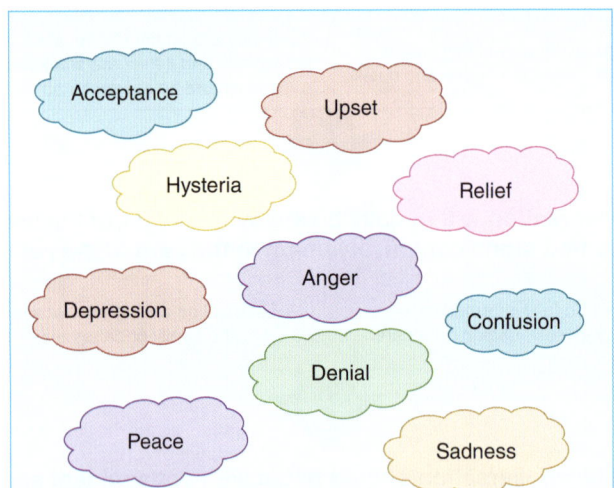

After a conversation with the family or bereaved, they may have more questions after for the nursing staff or medical team. Quite often, because there is a lot of emotion, information doesn't always stick or is retained by those receiving the news, or they don't always fully understand and may need things worded differently. This is an opportunity for nursing staff to help them understand or reiterate what has been said before.

Conversations don't always follow the same pattern every time. Every situation and every patient are different; however, this will hopefully give a rough idea and allow for some preparation of what to expect.

The grief process

Everyone will experience some sort of grief in their lifetime; it can look different depending on who is involved in any given situation. In terms of healthcare, there are many people who will be involved in a patient's care who will experience some grief around the time before someone dies, for example, anticipatory grief. We often think of grief as something that happens after death, but it can start a long time before someone dies (Taee, 2020). When someone receives a terminal diagnosis, grief can start right away, and these feelings can be just as intense and difficult as those after death. These can include feelings such as:

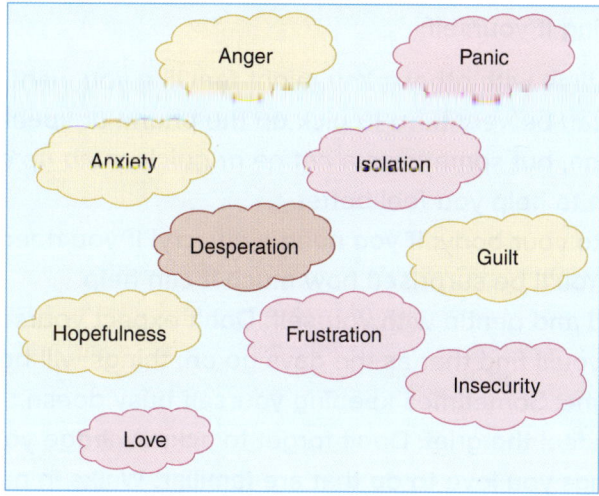

Grief can affect every person who's involved in the care of the patient, including the patient. Here, we look at some of the reasons why they might feel grief:

Patient	Grief for the life they will miss. Grief for the time will lose with family. Grief over missing children grow up. Grieving for the heartache they are putting their family through, leading to feelings of guilt. Feelings of 'why me?' Fear of losing control and dignity, grief of their loss of independence.
Caregivers/ family	The grief of missing the person. Grief for watching someone go through treatment and feeling helpless. Grief experienced because they feel lost without them. Grief of losing identity without them and having to live with only memories.
Healthcare providers	Grief of spending a long time caring for someone but having been unable to make them better. Grief of investing a lot of care and compassion and now experiencing loss. They may feel guilty that they are still here, and their patient is not. They might feel like they have failed because it was their job to make the patient better. There could also be trauma from abrupt loss, such as a sudden cardiac arrest.

(Source: Bruce, C.A., 2002.)

TIPS

Here are some tips that can help you deal with grief if you're experiencing it yourself:

- Spend time with others: You might feel like you want to be alone, and it can be very hard to pick up the phone or speak to someone, but sometimes a coffee or quick catch up can be enough to help you feel better.
- Listen to your body: If you need a cry, cry! If you need to sleep, sleep. You'll be surprised how much it can help.
- Be kind and gentle with yourself: Don't expect yourself to run at 100%; you'll find that as the days go on, things will become easier.
- Take time: Sometimes keeping yourself busy doesn't give yourself time to feel the grief. Don't forget to acknowledge your feelings.
- Do things you love to do that are familiar: Walks in nature, reading, crafts, whatever it is; do what you feel up to.
- Keep a journal: Writing down thoughts and feelings can help to keep track of them and make sense of what has happened.
- Stay active: Physical exercise, if possible, helps to enhance mood and can help with your sleeping pattern.

You can also find bereavement and grief support here:

Cruse Bereavement Support
https://www.cruse.org.uk
Sue Ryder
https://www.sueryder.org

CARE AFTER DEATH OR LAST OFFICES

While on placement, when a patient dies, you may hear the nurses or healthcare assistants talking about 'last offices'. If this is something you've never come across, you might be wondering what they are talking about. Last offices are caring for a person after death, and it is an enormous privilege. The nursing role extends beyond death, meaning that care is provided to the deceased person and support given to their family and carers. It is a term still used in hospitals, although many trusts are trying to move away from the term because of the association with the military and Christian religion (National Nurse Consultant Group [Palliative Care], 2011). Last offices only applies to the physical preparation of the body, whereas 'care after death' refers to the wider tasks carried out by nurses for families and carers as well as the preparation of the body, which is sometimes now called 'personal care after death'.

Care after death or last offices might include some of the following:

Respecting and honouring the spiritual or cultural wishes of the deceased person and their family/carers while ensuring legal obligations are met.	Preparing the body for transfer to the mortuary or for the funeral director, depending on where the body is situated.	Offering family and carers present the opportunity to participate and supporting them if they wish to take part.
Ensuring the privacy and dignity of the deceased person is maintained, taking cultural implications into account.	Considering health and safety of everyone who encounters the body is protected.	Taking the family wishes and cultural beliefs into consideration.
Honour the deceased person's and family's wishes for organ or tissue donation.	Being mindful that not all families are the same and individualised care is important.	Ensuring all the deceased person's belongings are returned to their relatives.

This whole process can be quite overwhelming if you've never experienced it before, especially if you've known the patient for some time. Here are some tips to help prepare and how to deal with it going forward:

TIPS

- **Grief.** It is only natural to be upset when a patient you have been caring for dies. It is important to remain professional so that you can support family, carers and relatives. But if you need to, take a moment away from the situation to collect your thoughts.
- **Compassion.** Be compassionate with yourself when you're in this situation. You're new to this, or this person's situation struck a

Continued

TIPS—cont'd

chord with you if their circumstances were like something that's happening in your personal life.

- **Participate.** If you can, ask to participate in caring for the deceased patient and getting them ready for the next part of their journey. It's the last thing you'll be able to do for your patient and can help give you some closure knowing you've sent them on their way.
- **Reflect.** Coping afterwards can be difficult, especially if it is the first time. Writing down a reflective account of the experience can help you to process things and gain clarity. It'll also help improve your practice next time.
- **Support.** Get support if you need it. You can talk to some of the other nurses or your supervisor on your placement. You could ask for a debrief. If you are struggling to cope, talk to your peers, practice supervisors, learning environment managers or university link lecturers so you can get some more support.
- **Exposure.** If you feel up to it and want to learn more, you could organise some time with specialist nurses such as palliative care teams, end-of-life care nurses, Macmillan nurses or the hospital bereavement team. By shadowing, you gain more of an insight and understanding into the area. This can help you going forward to compartmentalise if you understand the process better.

'Before being a nursing student, I had not experienced death personally. I had experienced grief personally; however, I had never seen death. During my time as a nursing student, I got to witness several patients dying and caring for them after. The first time that I had the opportunity to witness this, it wasn't what I expected. I expected it to impact me after; however, on several occasions I felt it didn't. For me personally, I felt empathy for the family, as I could empathise with them. However, the actual death of the patient was something that I didn't really have any emotion towards. Personally, I find it harder for the families to

communicate with them effectively, as there is no best way to approach the situation with a patient's family member.

Before performing last offices, I was nervous, as I wasn't sure what to do. However, once this was explained to me, I felt more relaxed around the topic. Overall, my first experiences with death were not what I expected. I expected to feel more attached to it then what I originally was, which has made me more confident for the future, and I am glad that I got to experience this while still being a student'.

Leah Richardson, second-year nursing student

SUPPORT FOR NURSING STUDENTS

Death affects everyone differently, and you are no exception. Caring for dying patients can take its toll emotionally. This section shares some tips on how to help you cope with death and consider what emotions you may go through and where to approach help if you need it.

Peer and family support

Opening up and talking to your student nursing peers can often be one of the best ways to process the death of a patient. Peers may have different perspectives from a friend outside of work because they may be able to understand the situation better and offer insight into their experiences (Westwood and Brown, 2019).

Speak to a mentor or a more experienced nurse who you trust on your placement who may have gone through a similar situation. They might be able to suggest some coping mechanisms that have worked for them in the past and, equally, what didn't work for them.

If you feel like you can talk to your family, then they are a good place to start too. If they don't work in healthcare, they might also be able to provide a different perspective to help you process how you are feeling.

If you feel like you need more help, then there are often counselling services within the hospital that are free of charge. You could also speak to the hospital chaplain. These services might be able to offer a unique perspective. This may come as a comfort as you talk through the situation, helping you work through your emotions and gain perspective and closure.

Just remember that when you do discuss whatever situation you've been in, the patient remains confidential, in line with the NMC code of conduct.

NMC

THE NMC SAYS

5 Respect people's right to privacy and confidentiality.

As a nurse, midwife or nursing associate, you owe a duty of confidentiality to all those who are receiving care. This includes making sure that they are informed about their care and that information about them is shared appropriately.

To achieve this, you must:

5.1 Respect a person's right to privacy in all aspects of their care.
5.3 Respect that a person's right to privacy and confidentiality continues after they have died.

Counselling

Some deaths are extremely traumatic; some can really take their toll on you emotionally, and you may feel you need further support. A trained counsellor will be able to help you with this. Many universities have these services that are accessible that are usually free or low cost. The hospital trust may also be able to offer some counselling. Your GP will also be able to refer you to services in the community; sometimes there is a waiting list for these. Private counselling is readily available but at a cost.

Burnout

Burnout is particularly prevalent in end-of-life care or palliative care nurses, as it is an emotionally demanding role which holds a high level of responsibility (Gómez-Urquiza et al., 2020). The key is to identify burnout or potential triggers for burnout early. It's incredibly difficult to have to manage your own emotions while comforting a family who is going through one of the most difficult times. Some signs of burnout to look out for are:

- Dreading going to placement to care for a particular patient.
- Feeling particularly emotionally drained.
- Inability to remain objective about the situation.
- Thinking about the patient or scenario constantly, even at home.

Learning to maintain boundaries while on placement can help with these situations, trying your best to separate yourself from the patient and their circumstances. Most of all, talking to someone you trust during placement to help decompress and allow you to compartmentalise will help too.

Grief

As mentioned before, it is normal to feel some sort of grief if the patient you are caring for dies. Whether it is a sudden or expected death, lots of emotions might be floating around, and you may be wondering if what you are feeling is normal. Whatever you are feeling, allow yourself space to feel. Perhaps do something that aligns with your faith, spirituality or values to allow yourself the space you need to process any difficult feelings you are having (Davidson, 2023). Remember, it's likely you won't have been the first person to feel the way you do. Don't be afraid to reach out for help if you need it.

Self-care

Nurses are notorious for putting everyone's needs before their own. Practice some self-care if you are feeling guilty, upset or angry about a patient's death. Be kind to yourself; self-care is so important. When you practice, you will start to become familiar with coping strategies that work for you, so you can practice them more often. If you are in such a position, try some of these steps to help give yourself self-compassion:

> **TIPS**
> - Flip the scenario: Imagine someone you care about is a nursing student and they are having a difficult time processing a death of a patient. What would you say to them?
> - Perhaps things such as 'Are you being too hard on yourself?' 'Are your expectations too high?'
> - Write them down, reflect and look back as often as needed.

Above all else, talk to someone about it. Below are some resources that can be accessed for further self-help:

- Headspace (www.headspace.com)
- Laura Hyde Foundation (www.laurahydefoundation.org)
- Nurse Lifeline (www.nurselifeline.org.uk/helpline) Tel: 0808 801 0455 (United Kingdom)
- Royal College of Nursing (www.rcn.org.uk): Wellbeing, self-care and resilience
- Samaritans (www.samaritans.org) Tel: 116 123 (United Kingdom)

CONCLUSION

Hopefully, this chapter has given you some idea of what to expect in terms of death and dying while on placement in whatever environment you might find yourself in.

Caring for patients in their final months, weeks, days and moments with the right support is a very rewarding area of nursing. It is one of the greatest privileges to be able to care for someone in their last moments and perform care for a person who has died by preparing them for the next part of their journey. It is a difficult part of nursing but necessary.

Final message: It is very important that you look after yourself when you are exposed to anything like the situations mentioned in this chapter. It can be emotionally demanding, and each situation will come with its own challenges. Some days may be harder than others, but in all circumstances, you should check in with yourself, assess how you are feeling, debrief and reflect, so you are able to process. It will build your resilience, but this can only be done if you look after yourself too.

Space for reader's own reflection:

_____

_____

_____

_____

_____

_____

_____

_____

_____

_____

_____

_____

_____

_____

_____

_____

_____

_____

_____

REFERENCES

Alzheimer's Society. 2023. This is Me. https://www.alzheimers.org.uk/get-support/publications-factsheets/this-is-me

Bloomer, M.J., Poon, P., Runacres, F., Hutchinson, A.M., 2022. Family-Centred Care at End of Life in Critical Care: A Retrospective Descriptive Study. Collegian vol. 29 (5), 574–580.

Bruce, C.A., 2002. The grief process for patient, family, and physician. J. Am. Osteopath. Assoc. 102 (9 Suppl 3), S28–S32.

Davidson, A., 2023. How Nurses can Cope with a Patient's Death. https://nursejournal.org/articles/how-nurses-can-cope-with-a-patients-death/#:~:text=Every%20nurse%20will%20have%20a,can%20grow%20from%20the%20situation

Gómez-Urquiza, J.L., Albendín-García, L., Velando-Soriano, A., Ortega-Campos, E., Ramírez-Baena, L., Membrive-Jiménez, M.J., et al., 2020. Burnout in Palliative Care Nurses, Prevalence and Risk Factors: A Systematic Review with Meta-Analysis. Int. J. Environ. Res. Public Health 17 (20), 7672. doi:10.3390/ijerph17207672

Gov.uk. 2022. Department of Health and Social Care. https://www.gov.uk/government/publications/nhs-continuing-healthcare-fast-track-pathway-tool

ICU Steps. 2023. End of Life in Intensive Care. https://icusteps.org/information/information-sheets/end-of-life

Macmillan Cancer Support. 2023. Difficult Conversations. https://www.macmillan.org.uk/coronavirus/healthcare-professionals/difficult-conversations#:~:text=Bring%20the%20person%20towards%20an,sympathy%3A%20I%27m%20sorry

Mannix, K., 2018. With the End in Mind. Anonymous Translator, first ed. Little Brown & Company, New York.

Murnane, S., Purcell, G., Reidy, M., 2023. Death, dying and caring: exploring the student nurse experience of palliative and end-of-life education. Br. J. Nurs. 32 (11), 526–531.

National Association for Hospice at Home. 2024. What is Hospice at Home? http://www.nahh.orb.uk/about-hospice-care/what-is-hospice-at-home

National End of Life Care Programme and National Nurse Consultant Group (Palliative Care). 2014. 'Guidance for Staff Responsible for Care After Death (Last Offices).

National Health and Wellbeing Team, NHS England and NHS Improvement. 2020. Our NHS People Understanding Different Bereavement Practices and how our Colleagues may Experience Grief. https://www.england.nhs.uk/wp-content/uploads/2021/01/Bereavement-Practices-Jan-2021.pdf

National Nurse Consultant Group (Palliative Care). 2011. Guidance for Staff Responsible for Care After Death (Last Offices). www.england.nhs.uk/improvement-hub/wp-content/uploads/sites/44/2017/10/Guidance-for-Staff-Responsible-for-Care-after-Death.pdf

NHS. 2022. https://www.england.nhs.uk/eolc/

NHS. 2023a. Advance Decision to Refuse Treatment (Living Will). https://www.nhs.uk/conditions/end-of-life-care/planning-ahead/advance-decision-to-refuse-treatment/#:~:text=As%20long%20as%20it%27s%20valid,own%20decisions%20about%20your%20treatment

NHS. 2023b. Advance Statement about Your Wishes. https://www.nhs.uk/conditions/end-of-life-care/planning-ahead/advance-statement/

NHS. 2023c. Changes in the Last Hours and Days. https://www.nhs.uk/conditions/end-of-life-care/your-wellbeing/changes-in-the-last-hours-and-days/

NHS. 2023d. What End of Life Care Involves. https://www.nhs.uk/conditions/end-of-life-care/what-it-involves-and-when-it-starts/

NHS Blood and Transplant. 2023. Organ Donation - Get the Facts. https://www.organdonation.nhs.uk/helping-you-to-decide/about-organ-donation/get-the-facts/

NHS Lothian. 2024. Palliative Care Guidelines. https://services.nhslothian.scot/palliativecare/palliative-care-guidelines/

Office for National Statistics. 2013. National Survey of Bereaved People (VOICES) - Office for National Statistics. https://www.ons.gov.uk/peoplepopulationandcommunity/healthandsocialcare/healthcaresystem/bulletins/nationalsurveyofbereavedpeople-voices/2014-07-10

Parry, M., Jones, B., Churcher, C., 2022. End-of-life simulation: a cross-field evaluation in an undergraduate nursing programme. Int. J. Palliat. Nurs. 28 (8), 388–395.

Resus Council, UK. 2023. ReSPECT. https://www.resus.org.uk/respect

Taee, K., 2020. Anticipatory Grief: Grieving before Someone Dies. https://www.mariecurie.org.uk/talkabout/articles/what-is-anticipatory-grief/271278

Taylor, J., 2022. End of Life Care and the End of Life Care Plan. https://www.theaccessgroup.com/en-gb/blog/hsc-end-of-life-care-plan/

The Queen's Nursing Institute. 2015. The Value of the District Nurse Specialist Practitioner Qualification. https://www.qni.org.uk/wp-content/uploads/2016/09/SPQDN_Report_WEB2.pdf

Thomas, K., 2023. Community Palliative Care https://www.goldstandardsframework.org.uk/cd-content/uploads/files/Library%2C%20Tools%20%26%20resources/ABC%20Palliative%20Care.pdf

Westwood S., Brown M., 2019. Preparing students to care for patients at the end of life. Nursing Times [Online]; 115: 10, 43-46.

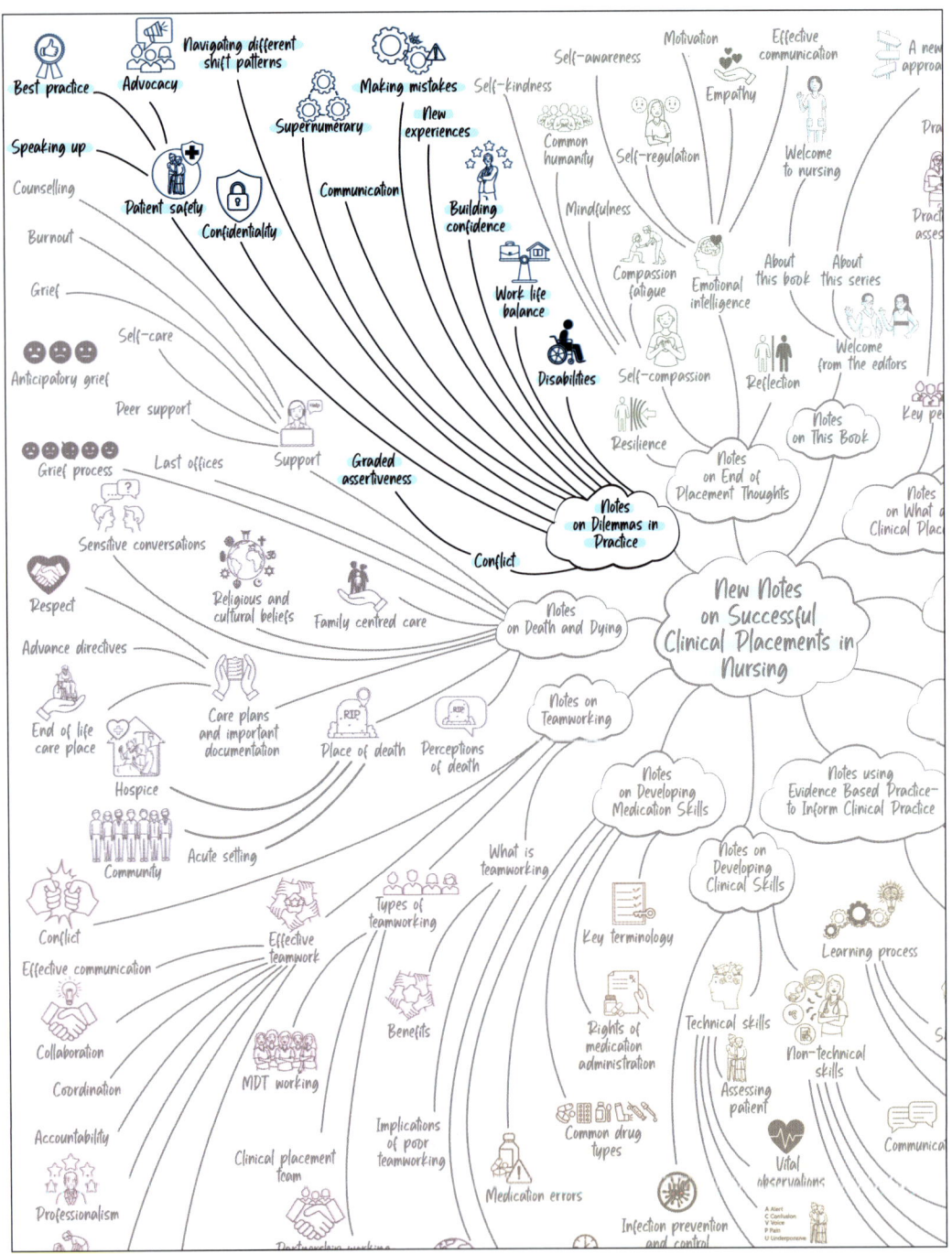

NOTES ON DILEMMAS IN PRACTICE

Brian Webster (he/him) ■ **Natalie Elliott (she/her)**

INTRODUCTION

Like many things in life, studying towards a nursing degree will bring challenges and worries. There will be times when you are unsure of a way forward or, indeed, if there is a way forward. There might be hurdles in front of you that you will need to navigate, either as an individual or with the support of peers and colleagues or, depending on the hurdle, the likes of university or practice placement staff.

For the purpose of this chapter, we shall call these 'dilemmas'. The definition of 'dilemma', according to the Collins Dictionary (2023), is 'a problem that seems incapable of a solution'. This of course can occur several times while studying for any degree but is particularly the case when studying a nursing degree and even more so when on the practice placement elements of your course. It could be that you witness poor practice, you are related to a patient in the area you are on placement or you have been a patient in an area you are on placement—the possibilities are too endless to grasp.

This chapter will aim to consider some real-life dilemmas that we have been able to collect from nursing students who have faced them while studying nursing at university. We will aim to respond to these dilemmas, giving possible solutions and justifications for them. It may be that some of these dilemmas simply do not have a solution, or there may be many solutions; therefore we will give options so that you can feel confident and knowledgeable to tackle any you might face in the duration of your clinical placements. The dilemmas will be focused on practice placement elements of nursing studies to ensure validity, appropriateness and professionalism. However, it is impossible for us to cover every dilemma that nursing students may face, but we have done our best to cover the more prevalent ones. If you do find that you come across something not mentioned in this chapter, please reach out to your university or practice placement area.

We will aim to map these to the most up-to-date evidence-based practice from peer-reviewed journal articles, other textbooks that are relevant, guidance and advice in policy and legislation and, most importantly, the Nursing and Midwifery Council (NMC) code. We hope you enjoy this chapter and, by the end of it, realise dilemmas can be overcome.

Before we start, make a list of some of the things that may be worrying you about your current clinical placement.

_____

_____

_____

_____

_____

_____

DILEMMA: I HAVE SEEN SOMEONE PERFORM A CLINICAL SKILL THAT IS NO LONGER BEST PRACTICE

Clinical skills often develop rapidly due to the demanding and dynamic nature of healthcare. With research continually evolving, it can be daunting for nurses to stay on top of the latest evidence while managing their clinical responsibilities.

It is important to be the advocate for the people we nurse; therefore you do and will have a duty to question and critique practice of skills that you are aware are not best practice, outdated or, indeed, dangerous. Unfortunately, this might not always be welcomed but is absolutely needed to ensure safe and effective practice. People might feel you are challenging their practice, which really you are, but this might come across as negative or aggressive, depending on your approach and style. This may cause conflict between yourself and others.

Conflict is a possible situation that you will undoubtedly come across in life, not just as a nursing student. Conflict can be simply a friendly disagreement or, at the more extreme end, a serious argument or dispute. It might end up meaning you feel someone or a group of people are portraying hostility towards you, and of course in a professional setting, this is unacceptable and inappropriate. Our regulator, the NMC (2018), have their publication, the code (Nursing and Midwifery Council, 2023), have their first standard as to prioritise people, and this of course is relating to the people we nurse, but also the people we work with, and the first substandard is to:

| NMC

THE NMC SAYS

1.1 Treat people with kindness, respect and compassion.

Let's look at some examples where nursing students have experienced conflict.

'You see/know a senior member of staff has made an error that has the potential to cause harm. You mention it; they dismiss you. What do you do? You feel inferior to their expertise, but you know it's an error, but do you question superiority?'

Anonymous nursing student

This example will be a real challenge for anybody, as it not only takes courage to mention it in the first place, but to then be dismissed will feel very challenging and demoralising. It's really hard but important to take a step back and, firstly, congratulate yourself for having the courage and compassion to advocate for the patients you look after. It is key that nursing students challenge wrong practice or even malpractice. The reasons it happens can vary; it could be down to human factors or human error, or it could be a lack of knowledge or understanding. Or hopefully, less often, it can just be a way of cutting corners or lack of acceptance of change.

'As a nursing student, I witnessed an experienced nurse giving an intramuscular injection using out-of-date practice. I was nervous about how to approach the nurse about this and the implications it may have on me. But I reminded myself of the NMC code, patient safety and the importance of evidence-based practice as opposed to ritualistic practice'.

Joy O'Gorman, registered nurse and PhD candidate

If you have pointed out someone's practice is wrong or questionable or they have made a clear error, it is really important to make note of this and then seek further assistance from someone senior to them or, if need be, someone from another area. Bickhoff et al. (2017) found a wealth of reasons why nursing students didn't, or wouldn't, report such incidences. Some reasons include a lack of confidence, feeling they are 'just a student', not wanting to rock the boat and a worry of the consequences if they did challenge the practice. The review suggested this was fairly widespread but that it was important nursing students acted as advocates for people and spoke up and spoke out to prevent harm and neglect. It is key for practice placement areas to create relationships between nursing students and the staff they work alongside in order that nursing students have the moral courage to advocate and defend people as patients' rights to good care (Bickhoff et al., 2017).

TIPS

Possible conflict solutions:

- Remain calm.
- Remember to be professional and respectful.
- Seek support/advocacy if needed.
- Possibly remove yourself from the situation if needed.
- Try to seek a solution.

DILEMMA: I AM ON PLACEMENT AND I KNOW ONE OF THE PATIENTS

'When I was on placement, my aunt was admitted to the ward I was placed on. I didn't know what to do, and I didn't really feel comfortable providing her with personal care. I wasn't sure what to do, as I felt it was a conflict of interest'.

Natalie Elliott, registered nurse

When a nursing student finds themselves in the situation of knowing one of the patients on their clinical placement, it can present unique challenges. Here are some steps that can be taken to navigate this dilemma effectively.

Firstly, it is important to disclose the information. Inform your practice assessor or practice supervisor about the preexisting relationship with the patient as soon as possible. Transparency is key in maintaining professionalism and ensuring appropriate guidance and support. Try to assess whether the existing relationship with the patient could potentially compromise your ability to provide unbiased care. Factors such as personal emotions, past interactions and the nature of the relationship should also be considered. Seek guidance from your practice assessor, practice supervisor or another experienced nurse on the placement. Highlight any concerns, seek advice on managing the situation and receive support in navigating any ethical dilemmas that may arise.

Setting boundaries is crucial to maintain professionalism and ensuring ethical care. You should refrain from discussing personal matters or engaging in activities unrelated to the patient's care.

Upholding patient confidentiality at all times is key, regardless of your preexisting relationship. You should not disclose any sensitive information about the patient to others, including friends or family, without proper authorisation.

This is a good opportunity to discuss your feelings, biases and potential challenges associated with knowing the patient. Developing self-awareness can help you manage your emotions and maintain professionalism in your interactions.

Collaborate with other members of the healthcare team to ensure comprehensive and effective care for the patient. By working together, you can leverage the expertise of others and mitigate any potential conflicts of interest.

Above all, you should prioritise professionalism and ethical conduct in your interactions with the patient. You should strive to provide the highest quality of care while respecting the patient's dignity, autonomy and confidentiality.

DILEMMA: I HAVE CONTACTED MY PLACEMENT, AND THEY HAVE TOLD ME TO TURN UP ON DAY 1 TO GET MY ROTA

Unfortunately, being advised to turn up on the first day and get your rota is all too common in practice placement allocation. This can feel disappointing and unfair, as it means that you are unable to plan. It can feel very unwelcoming. While it can be frustrating, it is important to understand this is not intentional. Clinical areas can be very busy places, and it can be difficult for staff to find the time to plan ahead. Aim to have a compassionate outlook, and if you feel you must challenge this, do so professionally and constructively.

In previous standards of education for nursing, there was a minimum amount of time (40%) a nursing student would need to spend with a mentor; however, in the new standards for education, this is no longer the case. There has been a move towards the introduction of practice assessors and practice supervisors as well as more professionals being able to be practice supervisors, not only registered nurses. The previous minimum amount of time with an allocated mentor could be one of the reasons why placement areas have historically wanted to wait until the nursing student has started before allocating their shifts. It's important to realise that this is no longer the case; however, in some areas, it still hinders nursing students from having early access to their rota. If you find that this is the case, then it's a good idea to refer to the latest standards and have a discussion with your practice placement area. Of course, working alongside your practice supervisor has benefits, but it should not be a barrier to early and reasonable access and notice of your working rota.

'I remember several, if not most, of my placements telling me just to turn up on a set day and not giving me much if anything more than that. It was really challenging to begin with as a first year when I lacked confidence, but as I grew as a student and a person, I would say to the area, "No, sorry. I need at least 2 weeks; I have children and a life". I remember once telling a placement that if they didn't give me a rota, I would give them the days I would be in, which they didn't like, and I soon got a whole month worth'.

Audrey, newly qualified nurse

Some practice placement areas may justify providing your rota upon arrival by stating they want to collaborate with you to tailor it for the best learning experience possible. It's essential to recognise that you have a voice in creating your schedule when working with placement staff. If you only receive your rota on the day of arrival, it can be challenging to plan anything in advance. If you find that this happens, then communicate this concern with the practice placement; they should be receptive and understanding.

The 'Nursing and midwifery e-rostering: a good practice guide' (NHS England and NHS Improvement, 2019) suggest that staff should have their rota 6 weeks before it is due to be worked, so you could use this example and argue the case for the same. If you find that a placement area is consistently challenging in regard to your rota and ensuring you have it ahead of time, you may wish to seek support from your university or union advisors. It's important to ensure that problems like this do not persist, and bringing it to light in a constructive way will reduce the incidence of it happening again for others.

DILEMMA: I WAS ASKED TO DO SOMETHING OUT OF SCOPE OF MY COMPETENCY LEVELS

WORKING WITHIN COMPETENCY LEVELS

'I came into this degree having no healthcare experience. My first placement in first year was before we had been taught any clinical skills (beside basic life support). As such, my first clinical placement in my first year was super overwhelming! Learning so many new skills was going to be so difficult ... or so I thought! It was actually the soft skills I struggled with the most, communicating with other professionals being the main problem for me.

My first placement was on the COVID ward at a large hospital. There was a lot to learn, it was exhausting and the imposter syndrome was rife! Nevertheless, I was learning a lot and enjoying it overall. However, after a couple of weeks, I was asked to cover a 'special' (this is what this ward called when a patient needed 1:1 support 24/7) for a patient with advanced dementia. I had already been told from my university that this is something students shouldn't be expected to do and that students aren't insured to cover such duties. At first, I said yes without hesitation. I could tell that this was an expectation of all people on shift, and I was too worried to speak up and say that I didn't think I should be doing this. Cant et al. (2021) discuss how having, belonging to and being part of a team creates a positive experience for nursing students, which may explain my hesitation to question the request. Why would I question it? I'm brand new to healthcare, to the hospital environment and, more specifically, to this ward. I wanted to blend in, to show that I'm a team player and to get stuck in. But at what cost?

On reflection, I did not have the skills or knowledge to complete this duty. I knew this, and the staff was also aware of this. However, I was expected to step up to the mark.

Situations like this happen all over the country—students filling gaps that they shouldn't be. I recognize that the likely reason I was asked to fill this duty was due to a staffing shortfall. Kalankova et al., 2021 studied the effect of rationed care on nursing students. One theme their study uncovered was, "I do what they ask me to do". Anecdotally, many of us have heard the stories or experienced "filling the gap" and having our supernumerary status stripped but not feeling like we can say no.

I've learnt since my first placement that this is a common experience and that many of us feel too nervous to say no. I've come up against similar scenarios since this placement 2 years ago, but because of my confidence increase, I've been brave enough to politely refuse and explain why. It's not been easy to say no, but nobody has ever questioned me or made me feel like less of a team player for doing so'.

Anonymous nursing student

This is a good example that several nursing students will be able to relate to. Many will have been asked to carry out tasks or been given responsibilities we know we should not have been given. It could be that the practice placement is not aware of the limitations and abilities of the nursing students they have on placement with them. It could be that they are also attempting to use the nursing student as an extra 'set of hands', so to speak. It is clear that there can be a learning experience from just about anything and everything we do on a practice placement, but the vital thing is having the ability to recognise that and subsequently then make a decision if this task, role or responsibility you are being asked to do or carry out is within your scope of practice (as a nursing student).

The best practice would be to seek support here. Your university will be able to give you support and advice on what your limitations and abilities are and should be while at certain points within your nursing education; for example, there might be certain skills appropriate in year 3 rather than year 1 of your studies. It will be important to have the confidence to speak up and speak out to say to your placement area either you'd like to seek support or advice first or, indeed, that you don't feel comfortable or confident. This is really important to speak up, even if this will cause conflict, as mentioned before, because conflict is easier to overcome than fitness to practice. Carrying out duties and tasks out of your scope is not safe for you or the people you are delivering care to, so always have that in the forefront of your mind. This works both ways. Delegation is an important part of healthcare practice overall. Nurses will delegate, and so might you. What is key regarding delegation is that it is appropriate and relevant. The NMC (2020) highlights the importance of these suggested delegated tasks to remain accountable to the delegator, so this is again vital to be at the forefront of your mind and learning. Anything you might delegate to another does remain your responsibility and accountability; therefore delegating tasks that are out of someone's scope of practice is inappropriate.

Would it have been more appropriate for the nursing student to have been observing the patient with a registered professional so that there could be learning and teaching happening alongside the observation? There is no doubt the observation was needed for the health and safety of the person, but to utilise a nursing student to do this (who might not know why or how or the underpinning evidence to such responsibility) could be seen as inappropriate and unprofessional. This is why it is key for nursing students to gain the confidence and courage to be able to challenge, appropriately

and professionally, but also for the practice placement to delegate appropriately and professionally and for good reason.

THE NMC SAYS

1.3 Avoid making assumptions and recognise diversity and
individual choice.

2 Listen to people and respond to their preferences and concerns.

2.1 Work in partnership with people to make sure you deliver care
effectively.

2.6 Recognise when people are anxious or in distress and respond
compassionately and politely.

4 Act in the best interests of people at all times.

Nursing students can also relate to the codes following standards relating to being asked to carry out roles, tasks and responsibilities they feel
are out with their scope of practice or do not feel comfortable doing,
even if these are within their scope of practice.

THE NMC SAYS

1.2 Make sure you deliver the fundamentals of care effectively.

1.5 Respect and uphold people's human rights.

2.1 Work in partnership with people to make sure you deliver care
effectively.

2.5 Respect, support and document a person's right to accept or
refuse care and treatment.

3.4 Act as an advocate for the vulnerable, challenging poor practice
and discriminatory attitudes and behaviour relating to their care.

4.1 Balance the need to act in the best interests of people at all
times with the requirement to respect a person's right to accept
or refuse treatment.

4.3 Keep to all relevant laws about mental capacity that apply in the
country in which you are practising, and make sure that the
rights and best interests of those who lack capacity are still at
the centre of the decision-making process.

There are many more elements of the code that also would be appropriate and important for nursing students to refer to, and those noted are only a small example. One way people in general can deal with conflict is through Socratic questioning (Carey and Mullan, 2004). Rather than simply refusing to carry out a role, task or responsibility or rather than asking why, this method will give the nursing student the ability to professionally challenge the person delegating to them. It is also a good way to challenge poor practice, again without causing conflict or hostility. Fig. 9.1 gives some examples of how to use Socratic questioning.

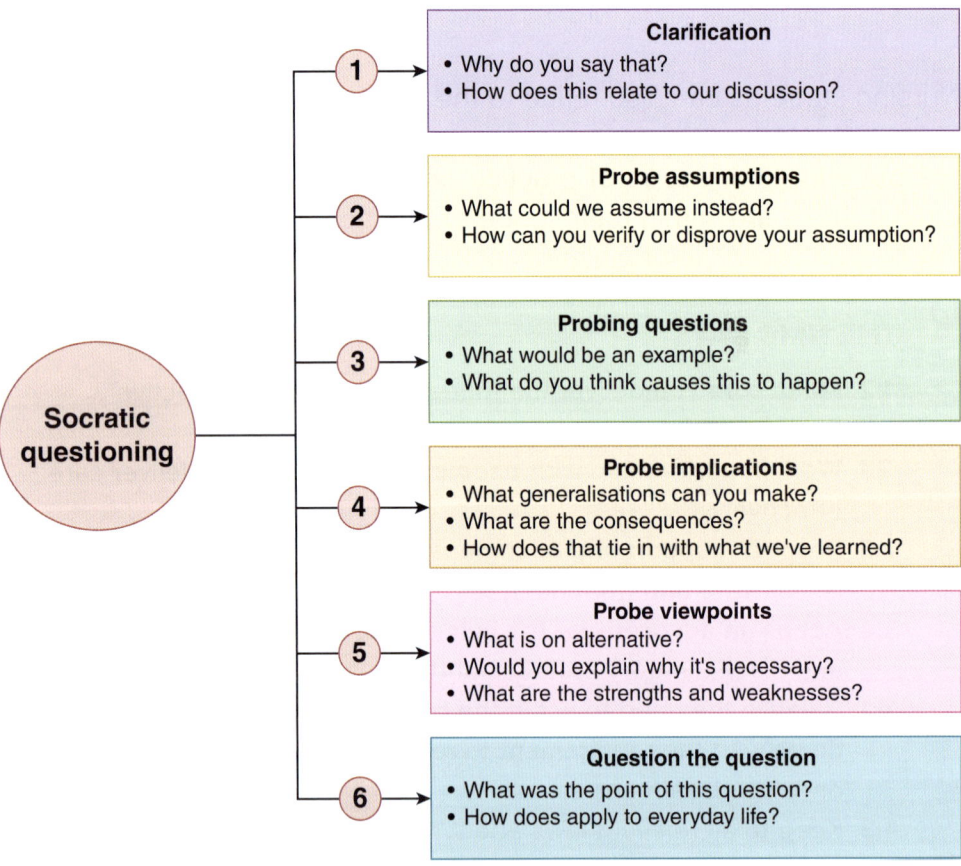

Fig. 9.1 Socratic questioning.

Using the example here, how could you apply the Socratic method to this scenario?

_____

_____

_____

_____

_____

_____

Applied here, the Socratic method could have meant that a question was asked about the relevance of the learning gained from this task, or the nursing student could have asked if the person who is delegating could go over the appropriate legislation beforehand so that the nursing student could have felt more confident and competent to carry out the role. This avoids refusing to carry out the task, role or responsibility at the same time as asking an appropriate and relevant question and gets the delegator thinking and questioning themselves and their practice.

DILEMMA: I HAVE NEVER WORKED A NIGHT SHIFT BEFORE. WHAT SHOULD I DO?_____

Staying physically and mentally well during night shifts is a challenge, but a little preparation and self-care can make it much easier, as will focusing on healthy eating and drinking and a good sleep routine.

The day before your nightshift, try to transition into your new sleep pattern. Try to stay awake as late as you can. This won't be easy, but try to find ways to keep your brain active while trying to avoid artificial stimulants (such as caffeine).

What things can you do to try to keep you awake?

_____

_____

_____

_____

_____

_____

It may also be helpful to let people know you're on night shifts, as good communication will minimise the disruption. Let those around you know that you are on night shift, and ask them not to contact you unless it is an emergency. It is worthwhile putting your devices on 'do not disturb' to reduce disturbances.

TIPS

You can buy notices for your front door that state you are a nightshift worker.

During your shift, it's crucial to prioritise staying hydrated and consuming nutritious food. Aim to drink at least one litre of water throughout your shift, as this supports cognitive function. Planning ahead is key; ensure you eat a nutrient-rich meal before your shift, and take your own food containing high-quality proteins and slow-release carbohydrates. While it may be tempting, try to resist junk food or takeaways to maintain optimal health and performance. While it may be a controversial topic, a 10- to 20-minute nap (if your area allows it) is optimum to help you quickly recover a bit of energy to get you through the last leg of your shift.

After your shift, try to not go straight to bed when you get home. It is unlikely that you would do this after a day shift. As far as possible, do what you would normally do at nighttime. If you usually watch some TV and have a light snack and then go to bed, and then do that after a night shift too. This will signal to your brain that it's time for bed.

If you're struggling with night shifts, please reach out for support. Seek assistance from those around you, whether it's family members, academic advisors, clinical peers or your university's wellbeing resources. Don't feel ashamed to discuss your challenges with your practice assessor or practice supervisor either. They can help, whether it involves adjusting your shift schedule or offering additional guidance to help you cope better.

DILEMMA: THE CLINICAL AREA IS SO SHORT STAFFED THAT THEY COUNT ME IN THEIR NUMBERS

 'Being used as a set of hands as in counted in the numbers, meaning lack of learning'.

Anonymous nursing student

As a nursing student, half your learning time is spent on clinical placements, where you have supernumerary status. This means you cannot be counted as part of the workforce but instead are treated as an additional part of the team on the basis that you are undertaking a placement to learn. This does not mean that you do not work while on placement—students are expected to learn through supervised participation in clinical work, with the level of supervision dependent on your stage of training and previous experience. The NMC standards for preregistration nursing programmes make it clear that placements should enable nursing students to learn to provide safe and effective care. Students are not merely there to observe, but they can and should add real value to care.

'On my placement, I was always tasked with handing out meals, every shift, every mealtime. I appreciate how important eating and drinking is, but it was obvious this was because the area was understaffed, and I wasn't learning anything from this. It was simply a hands-on task rather than a learning experience. When I reported it to the university, I was shot down, suggesting that I was downplaying the importance of hydration and nutrition, which I wasn't. I argued that if I was helping someone to eat or if I was learning about the different stages of diet, this would be a learning experience, but I wasn't. I was simply being made to hand out and collect meals. If I stopped to speak to a patient or even to help them, I was told to get a move on and hurry up, as the trolley isn't on the ward for long'.

Steven, second-year nursing student

The government agreed to introduce supernumerary status for nursing students in 1988, and it was gradually phased in over the following years. Before that, nursing students were seen as part of the workforce, with the employer having oversight of training. However, following a review by the UK's four national nursing boards in the 1980s, the government accepted this was unsafe for patients and students. The old model, it was suggested at the time, had led to students' learning needs becoming secondary.

If you are finding yourself being counted in the numbers in an area of practice, then it is key, like many of the responses to dilemmas in this chapter, to speak up. One way this can be done is via graded assertiveness. Fig. 9.2 gives an example of how to ask assertive questions.

Clarke-Romain (2023) highlights that graded assertiveness is a concept that emerged from the airline industry's probe into crash causes. It is a technique designed to help staff members escalate their concerns in a step-by-step manner. The concept was born out of the realisation that some staff members, despite recognising a problem, were hesitant to assertively communicate with pilots and other senior staff. This scenario is not uncommon in the healthcare sector, hence why this tool is also useful in the healthcare sector and may be the answer in challenging something you are struggling with.

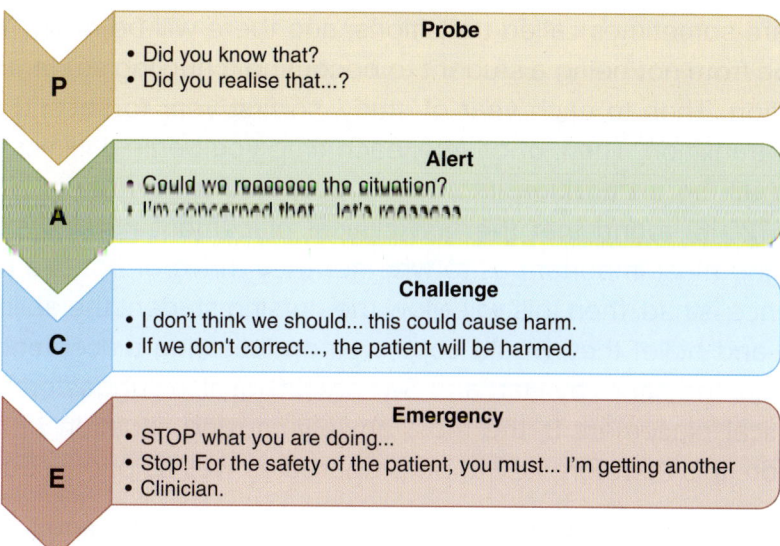

Fig. 9.2   Graded assertiveness.

The key is to tactfully employ assertive communication, prioritising what's right safely over the ideas and beliefs of others. Despite the daunting nature of this task, it's crucial to remember your primary role as a nursing student who is there to learn and gain confidence and competence.

Assertiveness should not be confused with aggression. The former is about self-respect and voicing your valid opinions, while the latter involves disrespecting others and denying them the chance to express their views. Graded assertiveness proves beneficial when team members have differing opinions about a situation or plan.

DILEMMA: I AM REALLY SHY. HOW CAN I INTEGRATE INTO THE TEAM?

Joining different teams is going to be something you will do on several occasions as a nursing student. While there will be times as a registered nurse that you may need to move to other areas to provide support and cover, this might often be only for a few hours or a day at most, so is not always as daunting as it will be as a nursing student who is joining an already established team.

These are sometimes called transitions, and there will be many. You will transition from not being a student to becoming a nursing student. That's a transition. Then to each year of study, so first year to second year is another transition. Then, of course, each time you begin a clinical placement, it will be a transition into a new area and a new team. Hart and Swenty (2016) found that the first clinical placement nursing students have is the most important as to whether they thrive or not. If a positive experience is had, then this will allow the nursing student the ability, confidence and belief they would cope well on following placements. That being said, the paper by Hart and Swenty (2016) also suggested that the first clinical placement is the most anxiety-causing situation in nursing education. It is therefore key to be prepared as well as prioritised.

The YouTube video *Advice for Nursing Students Transitioning to Nurses via ThinkTheory19* (2020) is a great resource for getting advice on transitions, with the following quote mentioning this video.

'I really struggled with transitions, especially as a nursing student, until I went to a webinar that was based on transitions in nursing student education. This webinar had several guest speakers who were able to give transition examples and advice, which really helped me in transitions. Now I am able to be moved to other areas of practice and such with no concerns. It has really helped me grow as an individual and as a nurse'.

Anonymous, newly registered nurse

DILEMMA: THERE ARE LOTS OF OTHER STUDENTS ON PLACEMENT WITH ME, AND I FEEL THE LEARNING OPPORTUNITIES ARE GIVEN TO THE OTHERS

'Preregistration nursing students must achieve set proficiencies each year. These are usually achieved while on placement: they not only

provide the evidence that you are a proficient practitioner but they are also what stipulates progression to the next year of your training. Being unable to achieve these proficiencies for whatever reason can lead some to find alternate ways to achieve this sign off. Some find ways to circumnavigate the system to achieve the result without achieving the desired skill. It is relegating the skills we are meant to have as an effective practitioner to a tick list. It doesn't give you a practiced skill and doesn't embed the purpose of the learning to build on.

I was unable to achieve one of my proficiencies on placement. Service pressures on the ward were such that I didn't manage to get it done and at the time didn't have the confidence to advocate for myself. I felt I had not experienced the skill, so I didn't feel I could have a professional conversation to get the sign off (one of the ways students achieve the proficiencies they haven't done), and there was not an opportunity to do a spoke placement (another way you can get this done).

My focus has always been on being a good and component nurse. I was not prepared to lie and find a way around it. The NMC is very clear about the standards we must achieve to proceed in our course, and skills are built upon skills, and I knew I had not achieved this. The cost was not progressing with the rest of my cohort into the next year and having to redo not only that placement but the entire practice placement module. The financial and emotional cost of this was huge; however, the benefit to my confidence that I made the right decisions and had integrity, even in the face of huge personal cost, was invaluable. During your nursing career, you will face many dilemmas. If you have high standards and practice with the small decisions, the big decisions and dilemmas will be easier to navigate'.

Anonymous nursing student

From this example, we can see there could be an issue of trust, malpractice, fraud and even gross misconduct if nursing students, indeed, along with practice supervisors and practice assessors, might sign off a proficiency that is expected to progress when, in fact, the proficiency has not been met to the appropriate and adequate standard. Although it would be difficult to gauge, this could be a problem much wider and deeper than we are aware of, as we are aware of the literature on 'failing to fail', which is where registered practitioners, for example, nurses, fail to fail their nursing students, as they lack the leadership, confidence and competence to do so, meaning we might end up having registered nurses meeting the needs of the proficiencies required to be a nurse on paper, but in practice, this might be a different case altogether.

As North et al. (2019) suggest in their literature review on the phenomenon of failing to fail nursing students, the assessment of competency of nursing students on practice placement is complex due to being carried out in often high-pressure environments, along with subjectiveness. The review found that it was key for universities and employers (such as the NHS) to be supporting supervisors and mentors to assess nursing students adequately and appropriately, for example, regular education and support on the competencies needed and the documentation style and how to complete this (North et al., 2019). North et al. (2019) also found that universities would and could overturn a decision made by a mentor and/or assessor, which led to a decline in trust, confidence and ability.

'Do you report a placement to your university for not giving you learning opportunities, leaving you alone for long periods, not doing your ePAD, etc., with the risk that you have to remain there and maybe be treated worse throughout the course?'

Tayloe, third-year nursing student

DILEMMA: I AM FINDING IT REALLY DIFFICULT TO JUGGLE PLACEMENT, LIFE AND UNIVERSITY

'Financial hardship meaning I almost had to leave the course numerous times despite student finance and bursary funding. Also having to work alongside placements due to the financial hardship, meaning burnout throughout the course'.

Anonymous nursing student

Personal issues are always going to happen in life. Everything about life is fluid and ever changing, so dedicating yourself to a degree, especially in nursing, will be a challenge, as life will throw up personal issues now and then. It could be a house move, a change in job, a pregnancy, a death or an illness. These things can be totally unexpected, but some might be planned, and it will be important for you as nursing students to be able to transition through these changes with the support and advice needed to be able to carry on with your studies while these changes are occurring.

'Not being paid for clinical practice. I understand why we don't, although there have been days when I've done more work than some of the staff on that ward and got not 1 ounce of appreciation for it. We should at least get a free meal from the cafe or be allowed to use the wards milk and coffee for a drink.'

Having to pay for our uniform if we damage the one we got (for free). I say this because we had the opportunity to have three uniforms when we started the course, although throughout the 2 years, I had put on some weight, and my uniform got incredibly tight. This made me so uncomfortable when working, and a staff actually referred to me as "the big one". My confidence levels were so low after this. I looked to ordering some more, and it was so expensive. I couldn't afford, it so I've had to just work with what I've got and be uncomfortable'.

Anonymous nursing student

What is important to appreciate is that nursing education can be flexible but also has limitations in total flexibility. It might be that you need to take some time away from your studies to transition through a personal change or issue, as it is just too much to be able to deal with all at once. That is ok. Or indeed, it might be you just need some alterations to your study. In the best-case scenario, it might be that you do not need either of these and just need some advice and minimal support with a personal issue or change. What is key is that the university and placement providers you have are supportive and compassionate about your circumstances and consider how they can help and support you.

DILEMMA: I'VE NEVER ENCOUNTERED SOMEONE WHO HAS DIED

Encountering a deceased patient for the first time can be a profound and challenging experience for nursing students. But it needn't be.

Before encountering a deceased patient, it's essential to mentally prepare yourself for what you may see. Understanding that death is a natural part of the healthcare journey can help alleviate anxiety. Take the time to learn about the process of death and dying, including the physiological changes that occur. Understanding the biological aspects of death can help demystify the experience and reduce fear or anxiety. Death is a complex biological process that involves the vital functions necessary to sustain life stopping. The exact mechanisms and manifestations of death will vary depending on the specific circumstances and medical conditions involved.

It would be helpful if you familiarise yourself with the process of postmortem care within the healthcare setting. Understanding the steps that occur after a patient passes away can clarify the experience and provide a sense of control. Postmortem care, also known as after-death care or last offices, refers to the procedures and protocols followed by healthcare professionals after a patient has died. These procedures will vary depending on the healthcare setting and cultural practices. Healthcare professionals will ensure that the deceased patient is treated with respect, dignity and privacy throughout the postmortem care process. This includes closing curtains or doors to provide privacy and covering the patient's body with a clean sheet. Any medical equipment or devices that were used to provide care to the patient, such as intravenous lines, catheters or monitoring devices, will be removed from the body. Careful attention is paid to minimising any discomfort or disruption to the patient's body. The body is carefully cleaned to remove any bodily fluids, blood or other contaminants. The body is then positioned in a comfortable and dignified manner, often with the arms crossed over the chest and the eyes closed. Overall, postmortem care in the United Kingdom is conducted with professionalism, compassion and respect for the deceased patient and their loved ones, recognising the importance of honouring the individual who has passed away.

It is important to reflect on your emotions and reactions to encountering a deceased patient. It's normal to experience a range of feelings, including sadness, discomfort and even curiosity. Finding a safe space to process your emotions can facilitate coping and growth. Also, self-care is important to prioritise. Engage in activities that promote relaxation, stress relief and emotional wellbeing. It's essential for nursing students to recognise and address any lingering emotional distress or trauma through self-care strategies or professional support if needed. You should seek support from their practice assessors, practice supervisors or other experienced nurses before and after encountering a deceased patient. Discussing your feelings and concerns with a trusted mentor can provide reassurance and guidance.

DILEMMA: I MADE A MEDICATION ERROR. CAN I STILL JOIN THE NMC REGISTER?

Encountering a medication error during a clinical placement can be a deeply distressing experience for nursing students. It's crucial to recognise that errors, while regrettable, are a reality of healthcare practice, and they present valuable opportunities for learning and growth. In the event of a medication error, the most immediate concern is ensuring the safety and wellbeing of the patient. Nursing students should promptly assess the patient's condition and notify the appropriate healthcare professionals, such as the responsible doctor or senior nurse, of the error. Open and honest communication is essential, as transparency fosters trust and collaboration within the healthcare team. It's vital for nursing students to take responsibility for their actions (duty of candour is about openness and honesty when things go wrong) and actively participate in the error management process. This includes documenting the error accurately and comprehensively, adhering to institutional protocols for incident reporting and implementing corrective measures to mitigate any potential harm to the patient. Moreover, nursing students should prioritise self-reflection and self-care in the aftermath of a medication error. Additionally, engaging in debriefing sessions or reflective exercises can help you process your feelings, identify areas for improvement and reinforce your commitment to patient safety. Ultimately, while medication errors are undoubtedly concerning, they serve as valuable learning experiences that contribute to the development of competent and conscientious healthcare professionals. By approaching errors with humility, accountability and a commitment to continuous improvement, nursing students can transform adverse events into opportunities for personal and professional growth.

NMC

THE NMC SAYS

14 Be open and candid with all service users about all aspects of care and treatment, including when any mistakes or harm have taken place.

DILEMMA: I HAVE A DISABILITY. HOW DO I MANAGE THIS ON PLACEMENT?

BROKEN CRAYONS

'Cliché as it may sound, the expression "broken crayons can still colour" applies to many people's lives everywhere. From a personal standpoint, I elaborate on the applicability of this expression. As a child, and even as I grew into adulthood, I was always told that I was slow, which is why I did not understand "simple" things that others understood. I heard this so often that it became a natural part of my existence, and I began to believe in the narrative. For numerous years, I clung to this and told myself I could not do or achieve certain things because I was slow. I even made sure that I chose a career involving no numeric calculations and no complicated diagrams that I may not understand. I became a dental nurse and loved my job. After that, I worked as an oral health educator and dental radiographer. I struggled, as I literally did not know my left from my right. I found coping mechanisms. For example, I have the letters "L" and "R", which represent left and right, respectively, pasted on the X-ray machine. I always had to study longer than average to understand what an author was trying to convey precisely. I also had to read tiny portions at a time and take frequent breaks between reading and studying to stop the letters from jumping to the next line and becoming jumbled.

I constantly craved to improve my knowledge base and educational qualifications, but I felt I needed to improve. I always want to be a nurse. I was always a nurse but wanted to be a mental health nurse. My journey to study mental health nursing was not linear. However, I have had a long-term plan. I began my first degree in 2018. I engaged in public health and health promotion. During this time, my mentor took a keen interest in me and asked whether I had a learning disability. I was not aware of the existing learning disabilities because, where I grew up, it was either you were brilliant or you were slow. When she mentioned dyslexia, I could not even spell the word to go and research it. It was Google Assistant that helped me with it. While writing this entry, I used my dictionary to spell the words. My question is, who decided to spell that word like that? It is hard enough using phonetics, but spelling it ... Oh well ... back to the story; I sometimes tend to wander.

So I went private. I was 35 years old when I was diagnosed with dyslexia, dysgraphia and dyscalculia.

Let me explain what they are.
1. Dyslexia is a learning disability that affects the abilities required for precise and fluid word reading and spelling.
2. Dysgraphia, a component of a learning disability or a sign of neurological illness, is the inability to write clearly.
3. Dyscalculia is a specific and enduring problem of number comprehension that can cause a wide range of issues in mathematics.

After the diagnosis, I received assistance. My favourite type of assistance was a ruler that I moved line by line while reading. In addition, using green paper to print my reading makes it easier to calm the words.

Continued

I am now a final-year nursing student, and my diagnosis has caused me to struggle with nursing. My weaknesses are anatomy, physiology and drug calculations. It is a struggle, but it does not deter my determination. I ensure that I use more time for planning and studying. Consistency is the key to me. The other thing is that, though I struggled, I received 90% in anatomy and physiology and consistently scored 100% in my final drug calculation exam. I need more time than an average person.

The big question is: what support exists for neurodivergent nurses in healthcare? I am anxious about it. Will I be given permission or help during the drug round as the university gives me time to complete my exam? Can I use my software and install it on computers? Will my colleagues be in oblivion like I was when I heard about learning disabilities? Although these questions boggle my mind, I am just focusing on my plan to graduate.

If you are a neurodivergent student on a nursing or any other educational journey, please do not give up or seek help. According to society's standards, you may be broken. However, being broken does not equate to uselessness. "Broken crayons still colour".

Recognising that one is not alone in confronting these challenges is crucial. Many individuals with neurodivergent conditions have forged successful careers in healthcare and other fields. The support and accommodation available for neurodivergent nurses and healthcare professionals can vary depending on the location and workplace. However, some resources and strategies can empower people to thrive in their careers. University support is vital; continue working closely with your university's disability support services for tailored accommodations such as additional time for exams. In your future workplace, don't hesitate to communicate with your employer about your neurodivergent conditions, as many workplaces have policies to provide necessary accommodations. Self-advocacy is critical; take a proactive approach in seeking support and maintaining open communication with supervisors and colleagues. Consider joining professional organisations, as they offer valuable resources and

> networking opportunities. Seeking mentorship from experienced nurses can provide essential guidance, and pursuing further education or certifications can enhance your skills. Your journey is a powerful reminder that everyone possesses unique strengths and capabilities, regardless of their challenges. Your determination and resilience have already led to remarkable academic achievements, and there's no doubt that you will make a significant impact as a mental health nurse. Maintain your determination, actively seek the support you require and always remember that "broken crayons still colour".
>
> **Sonney Atkinson, nursing student**

Navigating a clinical placement with a disability can present unique challenges for nursing students, but with careful planning, communication and support, it is entirely manageable. The first step is to assess your specific needs and requirements related to your disability. Consider how it may impact your mobility, communication or ability to perform certain tasks related to patient care. Once you have a clear understanding of your needs, it's essential to communicate openly and proactively with the clinical placement staff. Discuss any accommodations or adjustments that may be necessary to ensure your safety, comfort and ability to fulfil your duties effectively.

In many cases, healthcare institutions are legally obligated to provide reasonable accommodations for individuals with disabilities under anti-discrimination laws such as the Equality Act 2010. These accommodations may include physical modifications to the clinical environment, such as wheelchair ramps or accessible restrooms, as well as additional support from colleagues or assistive technologies to facilitate communication or task completion. By advocating for your needs and rights, you can help ensure that the necessary accommodations are in place to support your success on placement.

Most importantly, embrace your unique perspective and experiences as a nursing student with a disability. Your lived experience can contribute valuable insights and empathy to your practice as a healthcare professional. By embracing diversity and inclusion in healthcare settings, you can help foster a culture of respect, understanding and support for individuals with disabilities and enhance the quality of care for all patients.

DILEMMA: I GOT NEGATIVE FEEDBACK. WHAT SHOULD I DO?

'One of the biggest dilemmas for me which has been throughout my training is for nursing staff to support me to sign off proficiencies. There are a few reasons why this has been a dilemma.

1. *Nurses just don't have the time to give us on shift. We follow nurses round and learn as we watch; they struggle to be able to give us time to talk us through and give us quality learning time.*
2. *Some of the nurses don't understand the proficiencies or don't have the skill themselves. Under the new standards for nurses, we have now been given several new clinical skills to complete such as venipuncture, cannulation, ECG and chest auscultation. This, then, was difficult to find staff who was trained, and you weren't under their supervision to train you and then be able to keep this skill up by doing it over and over'.*

Amy Hnatyszyn, third-year nursing student

There will be times that you might receive feedback that you were not expecting or that you do not agree with. There will be times also that you receive 'negative' feedback. As registrants assessing and supervising nursing students, giving the appropriate and authentic feedback that is needed is a required part of signing a nursing student off or, indeed, not. It is vital that health and social care has a workforce that is capable and competent, so it will, unfortunately, be appropriate to sometimes give negative feedback to someone or indeed even fail them on their practice placement experience, as they have not met the required needs of the educational course.

Receiving such feedback might be difficult to digest, but, like another example in this chapter where we advise on raising concerns about practice, it is important to get this feedback so you can realise and appreciate where things might have gone wrong and, more importantly, how to improve and change them. Negative feedback, and even the extreme of failing a placement, does not mean you have failed as a nursing student or a future nurse. Failing is an important part of life.

When we fail at things It does not mean we can't then go on to success. The important thing to do will be to reflect. Reflection will allow you to see where you can alter and amend. Take the time to reflect on the negative feedback you have received and then set goals to overcome this or do this better the next opportunity you can. It might mean you change your approach, or you spend time learning about an aspect you weren't too sure about; you might even want to educate yourself on the element you failed or got negative feedback on. Take the time to work on this, and then it will be your opportunity to improve and grow moving forward. Barksby et al. (2015) have a new model of reflection for clinical practice called the REFLECT model, which is a helpful way to reflect on many situations.

The model comprises seven stages:

R: RECALL the events (stage 1): Give a brief overview of the situation upon which you are reflecting. This should consist of the facts, a description of what happened.

E: EXAMINE your responses (stage 2): Discuss your thoughts and actions at the time of the incident upon which you are reflecting.

F: Acknowledge FEELINGS (stage 3): Highlight any feelings you experienced at the time of the situation upon which you are reflecting.

L: LEARN from the experience (stage 4): Highlight what you have learned from the situation.

E: EXPLORE options (stage 5): Discuss options for the future if you were to encounter a similar situation.

C: CREATE a plan of action (stage 6): Create a plan for the future. This can be for future theoretical learning or action.

T: Set TIMESCALE (stage 7): Set a time by which the plan outlined in stage 6 will be complete.

Barksby et al. (2015)

DILEMMA: MY PLACEMENT IS OFFICE BASED; THERE ISN'T MUCH PATIENT CONTACT OR CLINICAL SKILLS TO DO ... WHAT SHOULD I DO?_

It is key that nursing students along with their supervisors and assessors are taking the steps that are necessary to ensure proficiencies are met and opportunities to do so are sought, created and facilitated. This is to ensure the nursing students registering with the NMC are safe and effective practitioners at the point of registration with the NMC as well as professional and responsible practitioners (NMC, 2023).

It could be that they seek the opportunity to visit alternative or linked placement areas; for example, if the placement area is community nursing, they might be able to link to the practice nurse in the surgery, or if a surgical ward placement, the nursing student is able to attend theatre or recovery to see the patient journey in more depth and detail, and also allow proficiencies to be considered in those areas. This must be considered with caution, though, as one visit for 1 day to an area might not give the longevity and exposure needed to be competent in a said proficiency, taking us back to the issue in question.

DILEMMA: MY PRACTICE ASSESSOR/SUPERVISOR IS HOSTILE TOWARDS ME. WHAT SHOULD I DO?_

'I sometimes find it difficult to work with members of staff such as healthcare support workers, as I find that they look down upon nursing students'.

Anonymous nursing student

Encountering inappropriate or unprofessional behaviour during your nursing studies can be disheartening and challenging to navigate. It's important to recognise that you deserve respect and support, and there are steps you can take to address these situations effectively. Firstly, it's essential not to internalise negative comments or perceptions of failure. Remember, you are investing in your education and skill development, and your worth is not defined by anyone else's opinion. If you feel your clinical skills are lacking, it's important to question whether you've received adequate training and support from your instructors.

'A nurse said to me once, "I hate having a student, no offence". This made me feel like a burden on her for the rest of the day. I felt like I couldn't ask questions, and I felt generally uncomfortable'.

Anonymous nursing student

Seeking support and advice is crucial when faced with unprofessional behaviour. Don't hesitate to reach out to your academic advisors, wellbeing advisers, student unions or the trade unions for assistance. If you don't receive the support you need from one source, escalate the matter until you find the right person who can provide guidance and assistance.

Building a strong support network around you is also vital. Talk to your family and friends about your challenges, and ask for their moral support. Additionally, accessing professional help, such as counselling services offered by your university or your GP, can provide valuable support in managing stress and navigating difficult situations.

Finally, learning from real-life case studies can provide valuable insights into how to address and overcome challenges related to unprofessional behaviour, as this can help you navigate these situations effectively and develop strategies for managing similar challenges in the future. Remember, you are not alone, and there are resources and people available to support you through these difficult times.

COMMUNICATION: A KEY THEME IN ALL DILEMMA RESPONSES

Communication is a key skill in many sectors of employment and in life in general. Communication in healthcare and, in particular, nursing, is a vital skill, ability and necessity to be able to practise efficiently and effectively. Without communication, care can go wrong, and we have unfortunately seen this in the well-known cases such as the Mid Staffordshire scandal (Holmes, 2013), which revealed widespread failures in patient care and safety. Investigations found systemic issues that included inadequate staffing levels, substandard patient care and a culture focused on meeting targets rather than patient welfare. Communication is not always easy or even as simple as some might suggest it is. There can be barriers for several reasons, such as spoken language or, indeed, lack of spoken language, for example, if someone has a speech impairment, but there can be other reasons such as hierarchy, lack of respect and lack of openness, meaning people don't communicate.

Within the NMC Code (2023), section 7 of the 'practice effectively' standard is to communicate clearly, which talks about the importance of adapting communication to suit the situation, for example, communication in a way people understand, using verbal and nonverbal communication and to regularly check back while communicating that the people you are communicating to are understanding you so that if not, you can go back over things.

NMC

THE NMC SAYS

7   Communicate clearly.

To achieve this, you must:

7.1 Use terms that people in your care, colleagues and the public can understand.

7.2 Take reasonable steps to meet people's language and communication needs, providing, wherever possible, assistance to those who need help to communicate their own or other people's needs.

7.3 Use a range of verbal and non-verbal communication methods, and consider cultural sensitivities, to better understand and respond to people's personal and health needs.

7.4 Check people's understanding from time to time to keep misunderstanding or mistakes to a minimum.

7.5 Be able to communicate clearly and effectively in English.

The code then goes into section 8, also within the same standard, 'practice effectively', which is about working cooperatively. This is key in communication, as communication is key to working cooperatively.

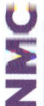

THE NMC SAYS

8.2 Maintain effective communication with colleagues.

'Some wards treat you as a healthcare assistant. I spent 14 weeks on a ward where every shift, I would be teamed up with healthcare assistants to start washes, breakfast, observations, etc. The sister and some of the nurses were way too intimidating to approach about this. As my course is 2 years, it's critical to learn as much as possible in the nursing area, as placements are less frequent but longer'.

Anonymous nursing student

The key thing when on a clinical practice placement is to be able to recognise a learning opportunity, or what could be one, versus being seen as a set of hands. This is an area that really requires you as a nursing student to be aware of your requirements for registration as a nurse and to pass your nursing education course.

There are going to be times during clinical placements, particularly on hospital wards, for example, where you must carry out several roles and responsibilities that you might deem as someone else's job, a task rather than a learning opportunity or, indeed, not relevant or appropriate to you as a nursing student. However, hopefully from your nursing education so far, you can appreciate what nursing is and is not. So, for example, Webster (2022) talks about getting the fundamentals of nursing right before considering or focusing on some of the skills and competencies, for example, chest auscultation and ECG interpretation. Someone's personal hygiene maintenance is just as important as their medication compliance, so if you are assisting a person to have a meal who is perhaps struggling with dexterity or functionality, this is a learning experience and will be able to allow you the ability to take part in assessment and possible referral if further assessment or support is needed. On the other hand, if you are being asked to hand out meals three times a day every day because someone is off sick while you are missing out on vital learning opportunities, this is not appropriate.

Cameron and Parkinson (2023) looked at nursing students who also worked as healthcare support workers in their spare time, and what will be key for you as a nursing student is to know which 'hat' you are wearing at any one time so you are in the area as a nursing student or as a healthcare assistant, and then consider the tasks being asked of you before using communication skills and abilities to converse with someone appropriate about your feelings and thoughts. If you feel you are missing out on a vital learning experience or opportunity, it is key to communicate this by reminding the teams you are working with the capacity you are there in as a nursing student, not as a member of staff such as a healthcare assistant.

CONCLUSION

It is clear from this chapter, and thanks to the amazing nursing student quotes, that nursing can be a challenging and testing degree, particularly regarding practice placements. There will be many dilemmas you face during your range of practice placements, and it will be key for you to see the learning opportunities when they arise but remain confident to challenge when you are missing out on learning experience and exposure.

During challenging times, take time to consider your options, and the most important thing will be to seek support and guidance if you feel you can't approach such challenges alone. This support might be from peers, university staff, practice placement staff or even trade union support or guidance, and remember, if one approach is not appropriate or agreed upon by you, don't worry about seeking further advice from another source. There will be times when bias comes into play, and this is when it might be more appropriate to seek support from an impartial source such as a trade union.

The key theme for this chapter is communication. It is about your ability and confidence to communicate effectively and professionally to ensure you can challenge and question when things go either wrong or don't seem to be right.

This chapter has exposed you to the possible wealth of dilemmas you might come across in your time as a nursing student, but we also hope you don't have a negative experience. You might not experience any of these or, indeed, all of these, but it is key you allow your studies to be the best you can, and to do this, you must ensure you get the most from your practice placements and challenges and overcoming such times, so you can thrive and really have a great time as a nursing student.

Space for reader's own reflection:

_____

_____

_____

_____

_____

_____

_____

_____

_____

_____

_____

_____

_____

_____

_____

_____

_____

REFERENCES

Advice for Nursing Students Transitioning to Nurses via ThinkTheory19. 2020. YouTube video, added by Brian Webster [Online]. https://youtu.be/jvoFbN429A4?si=ZzHJkl Cj3clWdygu [Accessed February 2025]

Barksby, J., Butcher, N., Whysall, A., 2015. A new model of reflection for clinical practice. Nurs. Times 111 (34-35), 21–23.

Bickhoff, L., Sinclair, P.M., Levett-Jones, T., 2017. Moral courage in undergraduate nursing students: A literature review. Collegian. 24 (1), 71–83. https://doi.org/10.1016/j.colegn.2015.08.002

Cameron, S., Parkinson, B., 2023. Nursing students' experiences of working as healthcare support workers. Nurs. Stand. 38 (5), 32–37. https://doi.org/10.7748/ns.2023.e11892

Cant, R., Ryan, C., Hughes, L., Luders, E., Cooper, S., 2021. What helps, what hinders? Undergraduate nursing students' perceptions of clinical placements based on a thematic synthesis of literature. SAGE Open Nurs. 7, 23779608211035845. doi:10.1177/23779608211035845

Carey, T., Mullan, R., 2004. What is Socratic questioning? Psychother. Theory Res. Pract. Train. 41 (3), 217–226. https://doi.org/10.1037/0033-3204.41.3.217

Clarke-Romain, B., 2023. Supporting nurses in acute and emergency care settings to speak up. Emergency Nurse. https://doi.org/10.7748/en.2023.e2162

Collins. 2023. Definition of dilemma [Online]. https://www.collinsdictionary.com/dictionary/english/dilemma [Accessed September 2023]

Hart, J.A., Swenty, C.F., 2016. Understanding Transitions to Promote Student Success: A Concept Analysis. Nurs. Forum (Hillsdale) [Online] 51 (3), 180–185.

Holmes. 2013. Mid Staffordshire scandal highlights NHS cultural crisis [Online]. https://www.thelancet.com/journals/lancet/article/PIIS0140-6736(13)60264-0/fulltext

Kalánková, D., Bartoníčková, D., Kirwan, M., Gurková, E., Žiaková, K., Košútová, D. 2021. Undergraduate nursing students' experiences of rationed nursing care – A qualitative study. Nurse Educ. Today 97, 104724. doi:10.1016/j.nedt.2020.104724

North, H., Kennedy, M., Wray, J., 2019. Are mentors failing to fail underperforming student nurses? An integrative literature review. Br. J. Nurs. [Online] 28 (4), 250–255.

NHS England and NHS Improvement. 2019. Nursing and midwifery e-rostering: A good practice guide [Online] https://www.england.nhs.uk/wp-content/uploads/2020/08/20190903_UPDATED_Nursing_Midwifery_E-Rostering_Guidance_September_2019.pdf [Accessed October 29, 2023]

Nursing and Midwifery Council (NMC). 2023. The Code [Online]. https://www.nmc.org.uk/standards/code/read-the-code-online/ [Accessed September 2023]

Nursing and Midwifery Council. 2020. Delegation [Online]. https://www.nmc.org.uk/standards/code/code-in-action/delegation/ [Accessed September 2023]

Webster. 2022. Fundamentals of nursing care [Online]. https://rcni.com/nursing-standard/students/clinical-placements/fundamentals-of-nursing-care-how-to-get-them-right-181036

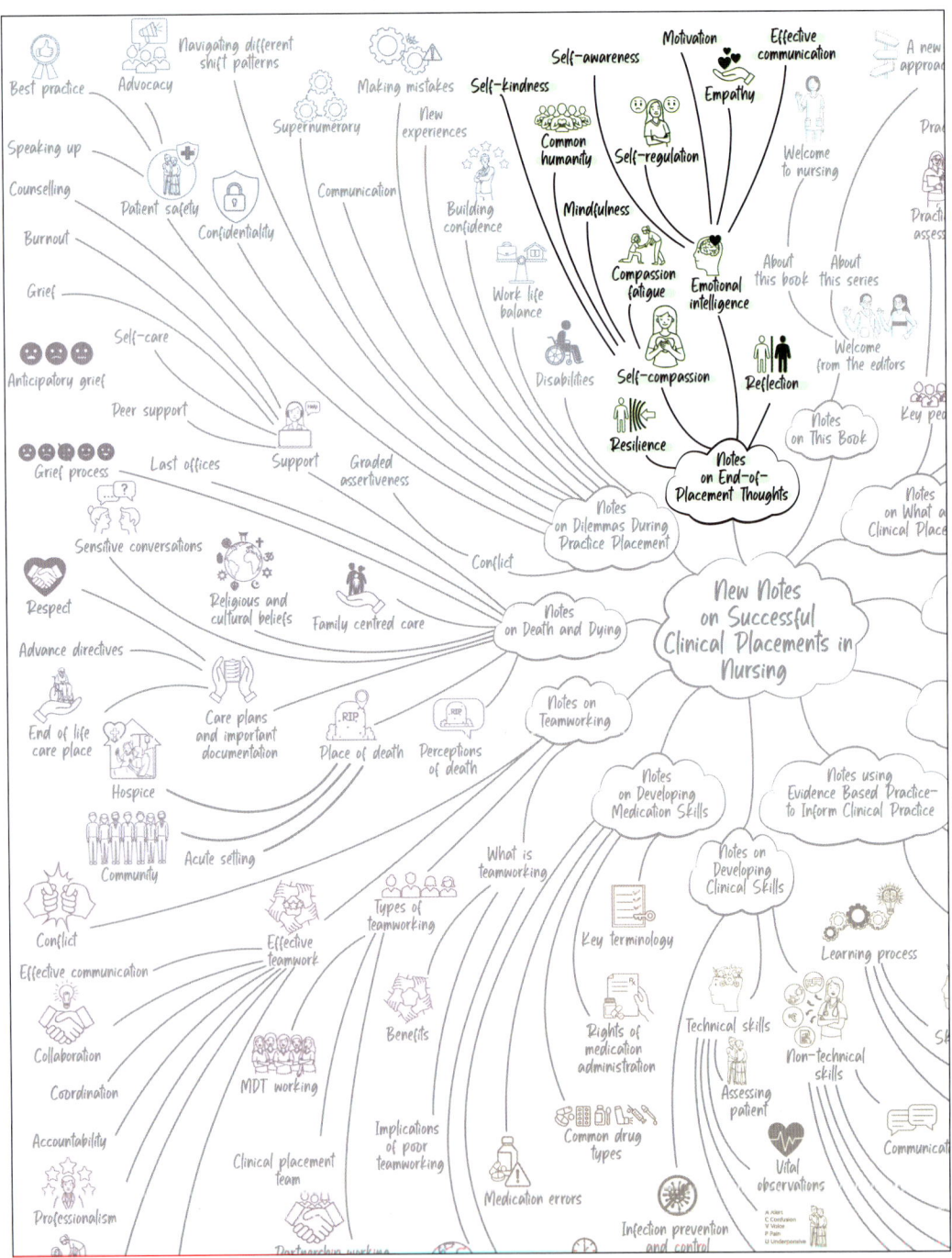

Best practice
Advocacy
Navigating different shift patterns
Making mistakes
Self-awareness
Motivation
Effective communication
A new approach

Speaking up
Supernumerary
New experiences
Self-kindness
Empathy
Pra

Counselling
Communication
Common humanity
Self-regulation
Welcome to nursing
Practi assess

Patient safety
Confidentiality
Building confidence
Mindfulness

Burnout
Work life balance
Compassion fatigue
Emotional intelligence
About this book
About this series

Grief
Disabilities
Welcome from the editors

Self-care
Self-compassion
Reflection

Anticipatory grief
Peer support
Support
Graded assertiveness
Resilience
Notes on End-of-Placement Thoughts
Notes on This Book
Key pe

Grief process
Last offices

Sensitive conversations
Conflict
Notes on Dilemmas During Practice Placement
Notes on What a Clinical Place

Respect
Religious and cultural beliefs
Family centred care
Notes on Death and Dying

Advance directives
New Notes on Successful Clinical Placements in Nursing

End of life care place
Care plans and important documentation
Place of death
Perceptions of death
Notes on Teamworking

Hospice

Acute setting
What is teamworking
Notes on Developing Medication Skills
Notes using Evidence Based Practice to Inform Clinical Practice

Community
Types of teamworking
Notes on Developing Clinical Skills

Conflict
Effective teamwork
Key terminology
Learning process

Effective communication
Benefits
Rights of medication administration
Technical skills
S

Collaboration
MDT working
Non-technical skills
Communicat

Coordination
Implications of poor teamworking
Common drug types
Assessing patient

Accountability
Clinical placement team
Medication errors
Vital observations

Professionalism
Partnership working
Infection prevention and control

A Allen
C Coolsaeen
V Voice
P Pain
U Underpinnine

NOTES ON END-OF-PLACEMENT THOUGHTS

Simon James (he/him) ■ **Natalie Elliott (she/her)**

INTRODUCTION

Once clinical placement has been completed, learning doesn't just end there. In fact, some people may argue that this is where learning truly begins. This is where nursing students should consider what they have learned, not just in relation to clinical skills but also thinking about the softer skills learned, such as conflict resolution and communicating with people.

At the heart of this chapter lies a profound recognition: clinical placements serve as more than mere training grounds for mastering technical skills; they are crucibles for the development of holistic nursing professionals. Throughout their placements, nursing students will be exposed not only to the intricacies of patient care but also to the challenge of confronting their own beliefs, values and capabilities.

Central to this exploration are four key themes that underpin the journey of self-discovery: self-compassion, emotional intelligence, resilience and reflection. These themes interweave throughout the fabric of clinical practice, guiding nursing students as they navigate the highs and lows of their experiences. These areas of learning will help make the most of learning opportunities, not only while on placement but for placements to come. It will also serve as a journey that transcends the boundaries of clinical practice and shapes the essence of compassionate nursing care.

SELF-COMPASSION

Self-compassion involves treating oneself with kindness, understanding and support during times of failure, inadequacy or suffering. For nursing students who often face intense academic pressures and emotionally challenging clinical experiences, self-compassion is crucial for maintaining emotional health and resilience.

Understanding self-compassion

'Self-compassion refers to being supportive toward oneself when experiencing suffering or pain—be it caused by personal mistakes and inadequacies or external life challenges' (Neff, 2023). It is the practice of extending compassion to oneself in instances of perceived inadequacy, failure or general suffering. It encompasses self-kindness, common humanity and mindfulness.

Self-kindness

Self-kindness is a crucial aspect of self-compassion, involving treating oneself with the same care, understanding and support as one would offer to our patients. For nursing students, who often face high levels of stress and sometimes self-imposed pressure, practising self-kindness can foster a healthier and more sustainable approach to both personal and professional life.

'As a student nurse, it is easy to be tough on ourselves. It can seem overwhelming on occasion, and you could be feeling "imposter syndrome". When I see my negative thoughts taking over, I count backwards from five to get my mind to stop. This is when I try to be kinder to myself by reflecting on what I've already accomplished. Self-compassion is essential; we as student nurses are compassionate and understanding with our patients. So why can't we be kinder towards ourselves? We need to channel our compassion and kindness inwardly and have more faith in our own capabilities'.

Kim Emberlin, student nurse

In contrast, self-judgement is the act of judging oneself (Linnett & Kibowski, 2020). It consists of forming opinions on your own performances and assigning meanings to those opinions which can produce feelings of insecurity, self-doubt, low self-worth, low self-esteem and not being good enough. If unrecognised and left to fester, these can lead to anxiety, anger and depression. At times, we can be our own worst enemies and harshest critics.

These negative thoughts and emotions could lead to feelings of being lost and isolated. With all the rigours involved within your course, it's not inconceivable that some of us will need a little more support than others. The majority of nursing students commencing their training will have just or recently left the school system. At this point, these young adults are undergoing major transitions in their own lives, from potentially not having to make decisions to the associated responsibilities of adulthood such as moving home, learning how to budget and survive on their own (Choo & Marszalek, 2019). This can lead to emotional distress; however, due to the perceived stigma of admitting any struggles, young adults are less likely to seek help. Always talk to your family, friends or whoever you feel comfortable confiding in. The nursing degree can be a rollercoaster of emotions—don't bottle it up!

It is easy to feel angry or remorseful at things you cannot do; instead, embrace your shortcomings and change your perspective. Accepting flaws and understanding that we are not all perfect allow us to be kinder to ourselves when considering our own limitations (Neff, 2023). Many nursing students can be overly critical of their own performance. You are not expected to know everything straight away ... so remember, do your best, but don't beat yourself about things you can't do ... yet!

 'Quite often, I would receive placement feedback from practice assessors and practice supervisors that I was too hard on myself and that I need to be kinder to myself. This often came from a place where I wanted to do my best for my patients. I tried to remind myself that I can't know everything, and that is okay'.

Natalie Elliott, RN

By integrating self-kindness into their lives, nursing students can create a foundation of emotional resilience, mental wellbeing and professional effectiveness. This practice not only benefits their personal health but also enhances their ability to provide compassionate care to others.

Common humanity

Common humanity is another key component of self-compassion that involves recognising that suffering and personal shortcomings are part of the universal human experience (Dreisoerner et al., 2021). For nursing students, understanding and embracing common humanity can foster a sense of connectedness, reduce feelings of isolation and enhance overall wellbeing.

Everyone learns in different ways, and we all have our strengths and weaknesses. Instead of focusing on the negatives, it's important to celebrate the wins and the positives, however small or insignificant they may feel. Creating an inclusive environment is something we can all be a part of.

'As a third-year part-time student, I was given the task to deliver a presentation detailing the knowledge and skills I had gained from my ongoing placement to my current employers. This task was set as part of my in-point assessment, which was to incorporate teaching and learning. I prepared a PowerPoint informing my audience of what the presentation would cover, and I had notes prepared. Although at the time, I felt relatively confident, this was the first presentation I had delivered face to face due to the restrictions of Covid and distance learning.

During my presentation nerves took over, I was very conscious of continuously referring to my notes and reading from the PowerPoint, which consequently led to missing valid information. Although some questions were asked at the end, and I was able to answer them confidently and without referring, I was very disappointed I did not cover the whole content prepared.

Feedback from the audience was very positive; they felt they had learnt from the information delivered and would implement it into

> *practice. While the feedback was positive, on reflection, I personally feel that more preparation and practice could have enhanced my performance'.*
>
> **Della Davies, student nurse**

Every student sets out with the intention of attaining the best possible grades during their course. However, the emotional stress this can generate can be detrimental and, in some cases, destructive (Neff, 2023). During the pursuit of perfection, it can be easy to focus on the mistakes or the shortcomings, and this is where self-criticism and self-judgement can creep in (Linnett & Kibowski, 2020).

> *'I recently had a setback when I received an essay result, showing that I hadn't passed. When I first saw my grade, I had a mix of emotions. Firstly, I felt an urge of panic, and I began to doubt that I could pass my last year at university. I kept reflecting on my mistakes that continued over a few days and found myself becoming stressed and evoking feelings of sadness.*
>
> *I confided in other students in my cohort, where there is an excellent support network, and one student pointed out that one unsuccessful essay does not define what I am worth as a person and to reflect on my academic success over the last 3 years. I was told to use my emotions and experience to bounce back, learn and grow to succeed. Having the support and after a discussion with my academic tutor, I was able to see where I needed to improve, I was able to think positively and I became motivated to learn from my errors.*
>
> *I reached out to the academic success team for guidance, and they discussed with me what I needed to cover to pass my resistance. There were plenty of resources and support available which helped me to stay on track. Mistakes are a natural part of a learning process that enables us to learn and become better'.*
>
> **Carly Glover, student nurse**

By embracing common humanity, nursing students can build stronger connections with their peers, patients and themselves. This understanding fosters a supportive and empathetic environment, enhancing both personal wellbeing and professional effectiveness.

Mindfulness

Mindfulness, stemming from Buddhism, is a skill which involves being aware of what is happening in the then and now of a situation (Dreisoerneer et al., 2021). However, there is no requirement to add any elements of spirituality or religion. Mindfulness is intended to make you take more notice and improve your awareness of your own mind, body and surroundings (Murphy & Shelley, 2019). For nursing students, cultivating mindfulness can enhance emotional regulation, reduce stress and improve overall wellbeing, which are essential for both personal and professional development. If you feel like you are running on autopilot, or your thought process keeps wandering in a different direction, then that indicates you need to work on your mindfulness (Murphy & Shelley, 2019).

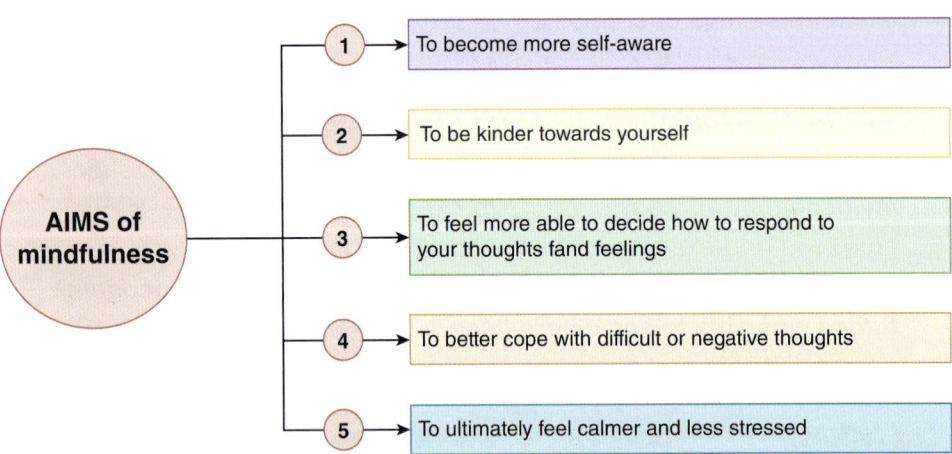

By incorporating mindfulness into their daily lives, nursing students can enhance their ability to manage stress, improve patient care and foster emotional wellbeing. Mindfulness not only benefits personal health but also cultivates a compassionate and focused approach to professional practice. Recognising the value of being present in the moment can transform both the personal and professional experiences of nursing students.

Importance of self-compassion

'Self-compassion should not be seen as an indulgence nor an approach that is anything less than focused on the betterment of patient care. Evidence is clear that healthcare staff members who prioritise their own wellbeing are subsequently better at supporting the wellbeing of their colleagues and also more able to provide compassionate care to patients. As there is an equally compelling and growing body of evidence to support the beneficial clinical outcomes for patients who believe they have been treated with kindness and compassion, it is obvious that self-compassion should be prioritised, role modelled and encouraged by placement teams and all those who assess and supervise students'.

Dr Sarah Tobin, RGN, RMN, Lecturer in Adult Nursing

The importance of self-compassion cannot be underestimated. Work/life balance is not only achievable but vital in order to prioritise your own health and wellbeing as a nursing student. It does not always automatically fall into place, and sometimes you have to make choices and put things in order of necessity. Being kind to yourself, switching off, spending time with family friends or just grabbing a long overdue coffee with a friend is the lifeline that can help to stay focused and maintain a positive mindset.

We may spend the majority of our time trying to cater to other's needs, and we sometimes forget to be kind to ourselves. We focus on promoting lifestyle changes (including consuming a healthier diet, exercising and relaxation techniques) to help patients improve their emotional wellbeing; however, we don't always remember to manage our own holistic health that well. Nurses and nursing students need to be kinder to each other and themselves in order to maintain and nurture their compassion levels.

Are you good at being self-compassionate? How do you practise this?

_____

_____

_____

_____

_____

Compassion fatigue and burnout

Mental health, along with physical health, can suffer if we do not practice self-compassion, which, unfortunately, can lead to issues at home and at work. Burnout is a very real concept and realisation in the nursing profession. Similar to burnout, compassion fatigue can occur if we give too much and don't give ourselves the time to unwind and relax. While nursing is an all-consuming but highly rewarding profession, it absorbs a lot of compassion, so we absolutely need to show some to ourselves! The problem with compassion fatigue and, similarly, burnout, is that all aspects of life can be affected.

Some of the signs to look out for are:

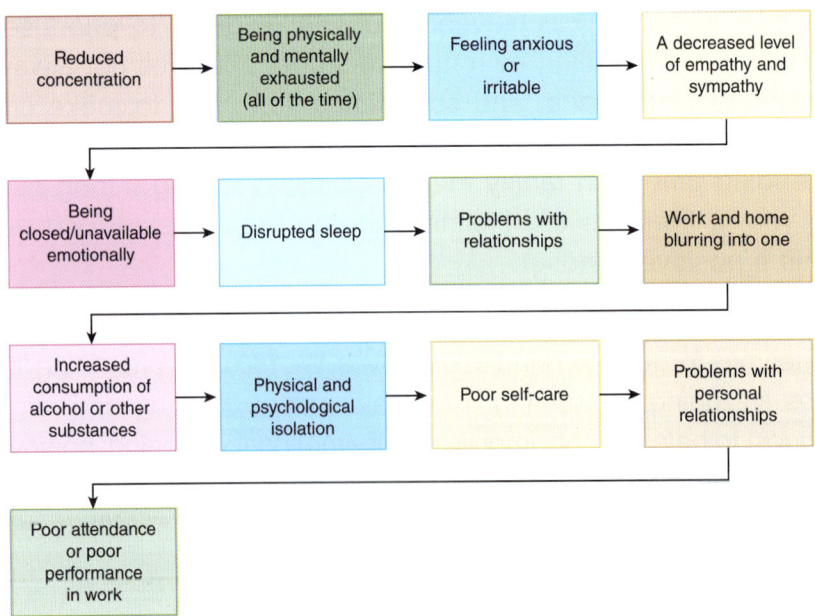

Strategies for developing self-compassion

It is important to remember that you are most definitely not a robot! Sometimes it may seem nurses and nursing students struggle to even stop for a toilet break due to the demands of our role. However, we are only human and do get tired; we can become emotional and feel hungry, and yes, we also need a bathroom break occasionally. Nurses have these needs, so it's not such a far-fetched idea that student nurses also have these requirements. In the roles we undertake, we need to look after those under our care, so we should be looking after ourselves too! Yes ... you may feel guilty for not being able to perform 10 tasks at the same time; however, rushing around leads to mistakes. Keep reminding yourself that the Nursing and Midwifery Council (NMC) code requires us to practise effectively and safely.

NMC

THE NMC SAYS

Preserve safety:

16.3 Tell someone in authority at the first reasonable opportunity if you experience problems that may prevent you working within the code or other national standards, taking prompt action to tackle the causes of concern if you can (Nursing and Midwifery Council, 2018).

19.2 Take account of current evidence, knowledge and developments in reducing mistakes and the effect of them and the impact of human factors and system failures (Nursing and Midwifery Council, 2018).

Self-care

Better self-care is the foundation of self-compassion. Sometimes it's necessary to be honest about where we are in our lives and the priorities we have at that time. Wherever you look, whether it be in books or through the media, work/life balance is important. We all have lives outside our career, and to make the most of 'work and play', we sometimes need to identify the draining elements. Many professionals have other life stresses to deal with, so finding that equilibrium where both areas flourish is vital.

'Although I like to push myself hard in work, I am a huge advocate of self-care and trying to find the little wins. The nursing degree is a very tough course, and you will be pushed to your emotional limits and, in some instances, your physical ones. You will inevitably identify your "triggers" and then work out and develop coping mechanisms. Once you feel on top of everything, it's time to find your "shimmer" and, most importantly, your "glimmer". You begin to shimmer when things are going right and you feel comfortable. Your glimmer is when your brain notices all the good little things. These glimmers will make you feel happy, feel at peace, bring you joy and make you feel grateful for where you are in life. Nursing can be demanding but really rewarding too. I can't stress enough the importance of taking time for yourself to find the things that give you a boost and get you smiling and loving life. So ... what are you waiting for ... .go find YOUR glimmer!!!!'

Simon James, RN,
national lymphoedema specialist practitioner

Take a moment to think about a recent experience. Can you identify any moments of 'shimmer' or 'glimmer'?

_____

_____

_____

_____

_____

_____

Switching off

In today's digital age, the constant connectivity afforded by technology can lead to information overload and increased stress levels, making it crucial to periodically switch off from digital devices. For nursing students, taking breaks from technology is essential for maintaining mental health and wellbeing. Constant exposure to screens and social media can disrupt sleep patterns, reduce attention spans and contribute to feelings of anxiety and burnout. Regular digital detoxes can enhance overall wellbeing, improve concentration and support a healthier, more sustainable lifestyle.

'As a result of the digital revolution within healthcare and the requirement to maintain national electronic health records, especially within the NHS (NHS, 2019; Welsh Government, 2023), there is evidence of the emerging prevalence of "technostress". Technostress is an advanced form of stress that detrimentally affects physical and psychological wellbeing in the workplace, especially within the nursing profession (Boywer-Davis, 2019; Lucena et al., 2021). It is now fundamental that the student nurse must be aware of the impact of IT use and digital wellbeing both in working practice and in their home life and embrace leadership opportunities in digital areas such as artificial intelligence (Agnew, 2022).

Technostress is a multidimensional concept, with Brod (1984) defining it as the "inability to adapt or cope with new computer technologies in a healthy manner" and Wang et al. (2008) subsequently defining it as "a reflection of one's discomposure, fear, tenseness and anxiety when one is learning and using computer technology". Technostress is also defined more generally as anything negatively impacting on attitude, thoughts, behaviours or body physiology that is caused either directly or indirectly by technology (La Torre, 2019).

Through continuous exposure to technology, technostress can lead to poor work performance, reduced job satisfaction and intention of leaving the role (Golz et al., 2021). Technostress not only affects professionals' working lives but also within their private lives, as they are also open to psychophysiological reactions such as headaches, fatigue or burnout symptoms; low emotional stability; anxiety and depression and consequently can lead to impulsiveness, compulsiveness and unregulated or addictive media use.

Continued

Evidence suggests that nurses who interact digitally have a higher level of technostress and are less digitally competent than those working in other professions (Golz et al., 2021; Peter et al., 2020). Lack of confidence using new digitalised systems and IT can lead to technostress; therefore the student nurse should identify any IT training needs and seek support from the IT department and include IT training as part of continued personal development, as strong leadership digital skills are required within the nursing profession, especially in areas such as artificial intelligence (Agnew, 2022)'.

Lisa Di'Iulio, RN, health and wellbeing coach

Creating boundaries

For nursing students, learning to say no and establishing clear boundaries is vital for cultivating self-compassion and maintaining a healthy balance between their academic, clinical and personal lives. The rigorous demands of nursing education can lead to overwhelming stress and burnout if students constantly overextend themselves by agreeing to every request or task. Setting boundaries means nursing students can protect their time and energy. By acknowledging their own needs and limitations rather than succumbing to the pressure of being perpetually available or perfect, self-compassion will be fostered.

Saying no when necessary empowers nursing students to focus on what truly matters and ensures they have emotional resilience. Establishing these boundaries is not an act of selfishness but a critical step towards sustaining passion and effectiveness for the nursing profession.

 'It can sometimes be overwhelming to cope with all the demands placed on you as a student nurse. You have placement and academic demands; however, you are also an individual outside of the sphere of university. You may have dependents, a relationship, work commitments, etc., to juggle alongside university. I am a huge advocate of trying to find balance wherever you can. The following strategies worked for me, and I still adopt to this day. Learning to perfect the art of saying no. As much as you may want to help others (you are

caring in nature, of course!), it's just as important to help yourself. If saying yes will place you under pressure or make your life that bit more difficult, then it is perfectly ok to say no or 'not right now'. JOMO (the "joy of missing out") can actually bring you some peace. I overcame the feelings of negativity and managed to switch FOMO to JOMO by ensuring that where I couldn't engage in whatever activity/ event it was that I was missing, I planned a meaningful activity for myself when I knew I had a little more time/energy. People won't judge you or dislike you. They may just have to ask someone else! Secondly, switching off notifications was a game changer! In this age of technology and social media, we are so available 24/7. I switched off notifications for social media, which meant I didn't feel pressured into responding to people immediately. I went on to the apps when I wanted to as opposed to feeling dictated by a "ping" on my phone. Thirdly, nourish your body! Nutrition and hydration are key and don't have to be expensive. I planned a menu each week and shopped around for the best prices ... even cottoning onto the reduction times in the supermarkets (7.30 p.m., FYI!). Batch cooking and freezing are a great way to be savvy with your time and money! Pick up a few recipe books from charity shops or ask for them as gifts from friends/ family. Perhaps there's a book share near you (our local supermarket has a book swap table) or free cooking classes locally (which can also be an opportunity to connect with others)? Taking nutritious meals with you to uni/placement helps your mind, body and purse! Lastly ... move your body. Get out in fresh air where you can. Spend time in nature. Stretch, walk, run, dance. I dance in the lounge before bed when I've had a bad/stressful day—immediate mood booster! And I try to listen to uplifting music every morning to help boost my mood and energy for the day ahead. Depending on where you live, try and get outside into nature; reset and reenergise your mind.

Be kind to yourself. This journey is a challenging one; however, it is worth-while. Speak out and seek support whenever you feel like you need it—there's a plethora of support available through charities, uni, friends and family. Don't suffer in silence, no matter what challenge you face'.

Chloe Scott, RN, CHC Nurse Assessor and Reviewer

Sleep hygiene

'Sleep hygiene' is the term used to describe healthy habits that you can practise during the day to help you get a good night's sleep. Sleep is essential for your physical and mental wellbeing. It allows your body time to recharge and your mind to process information. Without enough quality sleep, our brains are unable to function properly. Good sleep hygiene can help improve your sleep quality, which in turn can:

- improve your mood
- improve your concentration and memory
- prevent you from developing sleep disorders (such as insomnia)
- help you maintain a healthy weight
- lower your risk of developing serious health conditions (such as diabetes and heart disease)
- help your body fight off diseases

There are some really helpful apps and podcasts which can help with rest and meditation. These are:

- Insight Timer
- SnoreLab
- Calm
- Pillow
- Sleepo
- Bettersleep
- Headspace
- Twighlight (blue light filter)

 TIPS

USEFUL NUMBERS AND WEBSITES

National Sleep Helpline: 03303530541
https://thesleepcharity.org.uk/national-sleep-helpline/

NHS: Better Sleep: Every Mind Matters
https://www.nhs.uk/every-mind-matters/mental-wellbeing-tips/how-to-fall-asleep-faster-and-sleep-better/

Sleep Foundation
https://www.sleepfoundation.org/sleep-habits

EMOTIONAL INTELLIGENCE

'Emotional intelligence is important for students. This will help you not just listen to people's stories but listen and believe people even when their experiences don't match yours. Recognising emotion in yourself and others as a student is a key skill and can help you check in and clarify what you are hearing. Students may need to practice feeling emotion and moving through it rather than pushing it away because it's uncomfortable.'

Hazel Powell, Deputy Executive Director of Nursing and Patient Experience

Daniel Goleman conceptualised the idea of emotional intelligence, which is based on the balance of recognition and regulation (Meyer, 2023). The key components of emotional intelligence are self-awareness; self-regulation; motivation, empathy and communication skills (Meyer, 2023).

Self-awareness

Imagine you're a pilot preparing to take off in a complex aircraft. You have all the technical know how, but what if you were unaware of the weather conditions, your own physical state or potential equipment malfunctions? That's where self-awareness comes in. It's your weather report, your health check and your maintenance checklist rolled into one. In nursing, it can make the difference between a smooth flight and turbulence.

Self-awareness requires us to have a good understanding of our own emotions, behaviours, thoughts, strengths, weaknesses and motivations. Those who display a high level of self-awareness demonstrate the ability to not only recognise their own feelings but those of others around them, which allows them to perform more effectively in challenging moments. Acting with a high level of self-awareness generally leads to decision making based on personal goals and values rather than an emotional reaction to the situation.

> *'I think emotional intelligence is far more complex as we learn how to work in the systems around us. In terms of student nurses demonstrating this on placement, I think self-awareness to be the most important facet, as we don't start our courses the finished project, be that technically, scientifically or emotionally. Being aware of situations you find personal and knowing how to respond to those and reflect on them is really important'.*
>
> **Becky Nisbet, student nurse**

Why is self-awareness important for nursing students?

Enhancing clinical judgement: Clinical judgement is like the compass of nursing. It guides your decision-making process, helping you choose the right interventions for your patients. Self-awareness acts as the true north on that compass. It helps you assess your own biases, limitations and emotions that could otherwise cloud your judgement (Benner, 1984).

Patient safety: The NMC code (2018) places patient safety at the forefront of nursing practice. Being self-aware means you're constantly assessing your own readiness to provide safe care. Are you well rested? Are you emotionally stable? Are you aware of any personal biases that might affect your care? These questions are essential for maintaining patient safety.

Take a moment to write down anything that might impact your readiness to provide safe and effective care.

_____

_____

_____

_____

_____

Cultivating empathy: Empathy is a cornerstone of patient-centred care. Self-awareness allows you to tap into your own emotions and use them as a bridge to connect with your patients on a deeper level (Hojat et al., 2001). It enables you to understand and respond to their needs and concerns more effectively.

Benefits of self-awareness in nursing

Reduced medical errors: Self-awareness helps you recognise when you're not at your best (Brady and Goldenhar, 2011), reducing the risk of making critical errors in patient care (Halbesleben, 2006).

Ethical practice: You'll make ethical decisions with confidence, knowing you've considered all angles and potential biases.

Personal resilience: Self-awareness helps you manage stress and maintain your emotional wellbeing, ensuring a long and fulfilling nursing career.

Improved patient outcomes: When you're in tune with your own emotions and biases, you can provide care that is more patient centred and tailored to individual needs, leading to better outcomes. Self-awareness enables you to provide patient-centred care that respects diversity and individuality (Goleman, 1995).

Professional growth: Self-awareness is a lifelong journey. As you continue to develop this skill, you'll grow both personally and professionally, becoming a more competent and compassionate nurse. It's a stepping stone to becoming a better nurse. It helps you identify areas for improvement and take proactive steps towards growth.

Positive workplace relationships: Being aware of your own emotions and how they affect others fosters better teamwork (Weng et al., 2011) and collaboration among healthcare professionals (Shanafelt and Noseworthy, 2017).

In the challenging and dynamic world of nursing, self-awareness is your compass, your weather report and your maintenance checklist. It's the foundation upon which clinical judgement, patient safety and compassionate care are built. Embrace it, cultivate it and let it guide you toward becoming the skilled and empathetic nurse that every patient deserves.

Tips for increasing self-awareness

Now that we have discussed self-awareness and its importance, how can we increase our self-awareness?

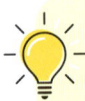

TIPS

- Take time each day to reflect on your clinical experiences. Ask yourself how you felt during patient interactions, what you learned and how your emotions influenced your decisions.
- Engage with your fellow nursing students and clinical staff. Seek their input on your practice. They can offer valuable insights into your blind spots and areas for improvement.
- After significant patient interactions or procedures, participate in debriefing sessions with your clinical team. Discuss your thoughts and emotions during the event to gain perspective and insights.

Self-regulation

Self-regulation is a fundamental component of emotional intelligence and is particularly crucial in the field of nursing. It refers to the ability to manage and control one's emotions, behaviours and impulses effectively. For nursing students and professionals, mastering self-regulation can significantly enhance their personal wellbeing and professional performance.

This is achieved by learning to manage but not suppress our thoughts, emotions and feelings relating to the given situation. Sometimes showing we are human is the best policy; however, our profession means that sometimes we need to be unwavering in the face of adversity in order to minimise the distress to our patients and their families. Often, humans exhibit subconscious actions through facial expressions, stance, tone of voice and language used, and sometimes we need to practise and train ourselves not to do it in order to break the cycle and change an unconscious habit (Purushothaman, 2021).

Motivation

Motivation plays a crucial role in emotional intelligence and can be broken down as follows: our personal drive to improve and achieve, commitment to our goals, initiative or readiness to act on opportunities, and optimism and resilience (Meyer, 2023). To maintain motivation levels, it's vital to cultivate a positive and optimistic mindset. It's key to view hiccups and setbacks as development opportunities rather than failures. Surrounding yourself with motivated friends and colleagues with positive outlooks can also boost you!

A significant element of maintaining and even improving your motivation reserves is to make a habit of reviewing your goals and achievements. This will also assist you in creating new goals to aid your professional development.

Empathy

Empathy is an amazing skill to have in healthcare and can be best described as the ability to take on another person's perspective in order to feel, understand and possibly share and then respond to the experience.

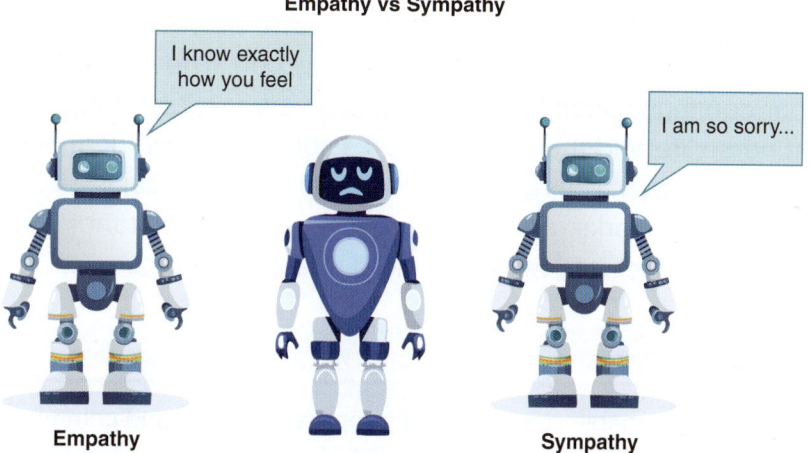

'Empathy is something that cannot be taught'. I'm sure you have already heard that in a lecture or five! Although nursing students should display empathy, this should not be confused for sympathy, as there is a fine line, which can build or harm a therapeutic relationship.

Empathy denotes an ability to relate with others' emotions while visualising yourself in their position and also is a measure of how much understanding and compassion we offer (Fernandez & Zahavi, 2020). Sympathy, however, includes compassion but can also be accompanied with feelings of pity towards the individual, which can contribute to a negative environment for our patients (Fernandez & Zahavi, 2020). There is an argument to suggest that empathy as a nursing skill can sometimes be draining to those offering it (Scheffer, Cameron & Inzlicht, 2022), whereas compassionate concern is considered to be a more positive and less demanding trait.

Effective communication

Effective communication is defined as the process of exchanging knowledge, information, opinions, thoughts and ideas in order that the message is conveyed clearly and interpreted correctly to its aim (McCabe & Timmins, 2013). Effective communication is not simply about sending and receiving information; there needs to be a comprehension of the purpose and the emotions behind the message.

When we communicate effectively, all parties can experience feelings of satisfaction and achievement and a sense of cooperation and concurrence. It feels like it should be straightforward; however, effective communication is a skill that needs to be worked on. The art of being clear with your communication is one which is a very useful commodity in the student nurse life and the nursing profession, be it at work, university or home. Barriers such as language, emotional and physical issues can put a spanner in the works, and this can lead to misunderstandings and, in some cases, conflict and the associated stress that comes with it.

NMC

THE NMC SAYS

7.2 Take reasonable steps to meet people's language and communication needs, providing, wherever possible, assistance to those who need help to communicate their own or other people's needs.

7.3 Use a range of verbal and non-verbal communication methods, and consider cultural sensitivities, to better understand and respond to people's personal and health needs.

7.4 Check people's understanding from time to time to keep misunderstanding or mistakes to a minimum.

In this section, we have considered the concept of emotional intelligence and how it runs through every part of our daily nursing life, from interactions to the way we perceive others and how others' views of us impacts us. The subject of emotional intelligence is a gentle reminder to be mindful of our own language, be it verbal, written or body, as it can have a number of different connotations and can affect the therapeutic relationship with the patients we look after and the colleagues we work alongside.

RESILIENCE

Resilience is more than just a buzzword; it's a crucial trait that can make or break a career in nursing. In the challenging world of healthcare, nursing students need to cultivate resilience to thrive amidst the trials and tribulations of their profession.

What is resilience?

Resilience isn't a one-size-fits-all concept; it's a multidimensional trait that encompasses the ability to bounce back from adversity, adapt to change and maintain a sense of wellbeing in the face of stress. Resilient individuals display emotional fortitude, cognitive flexibility and a sense of purpose, all of which are invaluable in nursing (Southwick et al., 2018).

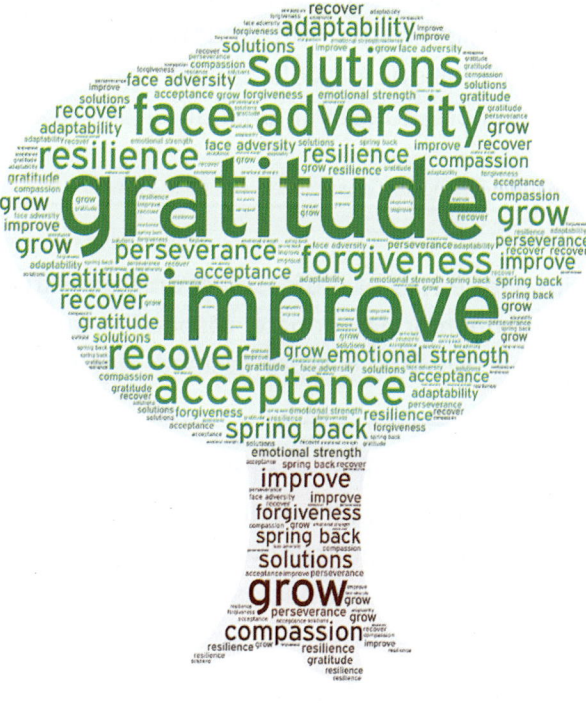

Why resilience matters

Nursing is one of the most emotionally and physically demanding professions (Mealer et al., 2017). Resilience helps students cope with the rigors of their studies and future careers, reducing the risk of burnout, which we have already discussed in this chapter. Moreover, nursing students often find themselves in high-pressure situations where quick decisions can impact patient outcomes. Resilience enables them to stay composed, think clearly and provide optimal care.

NMC

THE NMC SAYS

> 15 Always offer help if an emergency arises in your practice setting or anywhere else.

Another reason nursing students should build their resilience is that the healthcare landscape is constantly evolving with new technologies, research, skills and treatments. Resilience aids nursing students in embracing and adapting to these changes, ensuring they remain competent and up to date. Lastly, resilience enhances communication skills, which are crucial for building trust with patients and colleagues. Nursing students with higher resilience levels can navigate conflicts and emotional conversations more adeptly (Henshall et al., 2020).

NMC

THE NMC SAYS

> 9.3 Deal with differences of professional opinion with colleagues by discussion and informed debate, respecting their views and opinions and behaving in a professional way at all times.

It is important to remember that resilience is not about suppressing emotions or being immune to stress. It's not a 'toughen up and move on' mentality. Instead, it's about acknowledging emotions, seeking support when needed and bouncing back stronger.

TIPS

- Prioritise self-care, including regular exercise, healthy eating and adequate sleep. These basics provide the physical and emotional energy needed to face challenges.
- Developing resilience can be a collaborative effort. Students benefit from practice assessors and supervisors who can guide them through the challenges of their clinical placements.
- Mindfulness techniques and stress management strategies, such as meditation or deep breathing exercises, equip students with tools to stay grounded under pressure.
- Understand that failure is not the end but a stepping stone to success. Resilience is built through learning from setbacks and mistakes.
- Create a culture of continuous learning. Seek out new knowledge and skills; this will boost confidence and adaptability.

THE NMC SAYS

6.2 Maintain the knowledge and skills you need for safe and effective practice.

Some argue that the intense academic pressure placed on nursing students can hinder the development of resilience (Dyrbye et al., 2018). A system that overly emphasises grades and exams may inadvertently discourage risk taking and the ability to handle real-world nursing challenges (Carver, 2015). Balancing rigorous academics with opportunities for experiential learning and personal growth is essential.

We hope you can see that resilience is not a luxury but a necessity for nursing students. It empowers you to withstand the demands of your profession, provide exceptional care and adapt to a rapidly evolving healthcare landscape. By understanding what resilience truly entails and implementing strategies to nurture it, we can better prepare the next generation of nurses to face the challenges that lie ahead.

REFLECTION

You may have heard the word 'reflection' being mentioned on many occasions since you started your nursing journey. But why is it important for nursing students to do? What are the benefits of reflection, and how can we do it?

'Reflection during your clinical placement—love it or hate it ... it is absolutely crucial. Trust me, it's not just another assignment to tick off; it's your gateway to becoming a better nurse. But why is reflection so important for nursing students?

Without reflection, you are not evolving as a practitioner. Innovation in healthcare happens at an alarming rate; what you thought and did a day a week month or year ago is likely soon to be out of date. Reflection on the action and the learning and planning a way forward are all adding to your skill set. It also helps to keep you fresh and engaged with your role and helps to keep the passions for nursing alive'.

Karin Vertue, student nurse

Why reflect?

Reflection for nursing students on a clinical placement is not just a box to check; it's a transformative process that aligns with the NMC code and has a profound impact on your development as a nurse. It's about learning from experience, improving patient care, boosting confidence, enhancing critical thinking and strengthening interpersonal skills, to name a few benefits. Embrace reflection as a tool for growth and excellence in your nursing career.

1. Learning from experience:

Clinical placement is where theory meets practice. You're no longer just reading textbooks or listening to lectures; you're dealing with real patients and real situations. No amount of reading or listening is enough to cover every possible scenario. Reflection helps you dissect these experiences, understand what went well, what didn't and why (Schön, 1983). This deep level of thinking transforms every clinical encounter into a valuable learning opportunity and helps build your clinical judgement. It's not about dwelling on mistakes; it's about improving through self-awareness and recognising what you did well.

'Reflection for me is vital, as it helps me process information that I have experienced, whether it was a positive or negative experience, while on placement. I use reflection as a means to look back on something that has happened on placement, with a means to improving or developing my practice. Due to the fast-paced environments and the information that I have to process while on some clinical placements, I tend to reflect after I have finished my shift. Reflection varies for me, but I mainly reflect while driving home from placement or even in the shower when I get home.

Depending on how tired or stressed I am after placement, I am aware that may be how I reflect and view the experience as being viewed differently. On occasions, I have reflected the next morning over breakfast after taking the time to sleep and rest. I find that once rested, I can reflect in a different state of mind. There is no set structure to how I reflect, as I tend to just freestyle it. I will think about the event that happened, whether it is positive or negative. I then look at what feelings I experienced at the time of the event. I then tend to look at what I would have done differently and then make those changes in the future or be content with how the experience was. I believe that reflection is highly beneficial to me as a nursing student, as it improves my practice and gives me a deeper understanding of myself. Reflecting on experience in practice also gears me up for when I qualify, as reflection is a requirement by the NMC via revalidation.

A recent example of when I have used reflection was on my latest placement in an acute medical unit in a hospital setting. I was approached by a staff nurse to take a female patient from the assessment bay to another ward in the hospital and provide a handover to them. This was my first time going to a ward to hand over a patient on my own. I had the handover details in hand and went up to the ward with the patient and the porter.

Continued

On arrival to the ward, it was lunchtime and extremely busy at the nursing station. I approached the desk to speak to a member of staff to explain I was here as arranged for handing over the patient. I was informed by senior staff members that the bed available was for a male patient only, as they had moved patients around. In that moment, I stayed calm, as the female patient was now aware that there was an issue. I rang down to the acute medical unit I had just come from to confirm that the bed they now had available was a male-only bed. On ringing down, the staff on the acute medical unit stated that the matron was going to be contacting the ward, as the bed had previously been made available for a female. While waiting, I was now aware that the situation was becoming quite stressful, as I could see staff rushing about, and body language had changed. I waited patiently, talking to the patient and staying professional throughout, while advising staff that the bed originally had been held for a female patient by the bed managers. A call was made to the ward for me to return to the acute medical unit with the patient.

I spoke to the patient on the walk back, reassuring her and apologising for the confusion. After I had finished my shift, I reflected back on the situation. I was aware of my feelings of nervousness going to the ward for the first time to hand over. I was also aware that as a third-year student, having the opportunity to hand over alone was stepping out of my comfort zone, which is always good for growth. I reflected back on the feelings of anxiety I had entering the busy ward and being told that the bed was unavailable. I was content with how I handled the situation, staying calm and focused on what needed to be done without panicking. I was aware of my thoughts throughout the situation and managing the pressure in the moment. I was happy with how I handled the situation, staying calm in the busy surroundings, dealing with the circumstances surrounding the bed not being available and how I was able to navigate the concerns of the patient on returning her to the acute medical unit.

Ultimately, in what turned out to be an experience out of my control, I felt that I dealt with it in a professional manner with the skills I have developed over the past few years'.

Andrew Lelliott, student nurse

2. Aligning with the NMC code:

The NMC code (2018) places a strong emphasis on reflection. It's your professional duty as a nurse to reflect on your practice.

NMC

THE NMC SAYS

9.2 Gather and reflect on feedback from a variety of sources, using it to improve your practice and performance.

This means reflection isn't optional. Once you become a registered nurse, reflection will form part of your requirements for revalidation. Learning to do this early on in your career will set you in a good stead!

3. Improving patient care:

One of the main goals as a nurse is to provide safe and effective care. Reflecting on your clinical experiences helps you identify areas where you can improve (Levett-Jones & Hoffman, 2013). For instance, if you notice you struggle with communication during patient handovers, reflection can help you pinpoint why and work on it. Ultimately, this leads to better patient outcomes, which is the heart of nursing.

4. Boosting self-confidence:

Nursing can be challenging, and it's easy to doubt yourself. Reflecting on your successes, no matter how small, can be a confidence booster. It's like a personal high five. When you can say, 'I did this well', it reminds you that you're on the right track and capable of handling the demands of the profession.

5. Enhancing critical thinking:

Critical thinking is a cornerstone of nursing practice. It enables nurses to make informed clinical decisions, assess complex patient situations and provide evidence-based care (Alfaro-LeFevre, 2017). It empowers them to analyse, evaluate and prioritize information effectively. As Fero et al. (2010) highlight, critical thinking is essential for nursing practice, as it ensures safe and competent patient care. Reflective practice hones these skills by encouraging you to question your actions and decisions. It's not about accepting things at face value; it's about digging deeper and understanding the 'why' behind everything you do.

6. Strengthening interpersonal skills:

Nurses are at the forefront of patient care. Strong interpersonal skills are vital. Reflecting on your interactions with patients and colleagues can highlight areas where you can improve your communication, empathy and teamwork.

Tips on reflecting

If reflecting on clinical placement is a valuable skill for UK nursing students, how can we do it effectively? There is plenty of information out there which you can look to for more in-depth information, but we have summarised some top tips as follows.

TIPS

Consider using a reflective model or framework like Gibbs' reflective cycle, Borton's framework or Rolfe's framework. These models provide a structured approach to reflection, guiding you through the process of describing, analysing, evaluating and planning your actions.

'I use reflection as a tool to help me build new information, apply that knowledge to new experiences and reflect on and learn from past events while pursuing my nursing degree. Being a reflective learner, I can take a step back from what I am learning, analyse my experience and use that knowledge to improve my performance going forward. The reflective model I like to use is Gibbs' reflective cycle. It provides me with a framework for analysing the events and, because of its cyclical character, works effectively with potential repeated encounters. I can apply the model for understanding events, growing from mistakes, and analysing and reflecting on responses

to various circumstances. Using reflection, I can better recognise and value the good things that have happened during the event and find methods to enhance my work and care delivery by reflecting on my experience. When faced with difficult situations, it also helps me process and learn from the experience and pinpoint the positives'

Jessica Harrison, nursing student

TIPS

Keep a reflective journal or diary where you record your daily clinical experiences. Include details of patient interactions, procedures, challenges and successes. Reflect not only on your clinical skills but also on your personal and emotional reactions. Explore how your feelings and beliefs influenced your actions and interactions. Reflection is most effective when you're honest with yourself. This journal will serve as a valuable resource for future reflections. But remember, even if it is for your own private use, confidentiality is essential!

'Reflective journal writing while on placement has been promoted regularly from university. Placement can be an isolating and stressful experience but also exhilarating. You learn at such a rapid rate, and writing down experiences and feelings and the learning around them is incredibly helpful. It is also an effective tool to offload to. Being able to do this before going home means that we protect those around us. It can be shocking and upsetting for people not in nursing to hear some of the experiences we have. It is also important for us as nurses to have protected time away from work where we can be just us and not "the nurse". A journal helps bridge both those parts of your life without too high a cost on either'.

Karin Vertue, nursing student

TIPS

Think about any ethical or legal dilemmas you encountered during your placement. Reflect on how you addressed them and whether your actions align with the NMC code of conduct.

'I had a placement where a patient was at the end of their life and had stopped eating and drinking, but the family was insistent in continuing treatment and asking for IV fluids and for the patient to have a percutaneous endoscopic gastrostomy inserted. This got me thinking about the ethical dilemma of "do no harm" versus "medical futility"'.

Natalie Elliott, RN

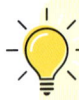

TIPS

Don't hesitate to ask your practice assessors, practice supervisors and colleagues for feedback. Their input can provide valuable perspectives and help you identify areas for improvement. It also doesn't need to be nursing staff that gives feedback; the wider multidisciplinary team and patients can give a unique perspective.

NMC

THE NMC SAYS

9.2 Gather and reflect on feedback from a variety of sources, using it to improve your practice and performance.

'Jihari's window talks about the four aspects of us and how they are viewed. How we see ourselves is different from how others see us, and our perception of how others see us is also different from how they really do. Developing professional relationships with peers and mentors who can see what we are doing and can positively but effectively give feedback is an important part of working in practice with others. Developing a mindset where you can separate yourself as a professional and your personal self enables you to accept feedback on your work and see it as an opportunity to develop as a practitioner'.

Karin Vertue, student nurse

TIPS

Use your reflections to set specific, actionable goals for your future clinical practice. What skills do you want to develop? How can you enhance your communication or time management?

'Having **SMART** goals is part of having a plan for continual growth. Do you have 10-year, 5-year, 2-year and 1-year goals? We know that plans change over time, but if you do not have something to work towards, that is not an effective use of your time. When on placement, you can become very focused on completing your proficiencies; however, this makes up only a small part of who you will be as a nurse. Look at other nurses around you, how they perform their tasks, maintain their growth mindset and learn from others, and then look at the areas you need to develop. Take time to speak to your practice assessor and the practice education team on placement. Look at opportunities to develop those areas that are not in your practice assessment document but that are just as important as a future nurse'.

Karin Vertue, student nurse

Take a moment to set yourself some goals for improvement.

_____

_____

_____

_____

_____

_____

TIPS

If you're unsure about how to approach reflection or need help with specific challenges, don't hesitate to reach out to your academic advisors, practice assessor, practice supervisor or colleagues. They can provide guidance and support.

THE NMC SAYS

13.3 Ask for help from a suitably qualified and experienced professional to carry out any action or procedure that is beyond the limits of your competence.

Now that we have given some of our reflection tips, take a moment to write down which ones you feel you'd like to try.

_____

_____

_____

_____

_____

_____

Remember that reflection is a skill that improves with practice. Over time, it will become a natural part of your nursing practice, helping you to grow both personally and professionally and allowing you to provide optimal patient care. But we really want to emphasise that it doesn't need to be all doom and gloom—remember that reflection can also be about looking at what you did well.

CONCLUSION

Hopefully, this chapter has shown that the journey through clinical placements is not simply about mastering clinical skills but also about developing a deeper understanding of oneself and that you will be presented with opportunities to develop essential qualities such as self-compassion, emotional intelligence, reflection and resilience.

Self-compassion emerges as a guiding light, reminding you to treat yourself with kindness amid the inevitable setbacks and pressures of clinical practice. Emotional intelligence serves as a crucial tool for effective communication and interpersonal relationships in the clinical setting. By honing your ability to recognise and manage your emotions, you can navigate complex patient interactions with empathy and professionalism. Through reflective practice, you can deepen you understanding of yourself and your practice. This also enhances self-awareness, which acts as a cornerstone for personal and professional growth. Building resilience becomes essential in the face of the numerous challenges encountered during clinical placements. By embracing setbacks as opportunities for growth and learning, you will emerge stronger and more resilient healthcare professionals.

The end of placement marks a significant milestone in the journey towards becoming competent, compassionate and resilient nurses. As nursing students, reflect on your experiences and lessons learned so you are poised to embark on future placements with newfound insight and determination.

Space for reader's own reflection:

_____

_____

_____

_____

_____

_____

_____

_____

_____

_____

_____

_____

_____

_____

REFERENCES

Agnew, T., 2022. Digital engagement in nursing: The benefits and barriers. Nur. Times [online] 118, 3.

Alfaro-LeFevre, R., 2017. Critical Thinking, Clinical Reasoning, and Clinical Judgment: A Practical Approach, third ed. Elsevier.

Benner, P., 1984. From Novice to Expert: Excellence and Power in Clinical Nursing Practice. Prentice-Hall.

Boyer-Davis, S., 2019. Technostress : an antecedent of job turnover intention in the accounting profession. J. Bus. Account. 12 (1), 49–63. https://www.proquest.com/openview/cdefe788ceef981a70d306ebe56cd322/1?pq-origsite=gscholar&cbl=2030638

Brady, M.S., Goldenhar, L.M., 2011. A qualitative study examining the influences on situation awareness and the identification, mitigation and escalation of recognised patient risk. Int. J. Nurs. Stud. 48 (11), 1436–1443.

Brod, C., 1984. Technostress: The Human Cost of the Computer Revolution. Addison-Wesley, Reading, MA, USA.

Carver, C.S., 2015. Resilience and thriving: Issues, models, and linkages. J. Soc. Issues 54 (2), 245–266.

Choo, P.Y., Marszalek, J.M., 2019. Self-Compassion: A Potential Shield Against Extreme Self-Reliance? J. Happiness Stud. 20 (3), 971–994. https://doi.org/10.1007/s10902-018-9978-y

Dreisörner, A., Junker, N.M., van Dick, R., 2021. Correction to: The Relationship Among the Components of Self-compassion: A Pilot Study Using a Compassionate Writing Intervention to Enhance Self-kindness, Common Humanity, and Mindfulness. J. Happiness Stud. 22 (5), 2409–2410. https://doi.org/10.1007/s10902-020-00306-9

Dyrbye, L.N., Shanafelt, T.D., Sinsky, C.A., Cipriano, P.F., Bhatt, J., Ommaya, A., et al., 2018. Burnout among health care professionals: A call to explore and address this underrecognized threat to safe, high-quality care. Natl. Acad. Med. 1–13.

Fernandez, A.V., Zahavi, D., 2020. Basic empathy: Developing the concept of empathy from the ground up. Int. J. Nurs. Stud. 110, 103695. https://doi.org/10.1016/j.ijnurstu.2020.103695

Fero, L.J., O'Donnell, J.M., Zullo, T.G., Dabbs, A.D., Kitutu, J., 2010. Critical thinking skills in nursing students: a comparison between freshmen and senior students. J. Nurs. Educ. 49 (3), 168–171.

Golz, C., Peter, K.A., Müller, T.J., Mutschler, J., Zwakhalen, S.M.G., Hahn, S., 2021. Technostress and digital competence among health professionals in Swiss psychiatric hospitals: Cross-sectional study. JMIR Ment. Health 8 (11), e31408. https://doi.org/10.2196/31408

Halbesleben, J.R., 2006. Patient Safety and Error Reduction in Surgical Pathology. Arch. Pathol. Lab. Med. 130 (5), 630–632.

Henshall, C., Davey, Z., Jackson, D., 2020. Nursing resilience interventions-A way forward in challenging healthcare territories. J. Clin. Nurs. 29 (19-20), 3597–3599. https://doi.org/10.1111/jocn.15276

Hojat, M., Mangione, S., Nasca, T.J., Cohen, M.J., Gonnella, J.S., Erdmann, J.B., et al., 2001. The Jefferson Scale of Physician Empathy: Development and preliminary psychometric data. Educ. Psychol. Meas. 61 (2), 349–365.

La Torre, G., Esposito, A., Sciarra, I., Chiappetta, M., 2019. Definition, symptoms and risk of techno-stress: a systematic review. Int. Arch. Occup. Environ. Health 92 (1), 13–35. https://doi.org/10.1007/s00420-018-1352-1

Levett-Jones, T., Hoffman, K., 2013. Enhancing nursing students' understanding of threshold concepts through reflective journals. J. Adv. Nurs. 69 (11), 2572–2581.

Linnett, R.J., Kibowski, F., 2020. A multidimensional approach to perfectionism and self-compassion. Self Identity 19 (7), 757–783. https://doi.org/10.1080/15298868.2019.1669695

Lucena, J., Carvalho, C., Santos-Costa, P., Mónico, L., Parreira, P., 2021. Nurses' Strategies to Prevent and/or Decrease Work-Related Technostress: A Scoping Review. Comput. Inform. Nurs. 39 (12), 916–920. doi:10.1097/CIN.0000000000000771

McCabe, C., Timmins, F., 2013. Communication Skills for Nursing Practice, second ed. Basingstoke: Palgrave Macmillan.

Mealer, M., Jones, J., Meek, P., 2017. Factors affecting resilience and development of posttraumatic stress disorder in critical care nurses. Am. J. Crit. Care 26 (3), 184–192. https://doi.org/10.4037/ajcc2017798

Meyer, H.M., 2023. Understanding emotional intelligence and its relationship to clinical reasoning in senior nursing students: A mixed methods study. J. Prof. Nurs. 46, 187–196. https://doi.org/10.1016/j.profnurs.2023.03.010

Murphy, S., Shelley, L., 2019. Fostering mindfulness: building skills that students need to manage their attention, emotions, and behavior in classrooms and beyond. Pembroke Publishers Limited.

Neff, K.D., 2023. Self-Compassion: Theory, Method, Research, and Intervention. Annu. Rev. Psychol. 74 (1), 193–218. https://doi.org/10.1146/annurev-psych-032420-031047

NHS. 2019. The NHS long term plan. https://www.longtermplan.nhs.uk/wp-content/uploads/2019/01/nhs-long-term-plan-june-2019.pdf

Nursing and Midwifery Council. 2018. The Code: Professional standards of practice and behaviour for nurses, midwives, and nursing associates. https://www.nmc.org.uk/globalassets/sitedocuments/nmc-publications/nmc-code.pdf

Peter, K.A., Hahn, S., Schols, J.M.G.A., Halfens, R.J.G., 2020. Work-related stress among health professionals in Swiss acute care and rehabilitation hospitals—A cross-sectional study. J. Clin. Nurs. 29 (15-16), 3064–3081. https://doi.org/10.1111/jocn.15340

Purushothaman, R., 2021. Emotional intelligence, first ed. SAGE Publications Pvt. Ltd.

Scheffer, J.A., Cameron, C.D., Inzlicht, M., 2022. Caring is costly: People avoid the cognitive work of compassion. J. Exp. Psychol. Gen. 151 (1), 172–196. https://doi.org/10.1037/xge0001073

Schön, D.A., 1983. The Reflective Practitioner: How Professionals Think in Action. Basic Books.

Shanafelt, T.D., Noseworthy, J.H., 2017. Executive leadership and physician wellbeing: nine organizational strategies to promote engagement and reduce burnout. Mayo Clin. Proc. 92 (1), 129–146.

Southwick, S.M., Bonanno, G.A., Masten, A.S., Panter-Brick, C., Yehuda, R., 2014. Resilience definitions, theory, and challenges: interdisciplinary perspectives. Eur. J. Psychotraumatol. 5 (1). https://doi.org/10.3402/ejpt.v5.25338.

University Hospital Southampton NHS Foundation Trust. Sleep hygiene - patient information. https://www.uhs.nhs.uk/Media/UHS-website-2019/Patientinformation/Other/Sleep-hygiene-3276-PIL.pdf

Wang, K., Shu, Q., Tu, Q., 2008. Technostress under different organizational environments: An empirical investigation. Comput. Human Behav. 24 (6), 3002–3013. https://doi.org/10.1016/j.chb.2008.05.007

Welsh Government. 2023. Digital and data strategy for health and social care: To improve the way we deliver modern health and care services through technology and use of data. https://www.gov.wales/digital-and-data-strategy-health-and-social-care-wales-html

Weng, H.C., Hung, C.M., Liu, Y.T., Cheng, Y.J., Yen, C.Y., Chang, C.C., et al., 2011. Associations between emotional intelligence and doctor burnout, job satisfaction and patient satisfaction. Med. Educ. 45 (8), 835–842.